Back Pain

Recognition and management

Back Pain

Recognition and management

Michael A. Hutson MA, MB, BChir, DObst. RCOG

Specialist Orthopaedic Physician, Park Row Clinic Nottingham and the London Bridge Clinic.
President, British Institute of Musculoskeletal Medicine (formerly Institute of Orthopaedic Medicine).
Principal lecturer and external examiner, Diploma of Sports Medicine, London University. Examiner, Diploma of Musculoskeletal Medicine and Diploma of Sports Medicine, Society of Apothecaries.

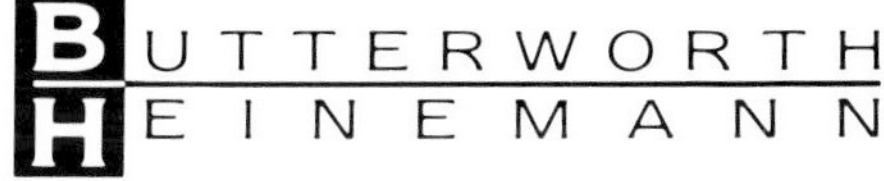

Butterworth-Heinemann Ltd
Linacre House, Jordan Hill, Oxford OX2 8DP

 PART OF REED INTERNATIONAL BOOKS

OXFORD LONDON BOSTON
MUNICH NEW DELHI SINGAPORE SYDNEY
TOKYO TORONTO WELLINGTON

First published 1993

British Library Cataloguing in Publication Data
Hutson, M. A.
I. Title
616.7

ISBN 0 7506 0578 2

Library of Congress Cataloguing in Publication Data
Hutson, M. A.
Back pain: recognition and management/Michael A. Hutson.
p. cm.
Includes bibliographical references and index.
ISBN 0 7506 0578 2
1. Backache. I. Title.
[DNLM: 1. Backache – diagnosis. 2. Backache – rehabilitation. WE 720 H981b]
RD771.B217H88 1993
617.5'64–dc20 92–48897
CIP

Composition by Genesis Typesetting, Laser Quay, Rochester, Kent
Printed and bound in Great Britain by Bath Press Ltd, Avon

Contents

Preface

> I suspect that the only books that influence us are those for which we are ready, and which have gone a little further down our particular path than we have yet gone ourselves.
>
> E. M. Forster, *Two Cheers for Democracy* (1951)

It is generally recognized that back pain contributes substantially to the workload of family doctors, physiotherapists, osteopaths and medical specialists. The statistics from reputable sources (for instance, the Department of Social Security, see DSS, 1990) support this view overwhelmingly. Despite the ability of clinicians and therapists, through their basic training, to recognize the benign nature of the vast majority of patients' back pains by exclusion of more serious 'non-mechanical' pathology, there continues to be a widespread dearth of knowledge of the practical methods of relating the pathoanatomical, pathophysiological, or pathoneurophysiological causes of common spinal lesions to their clinical presentation, and of the rational implementation of specific therapeutic procedures.

The majority of medical practitioners have received inadequate training in musculoskeletal medicine, a situation which is often apparent to patients who observe a lack of diagnostic skills and, frequently, a lack of interest in their condition, and who, correspondingly, are offered bland or inappropriate management strategies. A further problem for many patients is the heavy workload of NHS consultants – principally orthopaedic surgeons and rheumatologists – to whom they are usually referred if their back pains become persistent, thereby denying early specialist medical advice to all except the minority with very acute, usually very painful, lesions. As a result, physiotherapists and osteopaths often find themselves in a position of managing patients who have either not attended a physician of any type, or who have been referred with dustbin diagnoses such as 'low back syndrome'. Commonly, it falls to the therapist to make a definitive diagnosis, a situation which may be considered to be difficult without background medical knowledge and access to specific investigative techniques. Nevertheless, it has been shown that an experienced manipulative therapist may diagnose and localize joint lesions (in the cervical spine) as accurately by manual methods as may be effected by diagnostic nerve block techniques (Jull *et al.* 1988). Furthermore, the use of 'high-tech' investigations such as CT scanning and MR imaging for the vast majority of spinal lesions is costly and valueless.

The application of a structured appraisal by the therapist may lead to the use of simple, easily learnt, manual methods of treatment, thus overcoming the traditional response of rest, analgesics, localized heat applications, ultrasound and interferential which rarely satisfies the patient who has come to expect, and often benefits from, a more active approach. This book details these diagnostic examination techniques and therapeutic strategies in a form which, hopefully, enables the reader *to proceed from an understanding of basic concepts to a rational practical approach to back pain.*

It is appreciated that there are a number of short texts available to lay people on how to manage their back complaints; additionally, there are substantive texts on orthopaedic medicine in general, and on the narrower concept of manual treatment of spinal problems, for medical practitioners and therapists who have already gained a significant level of knowledge of musculoskeletal medicine. The author's experience of the subject has been gained over a 20-year period, initially from a base in general practice and, subsequently, from a specialist practice in musculoskeletal disorders in which he has worked closely with physiotherapists. His knowledge of the various strategies of doctors of different inclinations, for instance osteopathic physicians and orthopaedic surgeons, results in his awareness of the need for a text which might act as a practical guide to the subject from an *eclectic* background. From a base of diagnostic skills, problem-orientated management strategies are defined which utilize the facilities of the average consulting and treatment room complex – the basic requirements being an examination/treatment couch, and an interest in spinal manipulation and mobilization techniques. Guidance is given in respect of the application of injection treatment by medical specialists, and the type of patients for whom these techniques are applicable.

The individual chapters on cervical, thoracic, and lumbar and sacroiliac problems include a detailed analysis of the functional anatomy and biomechanics of each region, an examination routine which may be learnt and utilized in a short period of time, and a wide-ranging assessment of therapeutic techniques for the majority of spinal problems. The use of diagrams and clinical photographs augment the thrust of the text towards the practicality of the methods described. The circumstances in which referral to other health care groups – specialist medical practitioners or therapists such as osteopaths, chiropractors or relaxation therapists – are identified. Those conditions which require further investigation or surgery are specified, and a summary is provided of the nature of these investigative procedures.

Following resolution of an initial painful bout of back pain, the importance of stabilization of the dysfunctional spinal segment is stressed. In their review (following a literature search) of the results of spinal manipulation for back and neck pain presented in published papers, Koes *et al.* (1991) conclude that, although promising early results are demonstrated in a number of studies, recurrence rate is high on long-term follow-up. Regrettably, there is often no indication from many studies of the inclusion of a comprehensive rehabilitation regime following successful manipulative treatment for the acute phase (the conclusion being that such a regime was omitted). A comprehensive evaluation of this important rehabilitative phase is provided in Chapter 5, including the use of strengthening exercises, overall fitness regimes, and a practical response to the 'do I have to live with my back?' enquiry. It is the author's contention that the majority of patients are able to reduce the likelihood of recurrent problems resulting from spinal instability by appropriate therapeutic and rehabilitative regimes. Exercise schedules, which patients may undertake for themselves, and ergonomic principles are detailed.

This book is directed principally towards those physiotherapists who desire a clear and logical pathway through what may otherwise be considered to be a jungle of competing ideologies. Equally, the text is relevant to medical practitioners, to medical students in their later stages of training and to doctors in vocational training. The dual responsibilities of family doctors and physiotherapists have always been, and will continue to be, to work closely with other health care professionals in order to evaluate, and treat conservatively, the vast majority of mechanical spinal problems.

REFERENCES

DSS (Department of Social Security), Newcastle (1990) *Sickness and/or Invalidity Benefit: Spells of Certified Incapacity*, HMSO, London

Jull, G., Bogduk, N. and Marsland, A. (1988) The accuracy of manual diagnosis for cervical zygapophyseal joint pain syndromes. *Medical Journal of Australia*, **148**, 233–6

Koes, B.W., Assendelft, W.J.J., van der Heijden, G.J.M.G. *et al.* (1991) Spinal manipulation and mobilization for back and neck pain: a blinded review. *British Medical Journal*, **303**, 1298–303

Acknowledgements

I am grateful to Jean Oliver and Alison Middleditch for the use of the anatomical illustrations from *Functional Anatomy of the Spine* (1991, Butterworth-Heinemann, Oxford).

1
Fundamentals

> The physician must not think himself too important, for over him there is a master – time, which plays with him as a cat with a mouse.
>
> Paracelsus (1493–1541)

EPIDEMIOLOGY

Statistical surveys confirm the impression among the caring and healing professions that back pain in the community today is extremely common. Jayson (1987) has reported that between 6% and 7% of the population in the 45–65 years age group attend their general practitioners every year with back pain. The incidence in the younger and older age groups is only slightly lower. It is known, also, that approximately 50% of an osteopath's workload is accounted for by patients with back pain, of whom one-third have not previously consulted their doctor. Since only approximately 10% of patients with backache seek attention for their complaint, it can be seen that the incidence is very high, and the tolerance of the majority of the population is considerable.

Although community surveys indicate that the incidence of back pain is higher in females than males, industrial surveys demonstrate the reverse. In the year 1988–89, 35.75 million working days were lost in males, and 16.4 million working days lost in females in the United Kingdom; these figures do not include short periods of a few days lost which are subject to self-certification. Workers in heavy industry are more vulnerable than sedentary workers, although prolonged sitting at a desk creates its own problems, the ergonomics of which are addressed in Chapter 5. Porter (1982) has concluded that 75% of all miners over 50 years of age have experienced back pain, as a result of which most of them have been off work. 50 per cent of office workers over the age of 50 have experienced back pain, and half of them have needed to be off work. There is a relatively high incidence of back pain in occupations which demand a substantial amount of driving; added vibration causes greater risks, so that tractor drivers, for instance, have a high incidence. Bricklayers, too, often develop back pain owing to a combination of prolonged trunk flexion while laying bricks and the additional spinal stress caused by mixing cement. Handling patients is provocative; 16% of all sickness absence in nurses is due to back pain, and it is estimated that one in six nurses each year will suffer from back pain. In 1987, 750,000 nursing days were lost from this cause.

As for the load imposed upon the medical services in the UK, Jayson estimated (1987) that around 2 million adults in Great Britain consult their general practitioners each year with back pain; these numbers constitute 6.5% of all general practice consultations. Approximately 5% of all referrals to hospital are for backache. Between 20% and 30% of referrals to rheumatologists and orthopaedic surgeons are for backache; a substantial part of the workload of radiology and physiotherapy departments is for the same problem. Patients may wait an exceedingly long time on Health Service waiting lists to be seen by consultants whose interest is primarily in spinal disorders; in some regions in the UK in 1991 outpatient waiting periods had risen to three years.

According to statistics from the Department of Social Security in Newcastle (DSS, 1990), the incidence of back pain, as a proportion of all incapacities, continues to rise each year. In 1988–89, 12.61% of all incapacities were due to back pain. The financial implications of these 52.6 million working days lost each year are staggering: in 1987 the cost to society as a whole, including loss of industrial output, social security payments and Health Service costs was £2,000 million.

One final point is worthy of note from an epidemiological viewpoint. The incidence of low back pain decreases after the age of 55. The incidence of degenerative changes on X-ray, however, increases throughout a lifetime. The relationship between radiologically determined degenerative changes and back pain, therefore, is largely spurious. It would appear that, prior to the age of functional stabilization (perhaps around 60 years when the strains on the spine become less marked, and osteophytes have some protective and stiffening effect), the incidence of back pain is higher in the presence of moderately severe degenerative changes, although probably not appreciably higher in the presence of minor degenerative changes. As for whiplash injuries to the cervical spine, the longevity of symptoms is significantly greater in those patients with substantial pre-existing degenerative changes. What is abundantly clear, however, and emphasized throughout the text, is that the practice of basing a *diagnosis* on a patient with back pain primarily on radiological findings, although widespread, is seriously flawed.

APPLIED ANATOMY

Phylogenetically, the spine – a system of articulated segments superimposed one on another – has developed in such a way as to support man's ability to move with an upright posture. The curvatures in the cervical, thoracic and lumbar regions (Fig. 1.1) support the body weight which, effectively, rests on the sacrum and its

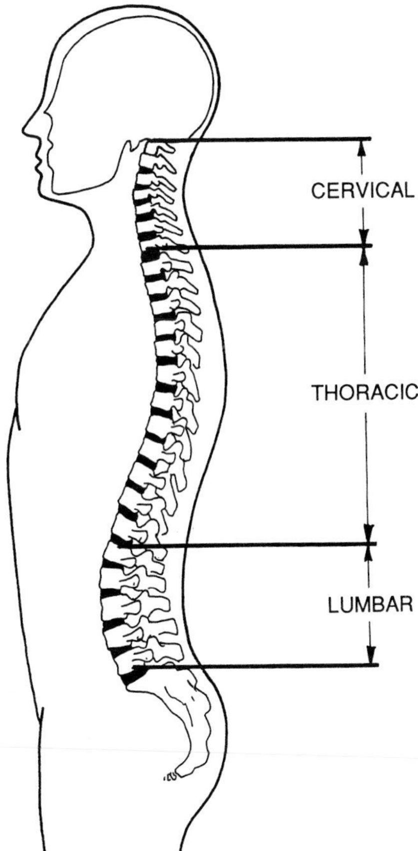

Fig. 1.1 The spinal curvatures are demonstrated – cervical lordosis, thoracic kyphosis and lumbar lordosis.

firm attachments to the pelvis. Marked natural variations in the degree of regional curvatures occur in different ethnic groups, particularly in the degree of lumbar lordosis. Although there are usually 24 separate segments, it is not unusual to find transitional variants, for instance at the lumbosacral junction; hemivertebrae and fused vertebrae also occur. It is not always easy to number the vertebrae clinically, however, as palpation of the spinous processes may be fraught with difficulties, not least because the mid-cervical and the mid- and distal lumbar vertebrae are partially 'hidden' to the palpating finger.

Each mobile (syn. 'motion') segment is composed of an anterior and a posterior pillar, each with different morphological and functional characteristics (Fig. 1.2). The **anterior pillar** of the spine has weightbearing and shock-absorbing functions: each vertebral body is connected via its end-plates to two intervertebral discs (except between the occiput and the atlas, and between the atlas and the axis). The **posterior pillar** comprises the apophyseal joints (correctly termed 'zygo-apophyseal', and colloquially known as 'facet' joints),

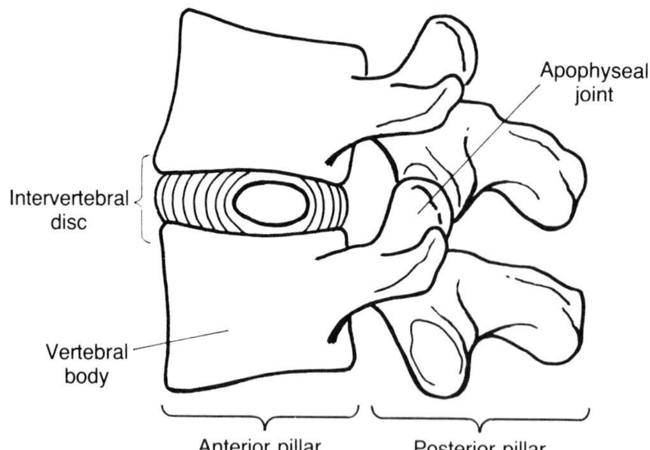

Fig. 1.2 The motion segment is composed of an anterior pillar and a posterior pillar.

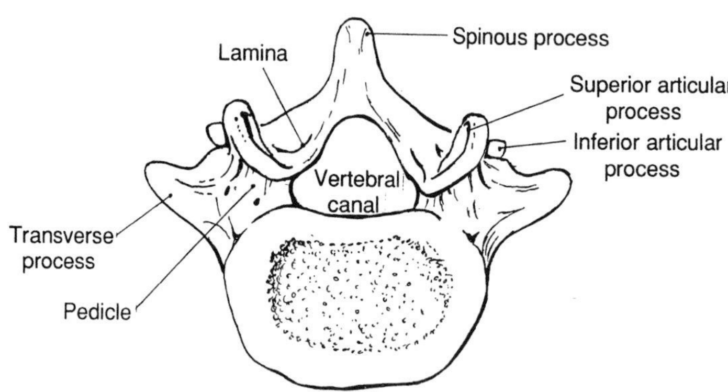

Fig. 1.3 The 5th lumbar vertebra. The elements of the posterior pillar – articular processes, spinous processes, transverse processes and laminae – are separated from the anterior pillar by the pedicles.

the neural arches, spinous processes and transverse processes which are separated from the anterior pillar by the pedicles (Fig. 1.3). The spinal cord is enclosed within the neural arch, and the apophyseal joints allow movements of varying degrees between adjacent vertebrae.

The intervertebral disc

Central to the supportive function of the spine is the intervertebral disc which is composed of an **annulus fibrosus**, connected superiorly and inferiorly to the cartilaginous vertebral end-plates and epiphyseal rings, and a **nucleus pulposus** (Fig. 1.4). The annulus is arranged as concentric rings of fibrocartilage which encapsulate the colloidal mucopolysaccharide material of the nucleus (Fig. 1.5). The anterior part of the annulus is the thickest; the posterior part is the weakest. While the annulus has elastic properties, the nucleus is capable of deformation because of its high (88%) water content, as a result of

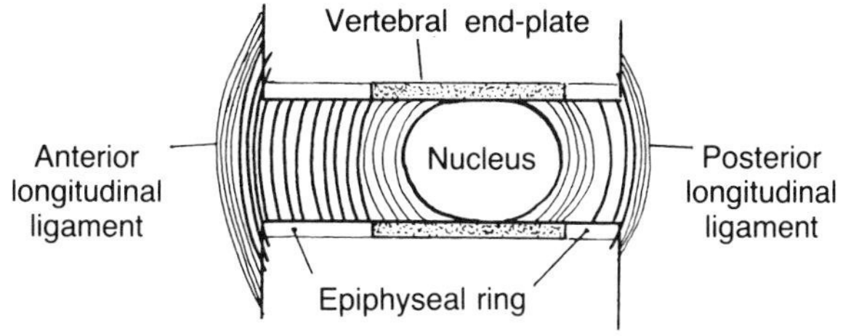

Fig. 1.4 The annulus fibrosus is connected superiorly and inferiorly to the cartilaginous vertebral end-plates and epiphyseal rings.

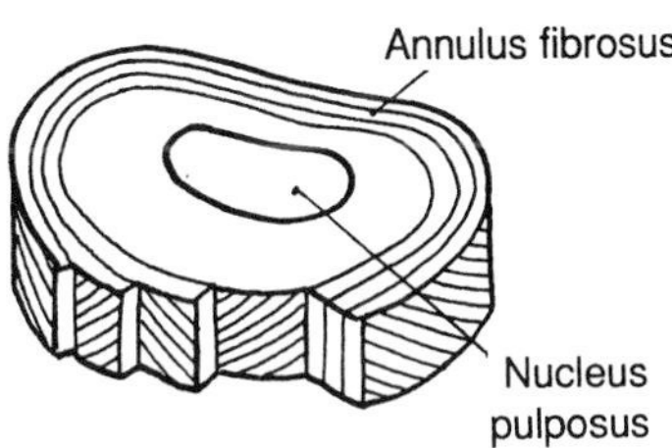

Fig. 1.5 The annulus is arranged as concentric rings of fibrocartilage which encapsulate the nucleus pulposus.

which axial stresses are distributed both superoinferiorly and peripherally to the annulus (Fig. 1.6). Deformation of the nucleus occurs also in response to angular loading stresses.

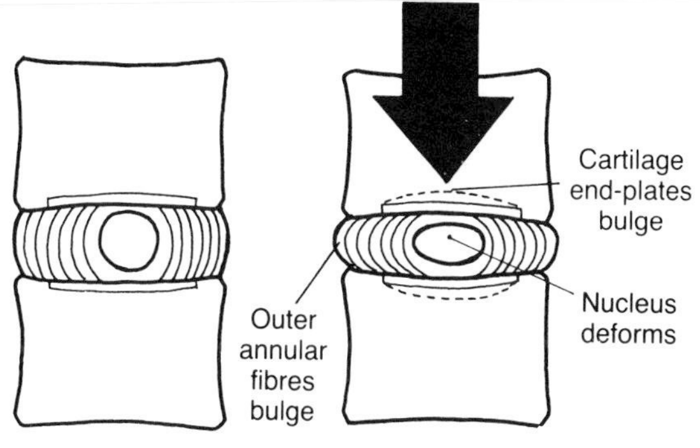

Fig. 1.6 Axial stresses are distributed both superoinferiorly, and peripherally to the annulus.

The disc becomes thinner by day, but water re-enters in the recumbent position. Consequently, flexibility of the spine is greater in the mornings in the young; however, the water content of the nucleus decreases with age. Morning stiffness in the middle-aged and elderly results from the combination of desiccation of the nucleus and degenerative changes in the apophyseal joints.

At low compressive loads, flexibility of the spine is maintained. With increasing compression loading, significant stiffness occurs, giving the spine enhanced stability. With high loading, end-plate fractures are more likely to arise than burst discs. Flexion and torsional loads are the most damaging to the disc.

The apophyseal joints

Although the facet joints, assisted by the muscles of the spine, transmit approximately 20% of the total compressive load, their principal function is to facilitate spinal movement. They are diarthrodial (synovial) joints which permit gliding movements, and are subject to the same types of stresses as the limb joints. As a consequence, it is reasonable to suppose that synovitis may develop as a response to trauma or excessive strain; osteoarthritic changes undoubtedly occur.

The orientation of the facet joints varies in the different regions of the spine, and this dictates the range of movements (Fig. 1.7). In the cervical spine the inclination of the facets is 45° to the transverse plane, permitting movements in all directions. In the thoracic region the facets demonstrate inclination of approximately 60° to the transverse plane and also 20° of internal rotation, allowing side bending and rotation. (Throughout the spine side bending and rotation are always coupled.) In the proximal lumbar spine the orientation is vertical, approximately 45° to the coronal plane, thereby allowing flexion and extension predominantly; at the lumbosacral junction the inclination is more coronal.

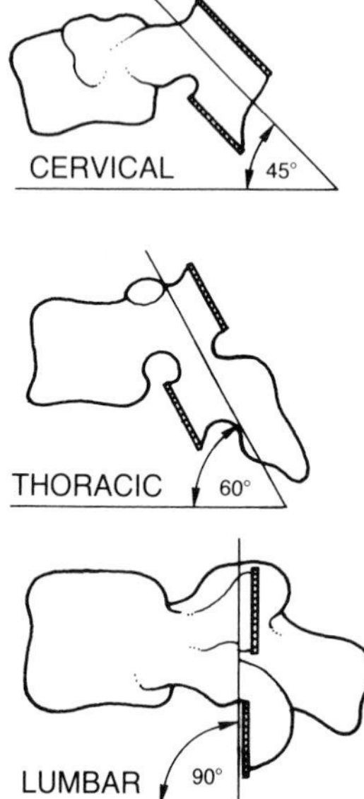

Fig. 1.7 The orientation of the facet joints in respect to the transverse plane is demonstrated in different regions of the spine. (After Cailliet, R., 1981, *Low Back Pain Syndrome*, 3rd edn, F.A. Davis, Philadelphia.)

The intervertebral foramen, spinal nerves and pain perception

At each segmental level the spinal nerve roots, invested by dural sleeves, emerge through an intervertebral foramen. In the cervical and lumbar regions the nerve roots are vulnerable to pressure in their passage through the root canals and at the intervertebral foramina. As a result of osteophytic hypertrophy of the facet joints, the walls of a foramen may encroach upon the nerve roots, giving rise to stenosis of the root canal (Figs 2.13, 4.16). A laterally placed disc fragment, usually in the younger age groups, may impinge upon the nerve root – the most common cause of sciatica under the age of 50.

Having formed from the dorsal and ventral nerve roots, the common spinal nerve gives off the sinuvertebral nerve which innervates the vertebral body, the posterior margin of the annulus fibrosus, the posterior longitudinal ligament, the contents of the epidural space and the dura mater (Fig. 1.8). It is probable that the sinuvertebral nerve is the transmitter of pain via nociceptor afferents from the region of the posterolateral margin of the disc. The common spinal nerve divides into anterior (ventral) and posterior (dorsal) primary rami, the latter providing a posterior articular (otherwise referred to as 'medial') branch to the facet joint. Cross-linkage over several segments occurs via ramifications from both the articular

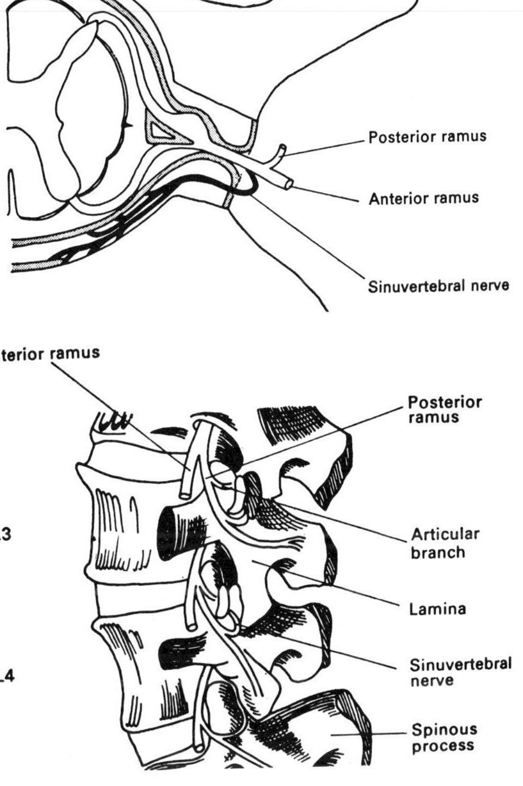

Fig. 1.8 The sinuvertebral nerve supplies the dura, the contents of the epidural space and the posterior margin of the annulus of the disc. The medial branch of the posterior primary ramus supplies the apophyseal joint. (From Hutson, M.A., 1990, *Sports Injuries: Recognition and Management*, Oxford University Press, Oxford by permission of Oxford University Press.)

nerves and the sinuvertebral nerves – of some relevance when injection techniques are used for facet joint lesions or nerve root entrapments.

Wyke (1987) has confirmed that nociceptive receptor stimulation is either by mechanical forces (for instance, pressure or distraction) or by chemical irritation (for instance, by chemical substances associated with inflammation or trauma). The afferent pathways, through which impulses are transmitted from nociceptive receptors, are composed of small myelinated and unmyelinated nerve fibres, 5 μm or less in diameter, whose cell bodies lie in the dorsal root ganglia. Perception of pain is modulated by both peripheral and central mechanisms. Peripherally, the centripetal projection of afferent activity from nociceptive receptor systems is continuously modulated by concurrent activity emanating from mechanoreceptors located in the same tissues (and which is transmitted by larger diameter nerve fibres in peripheral nerves). Of practical significance is the inhibitory effect on nociceptive transmission by stimulation of these mechanoreceptor afferent nerve fibres, for instance by massage, TENS (transcutaneous electrical nerve stimulation) and electroacupuncture. Excitatory mechanisms from higher neurological centres, on the other hand, may contribute to the prolongation of symptoms beyond the duration of the initiating stimulus.

Of some interest is the role of the autonomic nervous system in neurophysiological disorders of spinal motion segments (see 'Conceptual models of spinal disorders: dysfunction'). Physiologically, the autonomic (parasympathetic and sympathetic) nervous system exerts its effects on various systems of the body by its innervation of smooth muscle and exocrine glands; thus it controls sweating, blood vessel contraction and dilatation, and lachrymation, amongst other functions. The sympathetic trunks extend from the C1 level to the coccyx, and are composed of preganglionic neurones (the cell bodies of which are located in the T1–L2 segments of the spinal cord) and postganglionic neurones; synapses occur in the sympathetic ganglia. For the most part ganglia are located at each spinal level, though in the cervical region they are restricted to the superior cervical ganglion, the middle cervical ganglion and the stellate ganglion inferiorly. Rami communicantes convey pre- and postganglionic fibres to and from the ventral rami.

Ligaments

Running throughout the length of the spine over its anterior aspect is the **anterior longitudinal ligament**. Its function is to resist extension of the spine and, in combination with the annulus, to resist shearing movements of one vertebra on another. The **posterior longitudinal ligament** runs along the length of the posterior margins of the vertebral bodies, and is intimately associated with the posterior margins of the annuli. It resists flexion of the spine.

Associated with and strengthening the posterior columns are the posterior supporting ligaments – the ligamentum flavum, the capsular ligaments (of the facet joints) and the interspinous and supraspinous ligaments. These assist restriction of forward flexion of the spine. The **ligamentum flavum**, which is associated with the anterior aspect of the laminae and adjacent portions of the pedicles, is interesting in that it has elastic properties, containing 80% elastin and 20% collagen; perhaps this property prevents it from buckling into the spinal canal on spinal extension. The disposition of the ligaments between the spinous processes is as shown in Fig. 1.9. The supraspinous ligament ends at L5, though this region is further strengthened by the iliolumbar ligaments (which, together with the sacroiliac ligaments, are described in chapter 4).

The **intertransverse ligaments** are perhaps more appropriately considered to be part of the fascial planes, separating muscle groups; in the thoracolumbar region they merge with the thoracolumbar

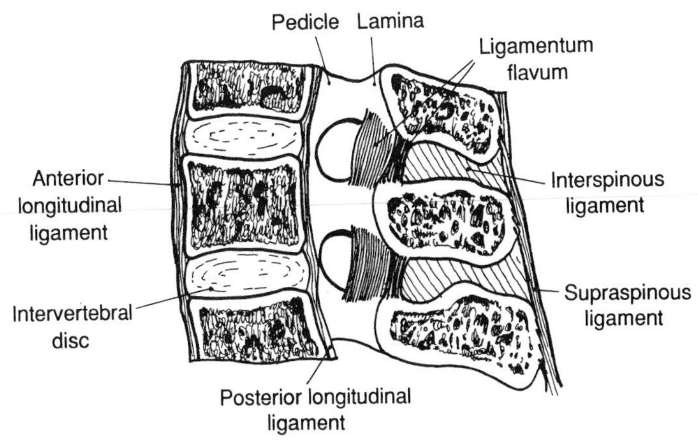

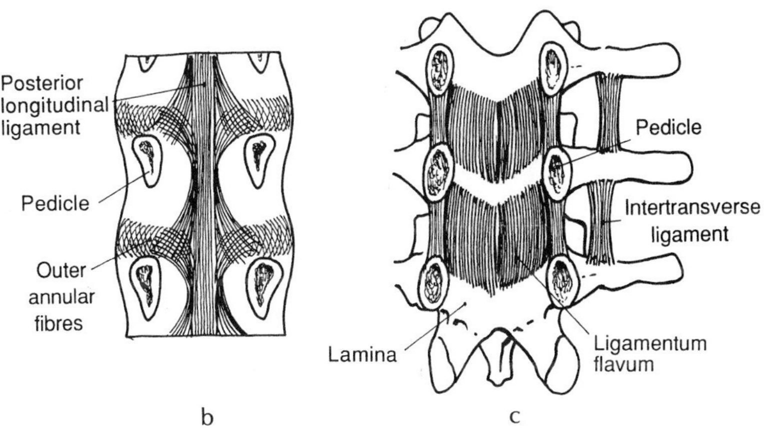

Fig. 1.9 The disposition of the ligaments in the lumbar spine is demonstrated. (a) lateral aspect; (b) posterior longitudinal ligament; (c) anterior aspect of ligamenta flava.

fascia which has attachments to both the abdominal muscles and the spine. Collectively, the posterior ligaments and the thoracolumbar fascia are referred to as the **posterior ligamentous system** which has an important role in the biomechanics of spinal movements, particularly lifting (see 'Biomechanics; lifting').

Muscles

In the neck is found a variety of strap muscles, which act either upon the head or neck independently, or upon both the head and the neck (Figs 2.7, 2.8). Although some muscles, for instance the sternomastoids, are readily defined and easy to palpate, the small muscles may be impossible to identify clinically; however, localized tension in the posterior muscles, when associated with spinal joint dysfunction, may be palpated when the neck is supported by the examiner in the neutral or extended position. Since there is considerable muscle activity in the

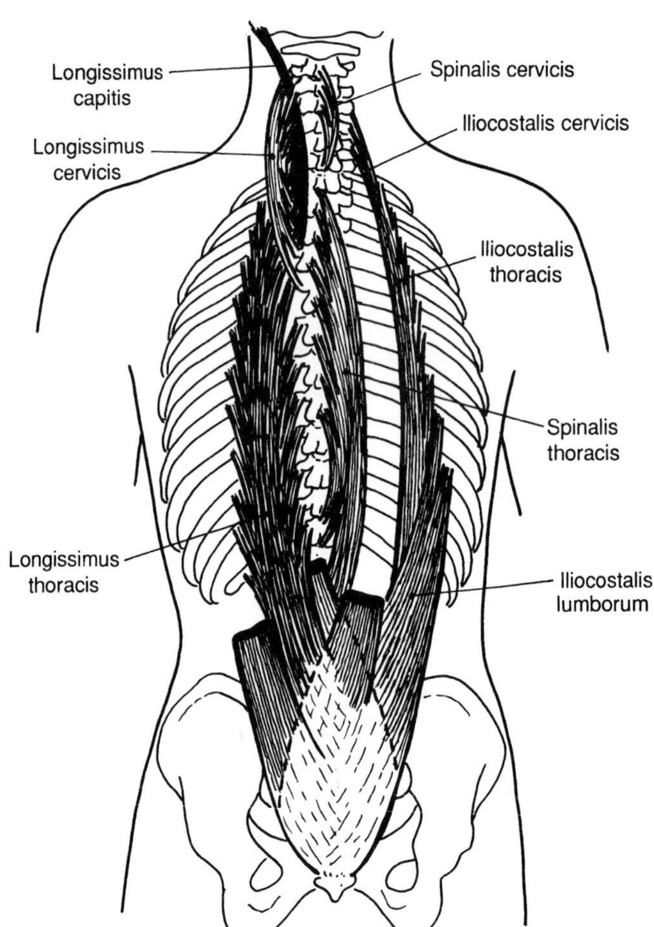

Fig. 1.10 The erector spinae are the most superficial and longest muscles in the spine.

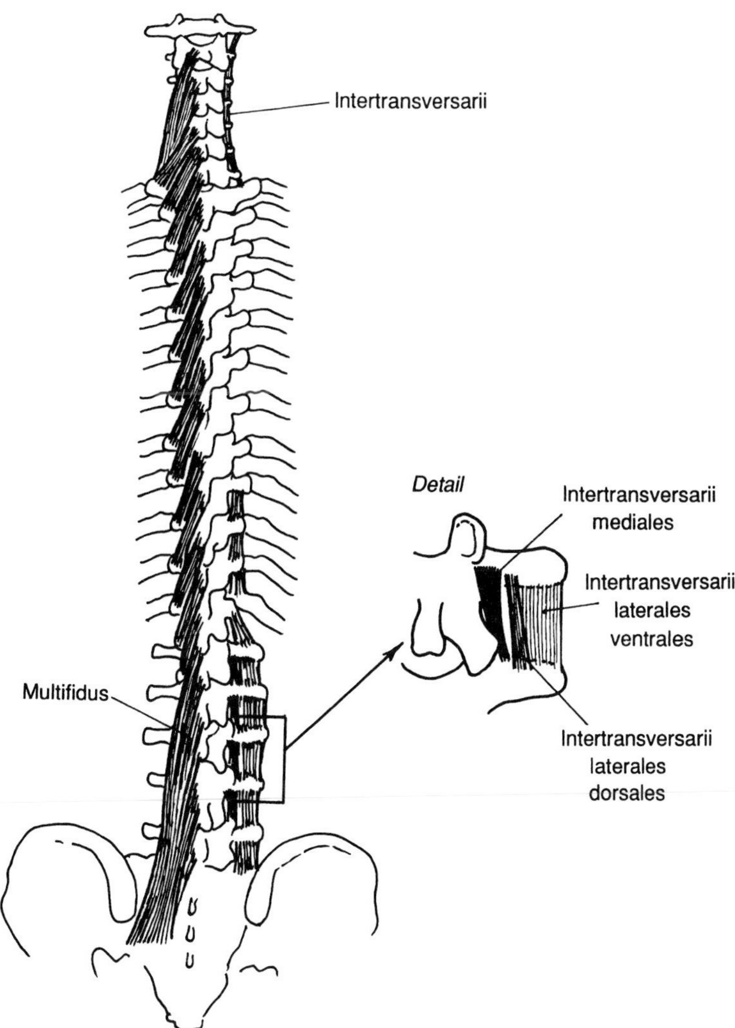

Fig. 1.11 The deep posterior muscle groups of the spine contain, *inter alia*, multifidus and the intertransversarii.

upright position to stabilize the head on the cervical spine, it is unusual for inadequate muscle function to be an aetiological factor in mechanical derangements of the neck. Chronic muscle fatigue, particularly in the trapezius and levator scapulae, commonly gives rise to myotendinoses, however. Accordingly, muscle strengthening exercises are not usually necessary during recovery from cervical spinal joint derangements except in exceptional circumstances, for instance in preparation for return to sports such as rugby; postural exercises, though, are frequently indicated.

The posterior muscles of the trunk may be classified according to the number of segments over which they act (Figs 1.10, 1.11). The erector spinae (iliocostalis, longissimus and spinalis) are the most superficial and longest, passing over at least seven vertebrae. In the second group, passing between two and seven vertebrae, are semispinalis and multifidus. The third group, passing from one vertebra to another, contains the intertransversarii, interspinales and rotatores. The principal action of the posterior muscles is to extend the trunk. The quadratus lumborum (Fig. 1.12*b*) is situated laterally and moves the trunk ipsilaterally on contraction.

The muscles which produce flexion of the spine are the abdominal muscles and the psoas (Fig. 1.12*a, b, c*). The recti abdomini, and the external and internal oblique muscles, act in concert to rotate as well as flex the trunk. If the rib cage is fixed the muscles act to lift the anterior part of the pelvis, and thereby assist in flattening the lumbar lordosis. The transversus abdominis is an important muscle in respect of normal spinal function. It is the deepest of the three muscles lateral to the rectus abdominis, and is attached posteriorly to the thoracolumbar fascia. It acts with the other abdominal muscles to increase the intra-abdominal pressure; and it also reinforces the strength of the posterior ligamentous system.

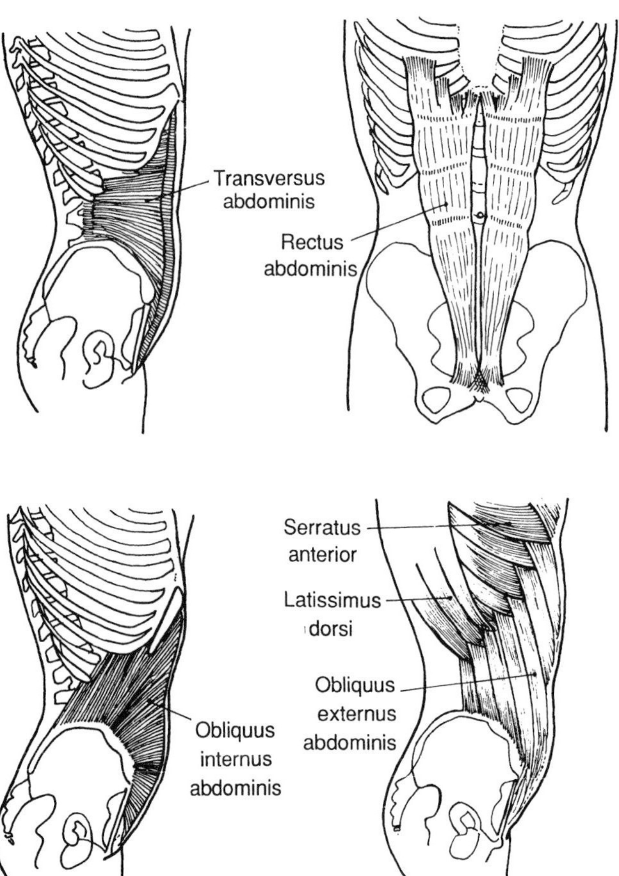

Fig. 1.12 The flexors of the spine and their relationships are demonstrated. (a) The abdominal muscles. (b) Transverse sections across the spine and the anterior abdominal wall. (c) Psoas and iliacus muscles.

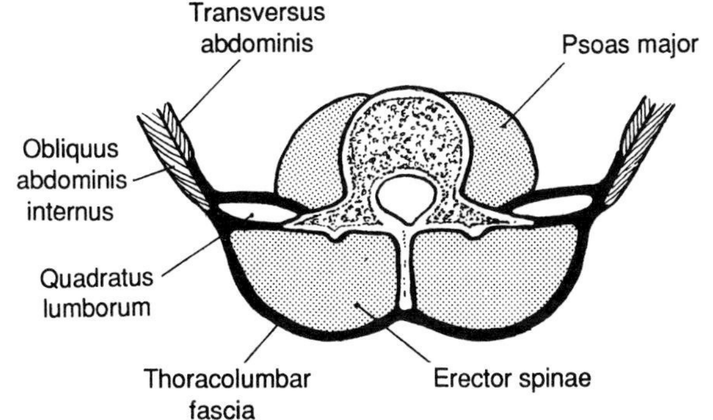
Transversus
abdominis
Psoas major
Obliquus
abdominis
internus
Quadratus
lumborum
Thoracolumbar
fascia
Erector spinae

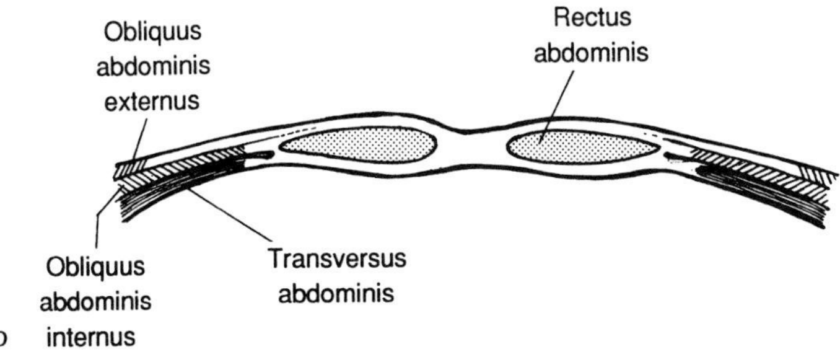
Obliquus
abdominis
externus
Rectus
abdominis
Obliquus
abdominis
internus
Transversus
abdominis

b

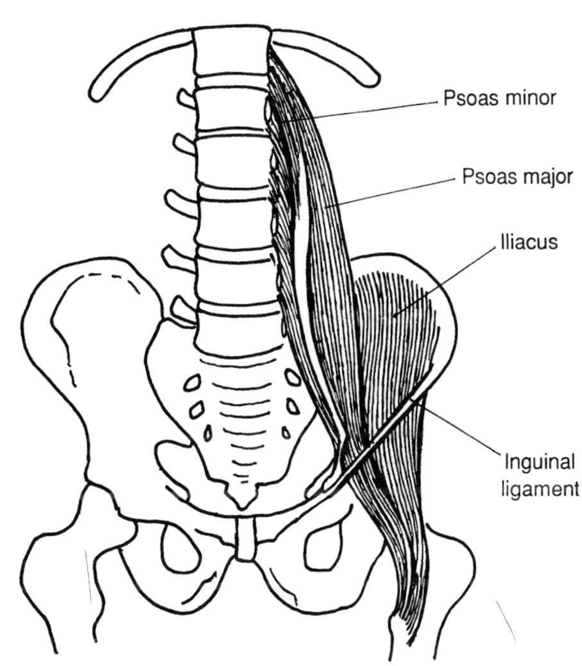
Psoas minor
Psoas major
Iliacus
Inguinal
ligament

c

MOVEMENTS

The basic movements of the spine are flexion and extension in the sagittal plane (about a transverse axis), side bending in the coronal plane (about an anteroposterior, syn. 'sagittal' axis) and rotation in the transverse plane (about a vertical axis, Fig. 1.13). Side flexion and

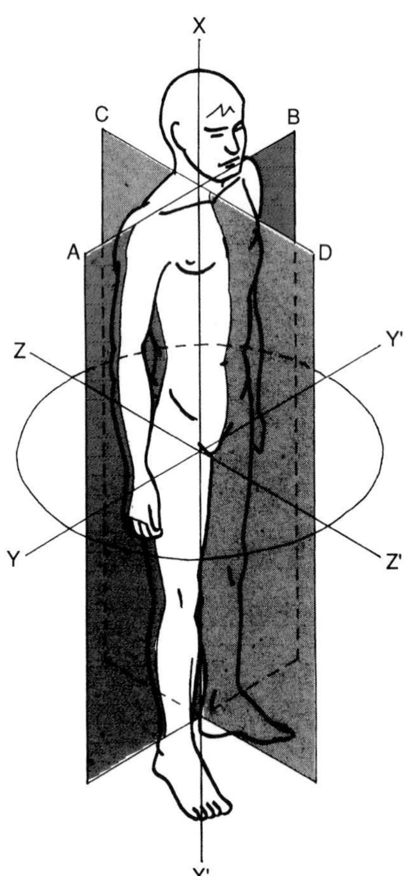

Fig. 1.13 Planes of the body and axes of movement.

rotation are always associated (or 'coupled') movements. The amount of movement at each vertebral level is dependent upon the inclination of the facet joints; overall, the amount of movement is greatest in the cervical and lumbar regions where the relative disc height compared with the height of the vertebral body is greater than in the thoracic spine (Fig. 1.14).

Extension

During extension the nucleus pulposus is driven anteriorly, and pressure is applied to the anterior fibres of the annulus, increasing

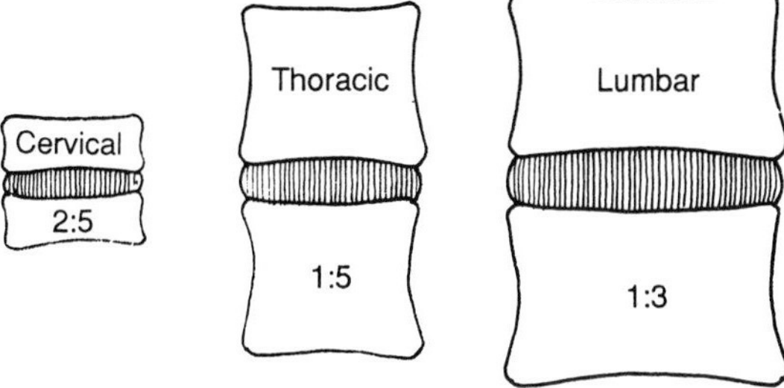

Fig. 1.14 The ratios of disc height to vertebral body height are demonstrated in the different regions of the spine.

their tension. The anterior longitudinal ligament is stretched; at the end of range there is impingement of the articular processes, and the spinous processes may touch. Posterior shear (syn. 'translation') of one vertebra takes place on the one below (Fig. 1.15).

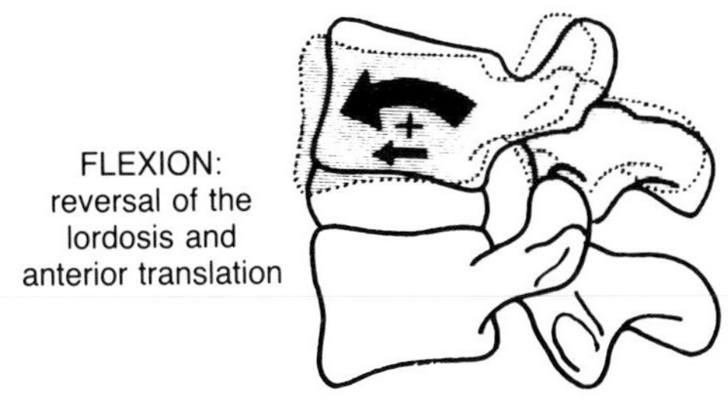

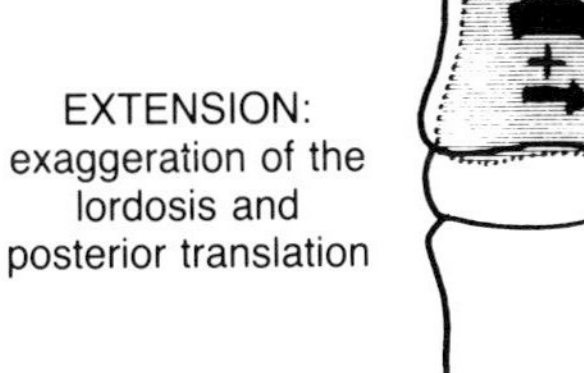

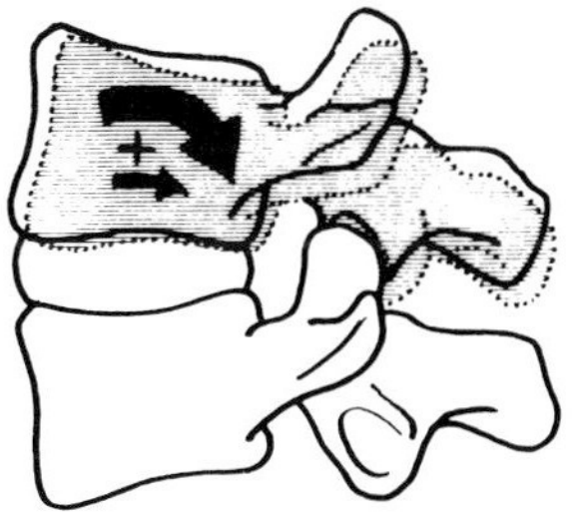

Fig. 1.15 Flexion and extension of a lumbar motion segment showing that the movements around a transverse axis are accompanied by translation (shear).

Flexion

In essence, flexion is a reversal of the lordosis of the lumbar and cervical spines. This is accompanied by anterior translation, in which the upper vertebra moves anteriorly upon the lower (Fig. 1.15). The nucleus is driven posteriorly, and pressure is applied to the posterior fibres of the annulus increasing their tension and creating self-stabilization. The inferior processes slide superiorly and away from the superior processes of the vertebra below. The result is maximal stretching of the capsular ligaments and also of the other posterior ligaments – the supraspinous, infraspinous and posterior longitudinal ligaments, and the ligamentum flavum. Initially, during flexion from the standing position, the extensor muscles exert control by eccentric contraction; once a critical point is reached, the final restraint is ligamentous tension. During flexion of the whole of the spine there is a significant degree of rotation around a transverse axis at the hip joints, and also some flexion of the head on the neck.

Side flexion

The articular processes slide, resulting in compression of the disc on the side towards which movement occurs. Contralaterally, the disc and the ligamentum flavum and the capsular ligaments are stretched.

Rotation (torsion)

Torsional stress is resisted by the facet joints and the ligaments (possibly 65%) and by the annular fibres of the disc (possibly 35%).

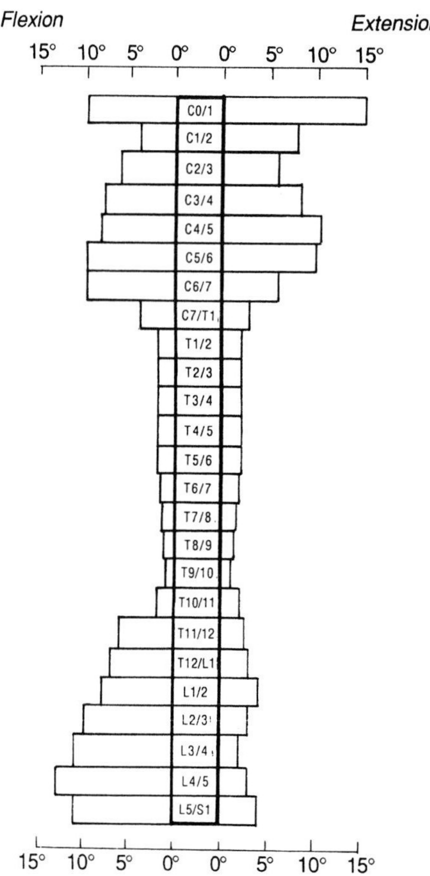

Fig. 1.16 Average ranges of segmental movement (flexion and extension). These are *average* values. Wide variations occur according to age, body structure pathology, etc.

In the thoracolumbar region the amount of rotation is significantly affected also by the degree of trunk flexion or extension; the effect of extension is to restrict the range of rotation. Globally, trunk rotation in the standing position is assisted by sacroiliac torsion and hip rotation, and also by movements of the shoulders.

The average ranges of segmental movements are shown in Figs 1.16 and 1.17, and are considered in greater detail in the following chapters.

Joint play

The preceding account of the global movements of the spine, to which individual segments contribute to greater or lesser degrees, refers to active movements under voluntary control. Segmentally, individual joints exhibit a further range of movements, known as joint play (after Mennell, 1960), which are not under voluntary control yet may be identified by specific examining techniques. Restriction in joint play is an important accessory sign, particularly when the examiner is faced with a patient who has minimal, if any, restriction in the range of

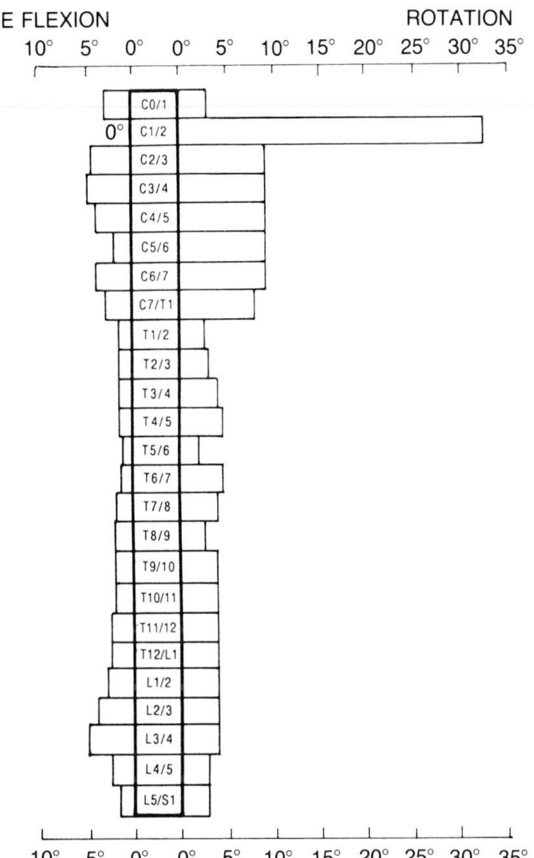

Fig. 1.17 Average ranges of segmental movement (side flexion and rotation). These are *average* values. Wide variations occur according to age, body structure pathology, etc.

active movements. Joint play reflects function and dysfunction of the spinal (apophyseal) joints, thereby providing the examiner with the facility to make a discriminant assessment of segmental function.

In common with the situation in the peripheral joints of the body, *spinal joint derangements* (from whatever cause) *are associated with loss of movement*; in the clinical setting, careful identification of the range of movement, both regionally and segmentally, is an essential examination requirement.

BIOMECHANICS

Disc tension

The complex of trabeculae in the vertebral body resists compressive, tensile and rotational stresses. Additionally, each intervertebral disc absorbs stress by deformation of the nucleus pulposus and distribution of forces to the annulus fibrosus (Fig. 1.6). The elasticity of the nucleus is dependent upon its water content; greater deformation occurs per given stress when the disc degenerates.

Pressures within the L3 disc have been measured by Nachemson and co-workers (1970), and have been shown to vary considerably according to posture and the level of physical activity (Fig. 1.18). The pressure in the standing (upright) position is four times that in the supine position. The standing pressure is increased by 50% in 20° of forward flexion. Various isotonic spinal flexion and extension exercises increase the pressure substantially – isometric exercises less so. It is clear, however, that muscular activity has a greater impact on intradiscal pressures than the effect of gravity alone. Of considerable significance, too, is the increased pressure within the L3 disc in the sitting position. When the degree of lumbar support is inadequate, and the sitting posture is prolonged, the adverse strain on the lumbar discs is substantial.

Postural characteristics

The lumbar lordosis has developed, phylogenetically, as a response to the upright posture. The centre of gravity of the body is aligned over the hips to accommodate prolonged standing. The line of weight, from below upwards, lies in front of the ankles, slightly in front of the transverse axes of the knees, and is considered to be very slightly behind the hip joints; it is well in front of the sacroiliac joints (Fig. 1.19). In the lumbar region the line of weight passes in front of the vertebral bodies at the convexity of the lumbar curve in 75% of individuals. Thus, the extensor muscles of the spine are usually active in counteracting gravity. A counterbalancing resistance is also required of the sacroiliac ligaments (both anterior and posterior sacroiliac, sacrotuberous and sacrospinous), and the gluteus maximus

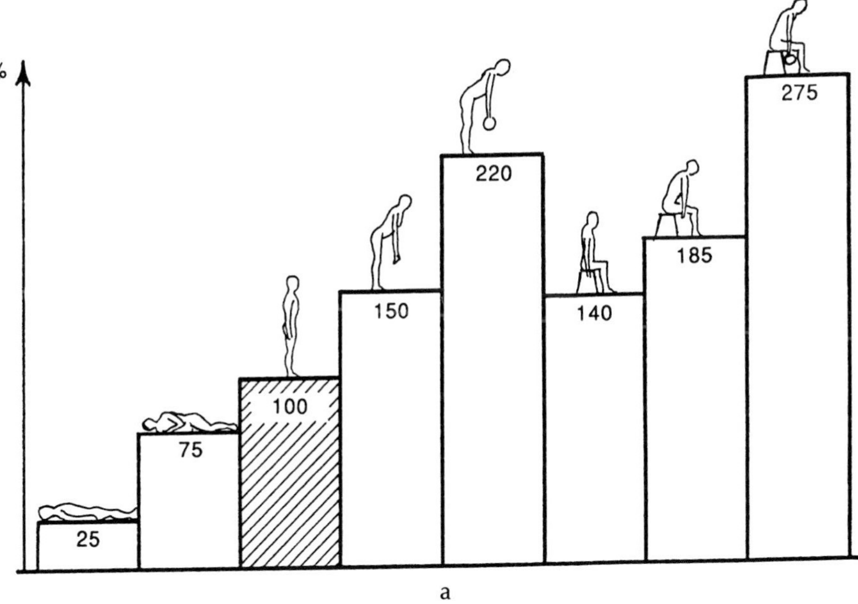

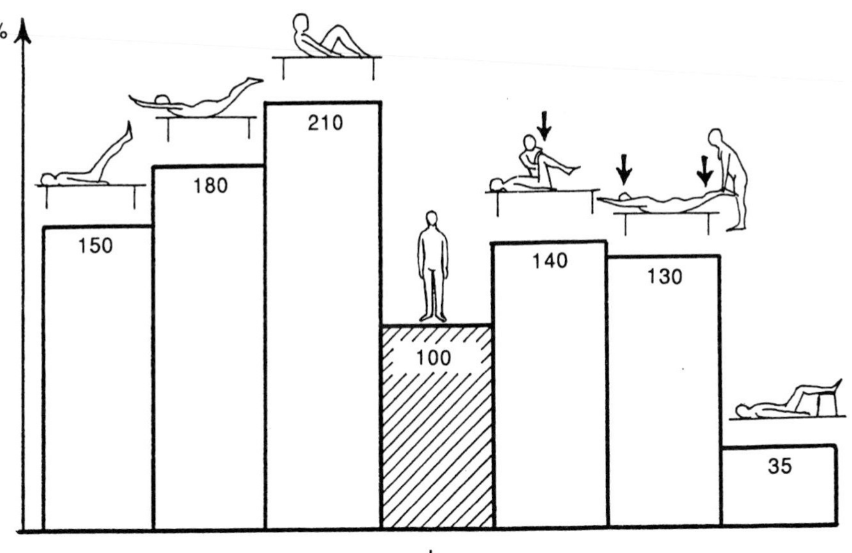

Fig. 1.18 Relative change in pressure (or load) in the third lumbar disc. (a) In various positions. (b) In various muscle strengthening exercises. (From Nachemson, A., 1976, The lumbar spine: an orthopaedic challenge. *Spine*, **1**, 59–71)

and hamstrings which assist in flattening the lumbar lordosis (Figs 1.20, 3.5).

The relative weakness of the abdominal muscles in the majority of the population allows increased forward rotation of the pelvis and increased hyperextension of the lumbar spine. In women it is aggravated by multiparity and by wearing high heels. Standing for prolonged periods is associated with an increased lordosis, and may give rise to discomfort in susceptible individuals, presumably caused

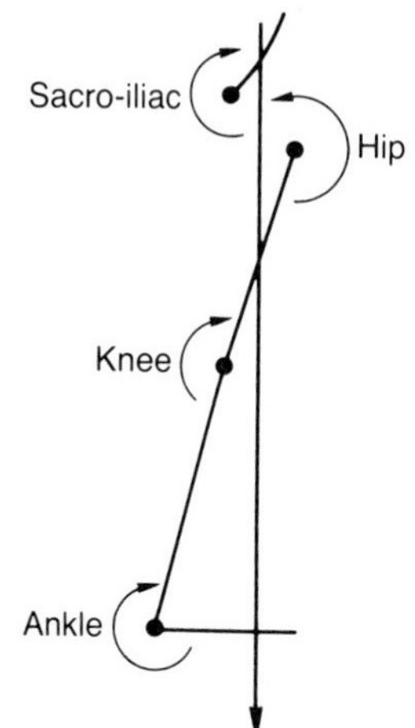

Fig. 1.19 In the standing position the line of weight falls well in front of the sacroiliac joints (from Evans, D.P., 1982, *Backache: Its Evolution and Conservative Treatment*, MTP Press, Lancaster.)

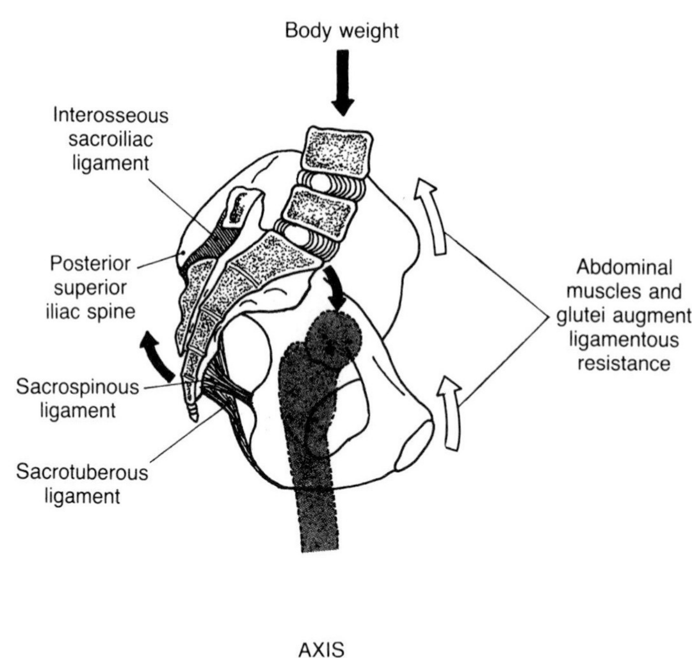

Fig. 1.20 The role of ligaments in weightbearing is demonstrated in this sagitttal section of the inner aspect of the left half of the pelvis. In the erect posture, the sacroiliac ligaments resist downward and forward movement of the sacral base. The sacrotuberous and sacrospinous ligaments resist the upward and backward tilting of the apex of the sacrum.

by the combination of excessive strain on the sacroiliac ligaments, fatigue in the spinal extensor muscles and irritation of the facet joints. Relief may be gained by flattening the lumbar spine, for instance by flexing one hip and knee and placing the foot on a rail or ledge for support. However, the main dynamic requirement is improvement of abdominal muscle tone. Unfortunately, for the majority of the population, there are relatively few daily activities which strengthen the abdominal muscles. The tendency, unless counteracted by specific spinal flexibility exercises and abdominal strengthening exercises, is for the extensor muscles acting on the lumbar spine to become relatively strong and to shorten.

Loss of extension at the hip as a result of osteoarthritis may be a contributory factor in the development of an excessive lumbar lordosis; apophyseal impingement is increased in the erect position. Loss of hip flexion too allows excessive stress to be applied to the 'static' connective tissues of the spine which must take up the slack on trunk flexion; hence a twofold adverse effect on the lumbar spine with osteoarthritis of the hip. This effect is particularly pronounced in the relatively young patient who wishes to engage in sports such as squash rackets which impose excessive flexion, extension and rotational strains upon the spine and hip joints. If the hips are stiff, and respond to impact loading ineffectually, the lower back (particularly the low lumbar facet joints and the sacroiliac joints) will suffer.

In the upper back, a pronounced proximal thoracic kyphosis is associated with 'round' (in comparison with 'square') shoulders, and hyperextension of the cervical spine. Aetiologically, there are probably a number of contributory factors, although relative weakness of the muscles which fix the lower scapula is a particular feature which must be overcome if posture is to be improved and tension reduced in the muscles (such as upper fibres of trapezius and levator scapulae) acting on the upper scapula.

Sitting

It is possible for the lumbar spine to hyperextend, and facet joint impaction to occur, if sitting is accompanied by outstretched legs (Fig. 1.21c). More often, however, the back 'slumps' during sitting, increasing the intradiscal pressures in the lumbar spine and stretching the posterior ligaments (Fig. 1.21a). To prevent backache in those occupations which demand prolonged sitting, particularly those requiring keyboard work or extensive car driving, consideration should be given to the choice of a seat with an adjustable lumbar support or to the use of a backrest. During prolonged sitting, there are considerable postural strains too upon the thoracic and cervical spines, and their supporting musculature; the primary fault, however, is often inadequate support of the lumbar lordosis. Further consideration is given to posture and ergonomics in succeeding chapters.

Bending and stooping

During flexion of the trunk from the standing position, the weight of the upper body is controlled by the spinal extensor muscles until a critical point is reached, usually at about 45° from the vertical. From then on the posterior ligamentous system tightens, relieving the strain

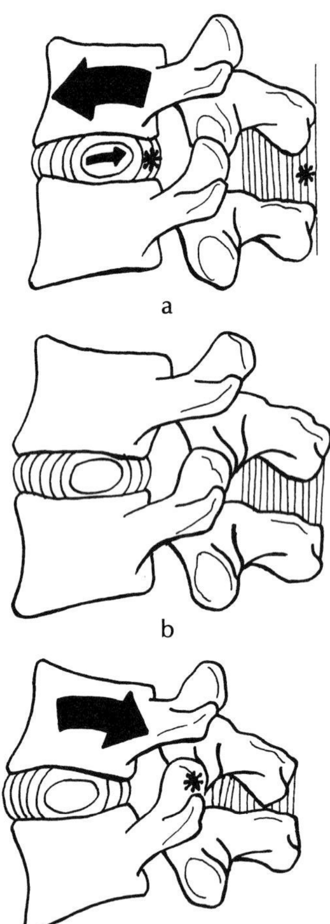

Fig. 1.21 The lumbar motion segments are demonstrated in different sitting positions. (a) Flexion. (b) Mid-range. (c) Extension. * = sites of stress.

on the back muscles. The elasticity of the ligamentum flavum is probably an important factor at this stage. The final phase of trunk flexion involves rotation of the pelvis around a transverse axis through the hip joints, and is under the control of the hip extensors. Reversal of this pelvi-lumbar rhythm is observed on recoil from the fully flexed position: initially, the pelvis is rotated backwards prior to the restoration of the lumbar lordosis. Shear in forward flexion, which is produced by contraction of the spinal extensor muscles, is reduced by the orientation of the lower two lumbar facet joints, and controlled overall by the tension in the thoracolumbar fascia.

In prolonged stooping, as may be found for instance during gardening, hyperextension of the lumbar spine is produced and maintained by the bowstring effect of the erector spinae. The sacrotuberous, sacrospinous and sacroiliac ligaments are strained in this position. In prolonged bending, however, as exhibited for instance by bricklayers, prolonged load-bearing in flexion is found and the 'creep' phenomenon occurs (progressive deformation of a viscoelastic structure under constant load). The anterior part of the disc is squeezed and the posterior ligaments stretched. Recovery from creep is far from instantaneous, as exemplified by the difficulty in straightening after prolonged spinal flexion.

In the elderly the strength of the quadriceps femoris muscles may be compromised, often in association with degenerative changes in the knee joints. Excessive strain may be imparted to the lower back if the quadriceps, when acting in concert with the glutei, are not strong enough to allow the recovery of the upright position from the semi-squat position adopted in picking up light weights from the floor. This is of some relevance during rehabilitation from, or prophylaxis against, low back strain.

Lifting

The force exerted on the lumbar spine is increased when lifting weights. This force is a reflection of both the mass of the weight being lifted and its horizontal distance from the vertebrae. When the weights are small, and particularly when held close to the body, the spinal extensor muscles are quite capable of balancing the forces. However, in weight-lifting (as a sport, or when heavy weights are lifted casually, or in heavy manual occupations) the forces generated demand additional muscle and ligamentous control. In the initial phase of a power lift the hip extensors rotate the pelvis. Subsequently, two biomechanical problems have to be overcome. First, the spinal extensor muscles alone are incapable of extending the spine to the upright position; secondly, should the force across the lumbosacral joint not be dissipated, then biomechanical analysis suggests that vertebral body and intervertebral disc failure could occur. Two different mechanisms are proposed to account for the calculated 30% reduction in forces which must occur across the lumbosacral joint.

A generally accepted theory is that increased intra-abdominal tension is produced by the contraction of the abdominal muscles. Conversion of the abdominal cavity to a semi-solid container produces unloading of the lumbar spine (Fig. 1.22). This is aided by fixation of the diaphragm and increased tension within the thoracic cavity. Weight-lifters usually use an abdominal belt in order to increase the pressure within the abdominal cavity and facilitate transmission of forces.

The second theory is that the posterior ligamentous system plays a crucial role. During contraction of the hip extensors and contraction of the abdominal muscles (maintaining lumbar flexion in the early stages of the lift), forces are transmitted with the assistance of the posterior ligamentous system. The posterior part of the thoracolumbar fascia plays a particularly important role; it contributes substantially towards absorption of forces to the extent that the weight may be brought closer to the body, allowing spinal extension to occur somewhat later in the lifting process. It would appear that

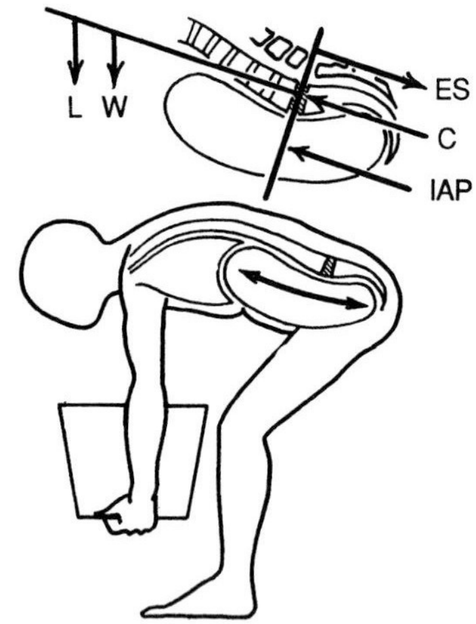

Fig. 1.22 Diagrams showing spine, thoracic and abdominal cavities during lifting, together with a force diagram demonstrating how the increases in intra-abdominal pressure (IAP) may relieve the intervertebral compression (C) which is equal and opposite to the tensile force in the erector spinae (ES) required to raise the load (L) and the upper part of the body (W). (From Troup, J.D., 1979, Biomechanics of the vertebral column. *Physiotherapy*, **65(8)**, 239.)

the thoracolumbar fascia continues to exert an anti-flexion effect during the final process of spinal extensor activity, even when the posterior ligaments are beginning to relax.

Whatever the mechanism, the importance of strong abdominal muscles, in addition to hip extensors, cannot be overstressed.

Relationship to shoulder and pelvic girdles

A close relationship exists, in biomechanical as well as anatomical terms, between the cervical spine and the shoulder. It is often found that patients with neck pain also complain of pain in the shoulder and upper arm. Pain in the arm may, of course, be due to nerve root irritation which arises in the neck, or to pain from other neck structures. A further association, however, appears to exist between disturbance of rotator cuff function and cervical spinal joint dysfunction. Although the exact mechanism is not understood, the answer probably lies in the common C5 neural pathway, possibly as a result of a 'facilitated cord segment'. The signs of cervical spinal joint dysfunction coexist with the signs of subacromial decompensation which often manifest as a painful arc on abduction of the affected shoulder, and weakness of the shoulder abductors. Sometimes, treatment to both regions is necessary; at other times, resolution of one condition appears to act as a catalyst to spontaneous resolution of the other. This association between cervical spinal joint dysfunction and subacromial dysfunction is seen sufficiently often for it to be considered a distinct entity, although a true C5 root palsy due to a C4/5 disc prolapse (one of the least common levels of entrapment) should be excluded.

A slightly different relationship exists between the lumbar spine, on the one hand, and the hip joint and the muscles acting over it on the other. Restriction of movement at the hip, usually due to osteoarthritis, places additional strain upon the posterior joints of the lumbar spine. In other patients tight hamstrings, which restrict trunk flexion by reducing rotation of the pelvis, may be an aetiological factor in injuries occurring in flexion: if trunk flexion is demanded by a particular activity, and it is not forthcoming from pelvic rotation, additional strain is imposed on those (spinal) structures resisting spinal flexion.

PATHOANATOMY

To some extent, degenerative changes in the spine are an inevitable accompaniment to ageing. The intervertebral disc loses some of its viscoelastic properties as a result of loss of its water content, and varying degrees of disc narrowing occur. Radiographically, this may be accompanied by marginal osteophyte formation and the spine is said to demonstrate the features of **spondylosis**. However, such radiological changes are no guide to the site of nociceptive afferent stimulation, nor to any *relevant* pathological changes which may be responsible for a specific episode of acute back or neck pain, or for chronic backache. Accordingly, it is useful to understand the nature of those pathological changes which are considered to make a significant contribution to the aetiology of disturbances of the spinal motion segment, yet which may be difficult to demonstrate radiologically (even with modern imaging techniques).

Severe compression of the spine, such as is found in pilots ejecting from jet aircraft, tends to give rise to vertebral body fractures. At lesser loads the vertebral end-plate is at risk of fracture, being less resilient than the disc. As a result of end-plate injury, however, disc prolapse (often at L5/S1) may arise at the site of weakness between the attachment of the annular fibres to the posterior margin of the plate. By contrast, the combination of axial and torsional loading is inclined to injure either the disc, or the facet joints, or both. A tear of the posterior annulus, which is a common finding, allows part of the nucleus to be driven posteriorly. Repeated torsion may give rise to disc degeneration which is accelerated if the facet joints are damaged also.

In childhood and adolescence a prolapse of a nucleus pulposus in the lumbar spine may occur superiorly or inferiorly, or relatively anteriorly, through a defective end-plate, and produce a localized erosion of the vertebral body; its radiological appearance is known as a Schmorl's node (Fig. 1.23). The characteristic feature of a prolapsed disc in adulthood is posterior protrusion (a 'central' disc prolapse), often developing into a posterolateral protrusion. Some of the nucleus may be 'extruded' through an annular tear (though the international terminology refers to an HNP – 'herniation' of the nucleus pulposus). In this text, however, the terms 'prolapse', 'protrusion', and

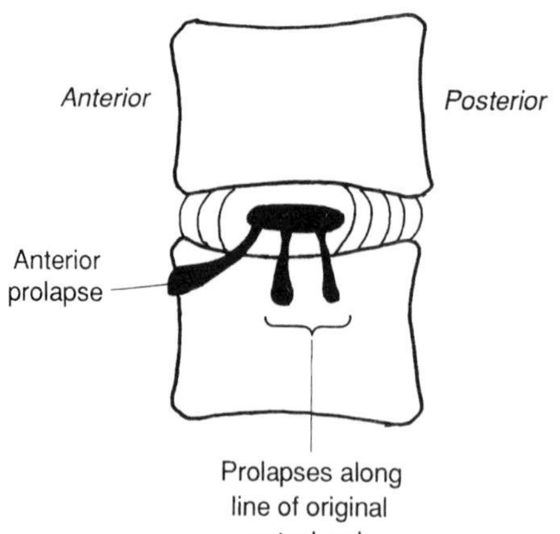

Fig. 1.23 A Schmorl's node is formed by vertical protrusion of a nucleus pulposus through a defective end-plate.

'herniation' are used synonymously. If **sequestration** occurs, a portion of the disc breaks away from the main body of the disc and comes to lie in the spinal canal, often compressing a nerve root (Fig. 1.24).

Irrespective of a history of frank prolapse of the nucleus pulposus, progressive degenerative changes in a motion segment may arise as a result of the combination of circumferential and radial tears of the annulus, and increasing laxity of the capsular ligaments of the facet joints. Narrowing of the disc produces further 'offsetting' of the articular processes posteriorly, giving rise to the clinically recognizable condition of **segmental instability**. Effectively, the vertebral

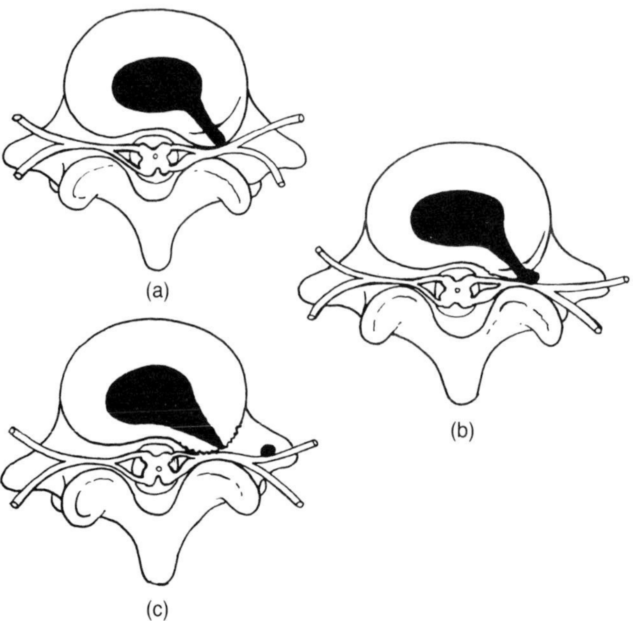

Fig. 1.24 Diagrams showing stages of disc prolapse. (a) Annular protrusion. (b) Nuclear extrusion. (c) Sequestration.

segment becomes destabilized, and *the loss of shock absorption* is accompanied by ligamentous incompetence.

On a functional basis, disturbance of a motion segment may best be considered in relation to the three-joint complex of facet joint – disc – facet joint, as structural abnormalities of one element of this complex will inevitably be accompanied by increasing strain upon, and eventually by pathological changes within, another element. Clinically, it is often possible to differentiate between lesions associated primarily with the disc anteriorly, and 'spinal joint dysfunction' which is due to disturbance in the posterior columns (the essential feature of which is facet overload). Under other circumstances, however, **acute segmental dysfunction** might be a more appropriate descriptive label as the clinical characteristics may suggest both a disc prolapse and accompanying facetal dysfunction. Whatever the clinical presentation, it is important that the examiner should fully evaluate the three-joint complex and, subsequently, consider the need for appropriate rehabilitation of *all* the supporting structures once the painful phase has resolved.

Consequent upon the progression of degenerative changes in the facet joints, the resultant osteophytic hypertrophy may give rise to lateral canal stenosis. The shape of the spinal canal is a determining factor in the development of nerve root entrapment resulting from degenerative changes (Fig. 1.25). In the trefoil spinal canal in the lower lumbar region the spinal roots are vulnerable to either discogenic or osteophytic compression. At this (distal lumbar) spinal level a spondylolisthesis may also reduce the diameter of the spinal canal. In the presence of bony hypertrophic changes, and thickening and buckling of the ligamentum flavum, symptomatic central canal stenosis may be precipitated by an additional event such as disc bulging. A claudicant picture may ensue, and differentiation from

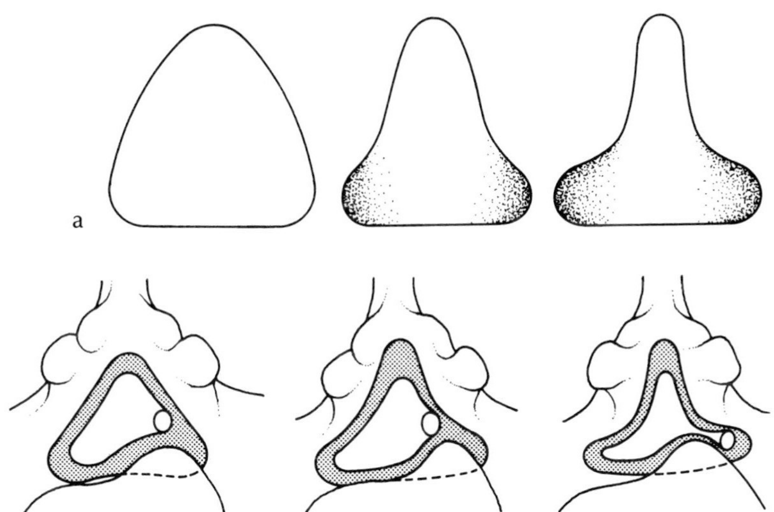

Fig. 1.25 (a) The variable shape of the lower lumbar vertebral canal. The trefoil canal has a deep lateral recess. (b) A nerve root is vulnerable to compression by a disc protrusion in a trefoil canal. (After Porter, 1982.)

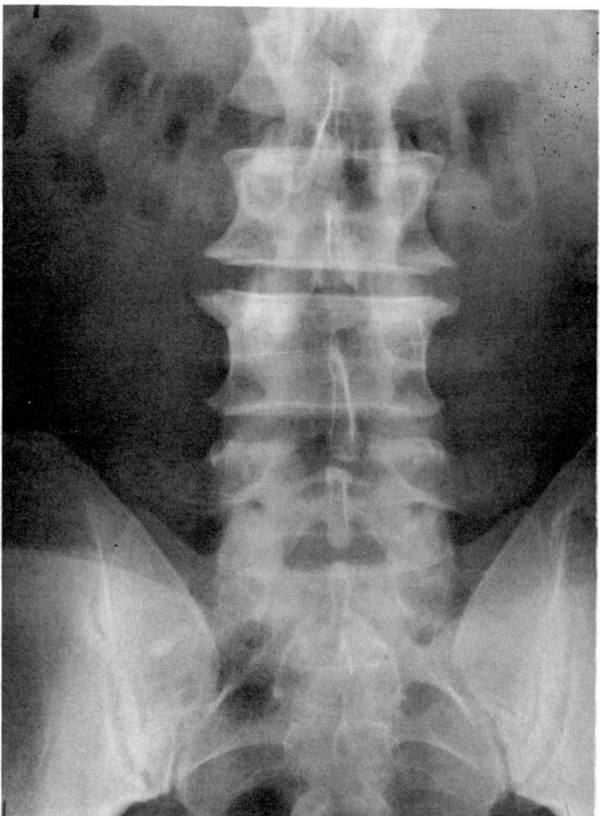

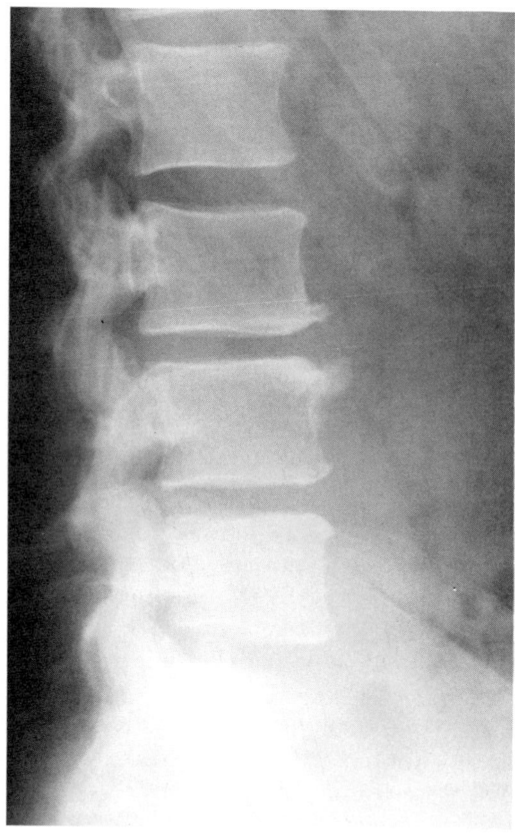

Fig. 1.26 The changes of spondylosis (disc narrowing and junctional osteophytes) are demonstrated on these anteroposterior and lateral X-rays of the lumbar spine.

intermittent claudication due to arterial insufficiency is necessary. In the cervical region central canal stenosis may give rise to a myelopathy detected by the presence of long tract signs in the lower limbs.

Osteoarthritis

Osteoarthritis of the apophyseal joints may be asymptomatic, though it is often associated with discomfort and stiffness following an unusual degree of exercise. Such symptoms are often felt after resting and, particularly, in the mornings – a typical response of joint degenerative disease.

Degenerative changes in the spine are probably universal by the age of 60, and advance in their severity with increasing age (Fig. 1.26). It is generally accepted, however, that the incidence of bouts of severe back pain or neck pain decreases after middle age, probably associated with increased stiffening of the spine and reduced inclination towards provocative exercise. Thus the correlation between radiological 'spondylosis' (sometimes, misleadingly, referred to as 'spondylitis' of the spine) and spinal pain is poor, and other sources or mechanisms of nociceptive afferent stimulation should be sought.

Other conditions, such as spondylolysis and spondylolisthesis, which are associated with specific pathological changes, are described in the relevant chapters.

Little reference is made in this book to 'pulled' or 'torn' muscles. Undoubtedly, muscle spasm is detectable in painful spinal conditions when it is secondary to underlying pathology or dysfunction. It is also reasonable to postulate that, following unaccustomed exercise, discomfort may arise from excessive eccentric muscle contraction in exactly the same way as it does elsewhere in the body. (Ligamentous stretching is another source of this temporary discomfort.) However, mid-belly tears of the spinal musculature are not a recognizable clinical entity, and the case for disruptions involving muscle attachments is unproved.

Trigger points

Trigger points (TPs) are usually considered to be tender areas in muscles, and commonly occur in predictable sites as *secondary* manifestations of disturbed spinal function. They may be considered to be areas of referred muscle spasm which disappear on successful management of the underlying dysfunction. Other authorities (for instance, Travell and Simons, 1992) consider that a trigger point is 'a hyperirritable spot, usually within a taut band of skeletal muscle or in the muscle's fascia, that is painful on compression and that can give rise to characteristic pain, tenderness, and autonomic phenomena'.

Myotendinoses (areas of 'myofasciitis' characterized by the presence of *primary* TPs) usually occur in muscles which are subjected to increased postural stress; for their management, specific therapeutic regimes to reduce both intrinsic tension and extrinsic stress may be required.

NERVE COMPRESSION

Dysaesthesiae in a limb may be caused by central (spinal) or distal nerve lesions: the differential diagnosis is extensive.

Spinal cord

Cord compression, for instance in the cervical spine as a result of cervical spondylosis, is painless but causes diffuse paraesthesiae in the lower limbs. Signs of an upper motor neurone lesion (spasticity, an extensor Babinski reflex and dyscoordination) may be apparent in the legs.

Nerve root

Traction on a nerve root which has been damaged, for instance by pressure from a disc, causes intense pain. The dura mater too is known to be mechanosensitive, and is also chemosensitive. Paraesthesiae and numbness in a dermatomal pattern result from pressure on the sensory fibres. A motor palsy may be detected if the corresponding motor fibres are involved in the root entrapment.

Nerve trunk

Pressure on the nerve trunk beyond the dural sleeve does not cause pain, but produces paraesthesiae on release of pressure. For instance, in the thoracic outlet syndrome, paraesthesiae may be caused by release of pressure on the brachial plexus by elevation of the shoulders. Similarly, release of pressure on the sciatic nerve after sitting causes intense paraesthesiae down the affected leg; sitting with the legs crossed may create pressure on the lateral peroneal nerve, following which paraesthesiae or even temporary muscle paresis may be apparent on standing, but not pain. In the upper limb, compression of the median nerve (in the carpal tunnel syndrome) causes paraesthesiae to be felt in the radial three and a half digits during the night. Historically, this situation has been considered to represent a release phenomenon, though it is perhaps more likely that the median nerve is *compressed* at night, either by swelling of the wrist joint, or by fluid retention. Some nerves, such as the ulnar nerve at the elbow, may definitely produce paraesthesiae *during* compression; and it is probable that the median nerve in the carpal tunnel may cause diurnal paraesthesiae if repeatedly compressed in jobs involving repetitive manual activities.

Peripheral nerves

Digital nerves and other nerves near their extremity cause more numbness than paraesthesiae if compressed (for instance, meralgia paraesthetica due to compression of the lateral cutaneous nerve of thigh).

CONCEPTUAL MODELS OF SPINAL DISORDERS

Structural concepts

Structural pathological changes in the middle-aged spine (at a time when the incidence of back pain is at its highest) are common, and have already been described. Some clinical conditions are undoubtedly associated with these pathoanatomical changes which may be detected by a variety of methods. For instance, compression of a nerve root by a protrusion of a nucleus pulposus may be identified by radiological imaging techniques (and subsequently confirmed at surgery); contraction of the protrusion, whether spontaneous or following surgical intervention, is usually accompanied by resolution of the radicular symptoms. Under other circumstances, for instance in segmental instability or in facet joint syndromes, the apophyseal joints are, undoubtedly, contributors to the symptomatology. Occasionally, diagnostic intra-articular injections, under fluoroscopic screening, are used to confirm the source of back and/or leg pain.

Dysfunction

The cause of back pain in a significant proportion of clinical cases, probably the majority, is **spinal joint dysfunction** (syn. somatic dysfunction) which may be diagnosed from the combination of the history and the specific examination findings. The exact nature of this lesion has been debated for decades. Structuralists consider that a mechanical lesion exists in a spinal segment, such as an annular tag, a meniscoid intrusion between apophyseal joint surfaces, or the locking of the posterior joints in a subluxed position.

Functionalists of an osteopathic inclination, on the other hand, are convinced of a *neurophysiological* disturbance which is independent of pathoanatomical changes; the concept of a facilitated cord segment has been propounded to explain the abnormal sensory and motor findings and the autonomic nervous system changes which are commonly associated features. Aetiological factors include trauma, fatigue and stress. Although these osteopathic concepts have been vehemently defended by their protagonists, there is no overwhelming evidence to support any particular view, and there is often little difference in proposed management strategies between the functionalist and structuralist ideologies.

A sensible approach to the dilemma of spinal joint dysfunction is to consider that the disturbance is centred primarily upon the apophyseal joint, and that *motion segment destabilization* (for instance, by disc degeneration and/or prolapse) is a presequitur in a large proportion of cases. In the thoracic spine the articulations with the ribs may play a part in the common type of dysfunction, though clinical identification of the different types of rib dysfunction (according to Bourdillon, 1992) is outside the scope of this text. Sacroiliac dysfunction is another lesion which enters into the differential diagnosis of low back and leg pain, and is addressed in Chapter 4.

Spinal joint dysfunction may be diagnosed by regional mobility tests, and by more specific segmental **mobility** tests and **stress** tests. In a proportion of cases there are other clinical signs relating to the texture and sensitivity of the skin, subcutaneous tissues and underlying muscles. Areas of hypoaesthesia or (more commonly) of hyperaesthesia may be found paravertebrally, or at a greater distance from the spine within sclerotomal segments. Trigger points and discrete patches of increased subcutaneous turgor (detected by 'skin rolling') suggest dysfunction in a nearby spinal joint. When trigger points and skin patches are generalized in the body, (that is, present to the right and left of the mid line, and above and below the waist), the condition of **fibromyalgia** should be suspected. The characteristics of this condition are widespread pain and tenderness, sleep disturbances, fatigue and agitated depression. Aggravating factors are stress, poor posture, postviral fatigue and cold and damp weather.

OTHER CAUSES OF SPINAL AND RADICULAR PAIN

Neoplastic

Secondary malignant deposits are more common than primary bone tumours. The likely sources are breast, kidney and prostate. A patient with back pain who gives a history of treatment for one of these primary malignancies should be suspected of having secondary deposits. If radiological findings are negative and clinical suspicions are high, scintigraphy (radioisotope bone scanning) should be performed.

Multiple myeloma is one of the commonest malignancies to affect the spine. There may be a generalized osteoporotic picture on X-ray, and the erythrocyte sedimentation rate (ESR) is high. Persistent thoracic spinal discomfort may be the presenting feature.

Osteoid osteoma typically presents as night pain. It may be associated with a fixed scoliosis in youngsters.

Tumours within the vertebral canal, such as neurofibromata, may present with neurological signs as a result of pressure upon the spinal cord, cauda equina, or nerve roots at the intervertebral foramen. Occasionally, highly malignant tumours such as Ewing's sarcoma give rise to nerve root pain (Fig. 1.27) following local invasion from their primary site in one of the pelvic bones.

Infective

Spinal tuberculosis is now rarely seen in Britain, though it should be considered in immigrants from areas in which it is relatively common. Pyogenic vertebral osteomyelitis is usually caused by haematogenous spread, and should be considered in the differential diagnosis of backache in people of poor general health, for instance in heroin addicts or in poorly controlled diabetes.

Occasionaly, discitis arises within a few weeks of discectomy. A physiotherapist who is responsible for rehabilitation following discectomy should refer the patient back to the surgeon if sudden severe back pain intervenes.

Visceral causes

Posterior thoracic pain may be associated with intrathoracic pathology: oesophageal carcinoma, for instance, should be suspected if there is coexistent dysphagia.

a

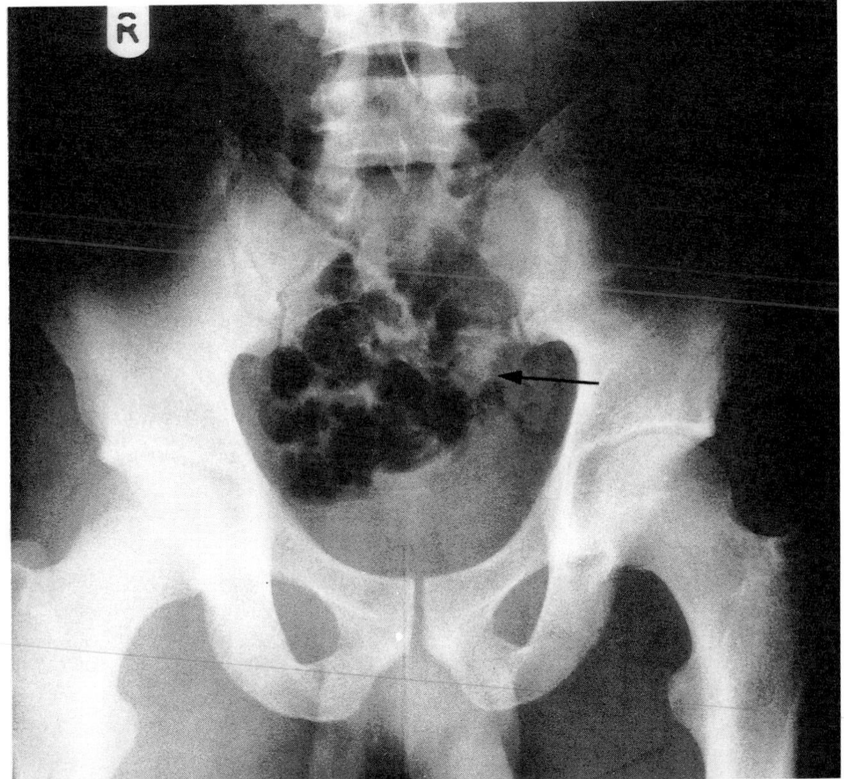

b

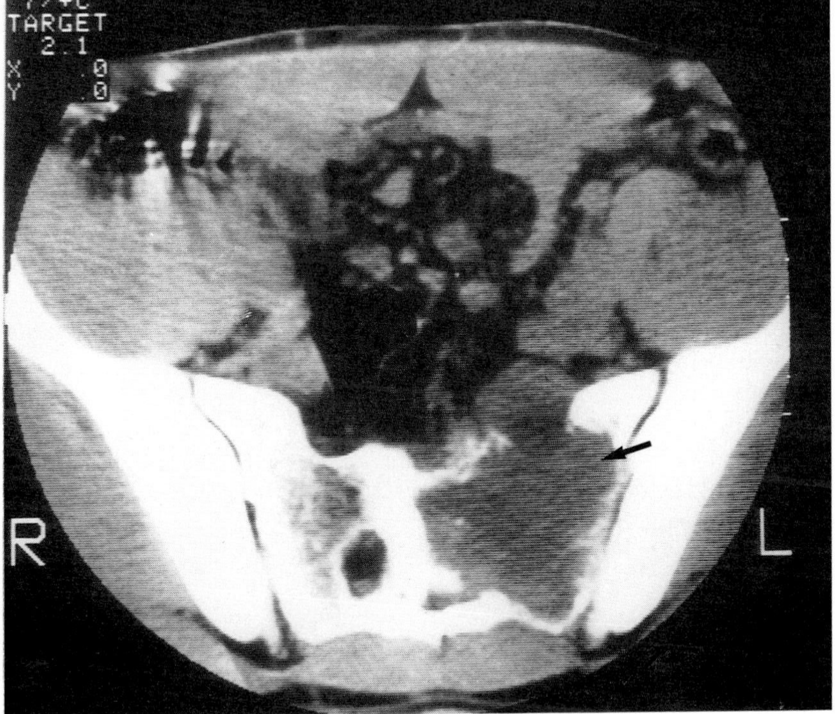

Fig. 1.27 The destructive changes seen on (a) X-ray and (b) CT scan of the sacrum are due to Ewing's sarcoma

Intra-abdominal pathology, such as renal and pancreatic carcinomata, may give rise to back pain as a result of retroperitoneal spread. Loss of weight is usually apparent. Abdominal examination is essential when abdominal pain is associated with back pain. Radiation of pain (referred pain) to the abdomen is not uncommon, of course, with spinal dysfunction in the distal thoracic spine; the site of the abdominal pain is usually distal to the site of the back pain.

Gynaecological pathology accounts for much backache in women. Although hopes may be raised that backache associated with the primary gynaecological symptoms may be cured by treatment such as hysterectomy, it is not uncommonly found that dual pathology exists, and backache persists following surgery. Perversely, the *onset* of backache may be associated with gynaecological surgery: the combination of the lithotomy position during anaesthesia, and a short period of postsurgical inactivity, may provoke spinal or sacroiliac dysfunction.

Inflammatory

Sacroiliitis is a feature of the early stages of a spondyloarthropathy, for instance ankylosing spondylitis, when low back pain, morning stiffness and often night pain are the predominant symptoms (Fig. 1.28). If the condition progresses, the whole spine may become involved and the typical stooped posture is seen, particularly if spinal

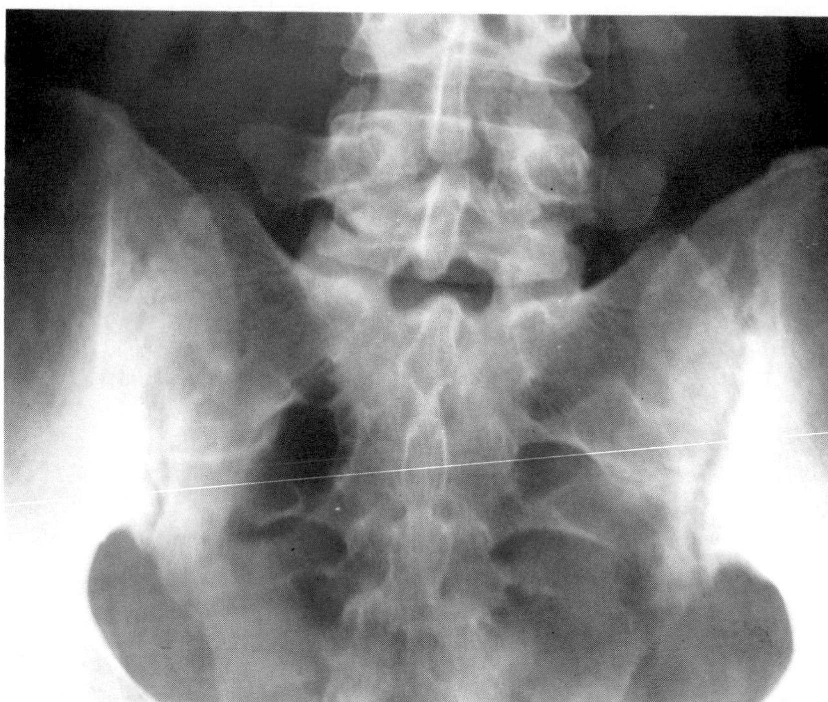

Fig. 1.28 The typical radiological features of sacroiliitis – erosive changes associated with sclerosis at the sacroiliac joints.

flexibility exercises are not undertaken. Sacroiliac fusion, a bamboo spine and gross thoracic kyphosis are features in the advanced case.

There is a high incidence of HLA B27 antigen in ankylosing spondylitis. In Reiter's syndrome sacroiliitis is associated with urethritis and iritis. In other patients there may be a connection with ulcerative colitis or Crohn's disease. Peripheral joints, particularly the hips, may be affected in the spondyloarthropathies.

Fractures

Trauma to the cervical spine, arising for instance from car accidents, or diving into shallow water, or scrum collapses in rugby football, may give rise to a vertebral fracture, or fracture-dislocation of the apophyseal joints. Although detailed analysis is outside the scope of this book, the possibility of spinal fracture and/or spinal cord injury should always be considered in circumstances in which:

- there is a history of axial compression loading, particularly with flexion and/or rotation;
- there is a history of severe whiplash;
- the signs and symptoms are those of a destabilizing injury.

A fracture of a lumbar transverse process may arise as a result of direct trauma; usually, healing is uneventful, and symptomatic treatment only is required, for instance by the temporary use of a light spinal support. Wedge compression fractures in osteoporotic thoracic and lumbar spines are common; postmenopausal osteoporosis is a likely cause in females. Back pain resulting from a spinal compression fracture usually resolves gradually over 6–8 weeks; more prolonged backache may be due to secondary facet joint disturbance. Referral to an appropriate specialist is indicated if sudden back pain occurs in a susceptible female, and the examination reveals marked pressure pain over the relevant spinous processes.

HISTORY

History-taking is an acquired skill which purports:

1 To accumulate sufficient relevant information to direct the subsequent examination.
2 To present a picture of the clinical problem which is compatible (or otherwise) with the examination findings.
3 To detect the behavioural response of the patient to his problem.

The perception of pain involves complex neurological pathways between the initial excitation of the nociceptive afferents and the cerebral cortex. The choice of therapeutic modality in an attempt to modify pain perception is as dependent on this behavioural pattern as it is upon the nature of the lesion.

The history given by the patient, whether spontaneous or on direct questioning by the clinician, should be meaningful and relevant. The directed part of the history-taking should not necessarily be a catalogue of standard questions. Some time may need to be spent on a particular enquiry in order to extract as accurately as possible the information that is sought, rather than merely the information that the patient chooses to impart. For instance, when a patient states that his back pain has been so bad that he has spent the previous three weeks flat on his back, it is of some considerable relevance to know whether the recumbency was imposed upon the patient by the severity of pain associated with getting up and walking, or sitting, or the recommendation of the attending general practitioner (in which case the patient may, or may not, have considered recumbency to be necessary, or even found it helpful).

The following are guidelines to the direction the history taking should take.

1 Longevity of symptoms

Have there been previous bouts of back pain? If so, how many, and when was the first bout?

2 Onset of symptoms

Did the symptoms arise suddenly and dramatically, or insidiously? Was there a history of direct trauma, for instance a bang on the head, or strain, for instance whiplash or bending and lifting?

3 Intensity of symptoms

Though pain is entirely a subjective phenomenon, its severity may be compared to other episodes or other painful illnesses experienced by the patient. A pain scale (for instance, the level of pain intensity between 0 and 10) is useful for monitoring the course of a condition. The attitude of the patient to his pain, and the behavioural responses are noted.

4 Change in symptoms

For instance, was the arm pain and dysaesthesiae preceded by neck pain and stiffness? Patients often forget or have been inclined to disregard preceding symptoms, either because they consider them to be of little relevance, or because a presumptive diagnosis (by a referring doctor, for instance) has appeared to diminish their importance.

5 Site of pain

Patients are often vague, even when entirely genuine and not in the slightest neurotic, about the site of their pain. This is understandable as pain that is well localized to the lesion is often accompanied by **referred pain**, which tends to be much more diffuse. Even **radicular pain** which is often considered to follow strict dermatomal patterns (as a result of nerve root irritation) cannot always be described with great accuracy by the patient.

An example of referred pain is 'sciatica' when the nociceptive source is to be found in the ligaments, muscles and apophyseal joints of the lumbar spine. Past research has demonstrated that:

- Injections of hypertonic saline into the lumbar apophyseal joints under radiographic control provoke pain which spreads to the buttock, then the thigh, and even as far as the calf (Mooney and Robertson, 1976).
- Injections of hypertonic saline to the interspinous lumbosacral ligament are painful all the way down the posterior aspect of the leg (Kellgren, 1939).
- After injections of hypertonic saline into the lumbar paravertebral muscles, different pain patterns are found (Fig. 1.29) depending upon the exact site of the injection (Feinstein *et al.*, 1954).
- Sacroiliac pain may also be felt in the posterior aspect of the leg as far as the heel, thus entering into the differential diagnosis of 'sciatica' (Hackett, 1956).

From the cervical spine, referred pain is common. In a small study of normal volunteers by Dwyer *et al.* (1990), constant patterns of referred pain in the neck and shoulder region were detected following noxious stimulation of the cervical apophyseal joints with contrast medium under fluoroscopic screening (Fig. 1.30). Following whiplash injury, occipital headaches (which are much more likely to be due to proximal cervical spinal joint derangement than a postconcussional syndrome) are almost invariable.

Cardiac pain may be mimicked by dysfunction at the cervicothoracic junction or the proximal thoracic spine. From the transitional area at the lower end of the thoracic spine – the thoracolumbar junction – symptoms may be referred to the iliac fossa or groin, suggesting a visceral cause to the unsuspecting observer.

In any one individual, the fields of referred pain (sometimes called sclerotomes) from spinal motion segments overlap considerably; the patterns exhibited by different individuals also vary considerably, but they are consistently different from dermatomal patterns.

Cyriax (1982) considered that extrasegmental referred pain is primarily due to pressure on the dura mater.

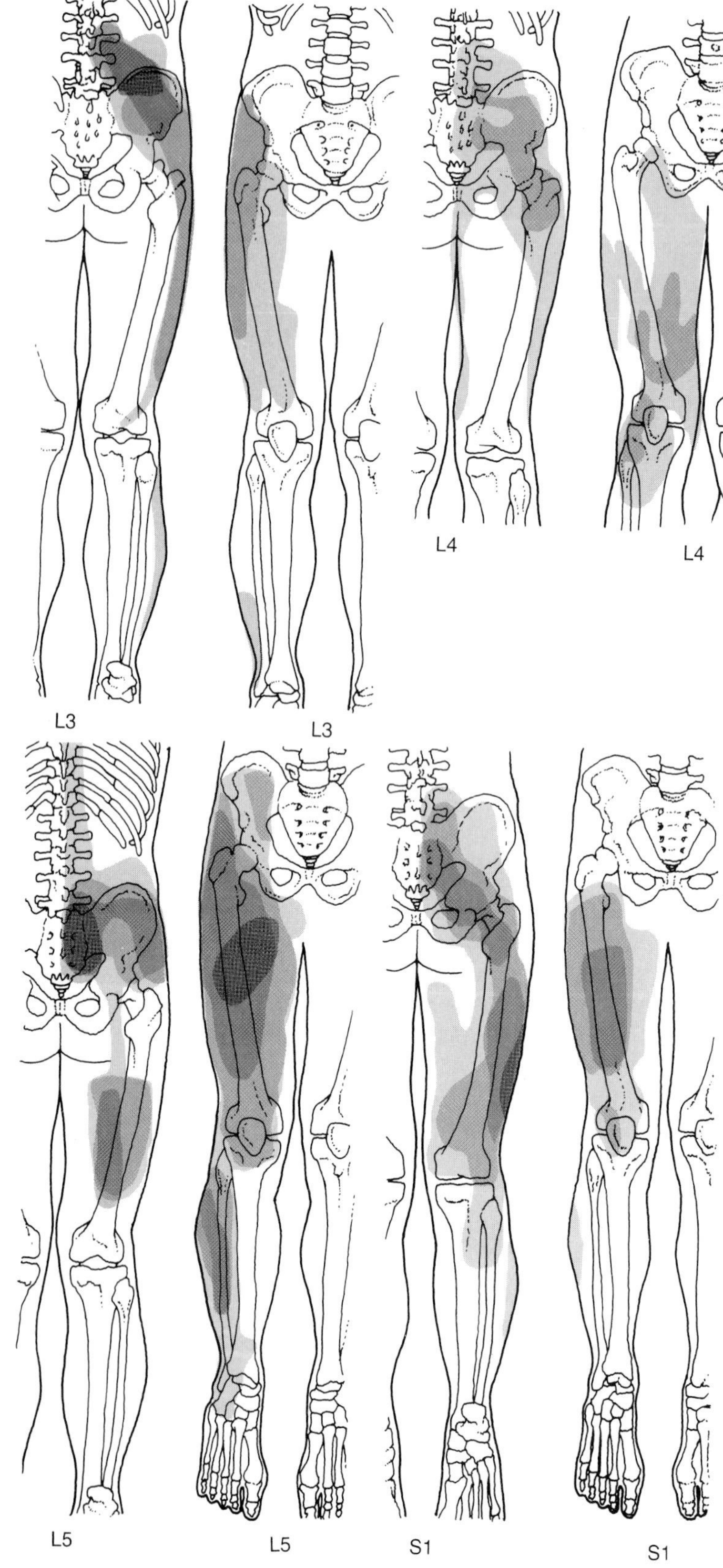

Fig. 1.29 The distribution of pain following the stimulation of interspinous tissue by hypertonic saline injections between the L3 and S1 levels. (From Feinstein *et al.*, 1954.)

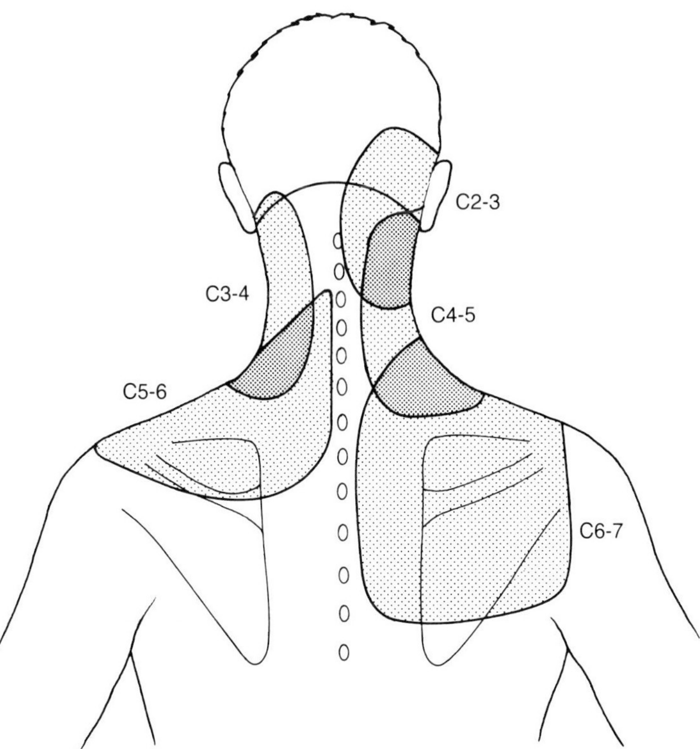

Fig. 1.30 A map of the characteristic areas of pain referred from cervical apophyseal joints of C2/3 to C6/7. (From Dwyer *et al.*, 1990.)

6 Accompanying symptoms

Are paraesthesiae and numbness present? If so, what is their distribution? Often, patients take sufficient interest in these symptoms, which are usually felt in the extremities of the limbs, to be able to locate them accurately and to state, for instance, that their 'pins and needles' are felt in the index and long fingers, compatible with a C7 root entrapment; but sometimes 'it's in all the fingers' may be due to a single nerve root entrapment too. Although paraesthesiae and numbness are commonly due to nerve root compression, small areas of hypoaesthesiae may be present, either paravertebrally or peripherally, in association with referred pain secondary to joint dysfunction.

Symptoms which suggest the involvement of the autonomic nervous system, such as dizziness, tinnitus and headaches, are often volunteered by patients, but sometimes need to be enquired about specifically.

7 Terminology

The patient's knowledge of anatomy may be poor, and he is likely to use colloquial expressions. When pain is felt 'in the hip' it usually means the buttock or greater trochanteric region. Patients rarely volunteer 'the buttock'. When pain is felt 'in the shoulder' it often means the supraspinous region of the scapula.

When pain is felt 'in the back' (from a lesion in the cervical spine) it is often felt along the medial border of the scapula.

When pain is felt 'in the back' from a lesion in the thoracolumbar spine it could be anywhere from C7 downwards, and the patient should be asked to point out the site again when undressed.

8 Relationship to activity

The relationship to the following activities or postures should always be determined.

In **low back pain**:

- Standing
- Walking
- Sitting – at home, in the office, in a car
- Lying
- Bending, including domestic chores
- Coughing/sneezing/straining = impulse pain
- Sport/recreational activities, e.g. squash, gardening
- Working

Further information from direct questioning is often required, for instance the effect of lying on one side or the other, or lying in the supine or prone position.

In **thoracic pain**:

- Coughing
- Deep inhalation
- Twisting
- Bending
- Sitting
- Lying
- Sporting activities, e.g. golf, squash
- Working

For **neck and arm pain**:

- Sleep patterns
- Number of pillows
- Position of the arm(s) at night
- Rotation of neck
- Looking up
- Sporting activities, e.g golf, swimming (different strokes)
- Car driving
- Sitting, reading or knitting
- Working

9 General health enquiry

Enquiry should be made, for example, about loss of weight, appetite, gastrointestinal function, genitourinary function.

10 Past health

A history of surgery should be asked for, and also details of any malignancies, previous bouts of back, neck, or joint pain and frequency of visits to the GP.

11 Effect on lifestyle

Is the patient able to continue at work, do the shopping and housework, and engage in sporting or recreational activities?

EXAMINATION

It is important not to lose sight of the purpose of the examination: following history-taking, the examination should lead the examiner towards a *diagnosis*. Naturally, there are occasions when further investigations are deemed to be helpful; but an attempt at making a specific diagnosis, however presumptive, should be made. The concept of 'syndromes' should be abandoned; their protagonists consider that, as there are gaps in the current understanding of spinal pathomechanics and pathoneurophysiology, specific diagnoses are often impossible. Should this philosophy be extended to the rest of medicine, on the basis of a shortfall in our understanding of disease and injury processes, little progress would be made in the evaluation of management strategies. Medicine is indeed as much an art as a science; and, in respect of the examination of a patient with spinal pain, the art is to collect, then collate sufficient pieces of the jigsaw to make up the whole picture (or 'diagnosis'). The distinct lack of scientific corroboration of the nature of spinal dysfunction, which is the cause of back pain in the majority of cases, should not prohibit the establishment of a working diagnosis.

Examination techniques are designed:

1 To exclude conditions such as malignancy, the management of which is outside the scope of this text.
2 To determine the exact site and nature of the spinal disorder:
   - Is there a disorder of the anterior pillar such as disc protrusion?
   - Is there a disorder of the posterior pillars such as spinal joint dysfunction?
   - Is there a disorder of both – segmental instability?
   - Is there a disorder of the supporting structures such as the pars interarticularis, e.g. spondylolysis, or of the spinal canals e.g. spinal stenosis?
   - Is there entrapment of a nerve root?

The spinal examination should include:

1 Posture

Is the neck, for instance, or the thoracolumbar spine held in a 'natural' position? If not, is there an obvious torticollis, or pelvic tilt, or kyphos, or loss of normal lordosis?

2 Mobility tests

Although 'global' tests of mobility, that is the range of active or passive movements in the standing position, beg the question – what is the normal range for this patient? – an assessment of the **degree of comfortable movement** may be made. In respect of rotation and side flexion, a comparison with the other side should be established. For movements in the sagittal plane, particularly forward flexion, the patient is usually aware of the pre-existing 'normal' range. A significant observation is the feeling of the **end-point**; is the end of range accompanied by pain and muscle tension, or the feeling that a natural state of tissue tension has been achieved (the taking up of the 'slack')? Reassessment during treatment is of major importance, so that comparison with the initial findings may be made.

Assessment of thoracic rotation should be performed with the patient sitting to reduce pelvic movement. Specific mobility tests for the sacroiliac joint may be performed in the standing position, as well as sitting or lying.

3 Joint play assessment

This reveals further information on the degree of segmental mobility and reflects facet joint function. The examination is usually conducted in the supine or prone positions. Both hypomobility and pain at the end of range are indicators of dysfunction. In relatively minor degrees of dysfunction, reduction in joint play (sometimes referred to as joint blockage) may be the only detectable abnormality on mobility assessment. In the presence of gross muscle spasm, on the other hand, usually caused by disc prolapse, it may be impossible to detect segmental disturbance (other than a gross loss of mobility over several segments).

Spinal joint play assessment is comparable to joint play assessment at peripheral joints: loss of mobility, pain on movement, and localized tenderness are sought. Additionally, localized muscle hypertonus is a feature of spinal joint dysfunction.

4 Dural tension tests

These are designed primarily to detect nerve root irritation or entrapment by provoking discomfort on stretching the dural sheath.

The **straight-leg raise** test stretches the L5 and sacral nerve roots and their sheaths.

The **slump test** stretches the dura throughout its length, utilizing total spinal flexion.

The **femoral stretch** test stretches the L3 and L4 nerve roots.

Passive neck flexion alone may reproduce pain in the thoracic or lumbar spine by stretching the dura mater over a prolapsed intervertebral disc.

Dural tension in the cervical spine at the C5 or C6 nerve root level may be detected by specific **adverse neural tension** tests.

5 Skin signs

Skin rolling is a further sign of spinal joint dysfunction. Localized patches of tenderness and subcutaneous turgor (sometimes referred to as trophoedema) may be palpable in the paravertebral region adjacent to a disturbed segment. Although skin rolling may be 'positive' in any spinal region, it is a particularly useful sign in lesions of the thoracic spine.

Skin pinching and **skin drag** are further tests, both of which detect altered sweating resulting from a disturbance of the autonomic nervous system.

6 Muscle signs

Isometric contraction of the paravertebral muscles (for instance, resisted side flexion of the trunk) is almost invariably painless, even during a bout of acute back pain. An exception is painful ipsilateral contraction in the presence of a fractured transverse process. Diagnoses of acute (or chronic) muscle tears of the spinal extensors are almost invariably flawed.

Weakness of muscle groups such as the abdominals, which play an important role in the biomechanics of the lumbar spine, may be detected by appropriate tests.

Trigger points (TPs) are felt as localized areas of tender muscle spasm deep to the skin and subcutaneous tissues. They may be detected some distance from the site of the primary disturbance. Pressure on a TP causes considerable pain, reproducing some or all of the patient's complaints. It is often accompanied by a grimace and a sudden movement by the patient – the 'jump' sign of Travell and Simons (1992). Discomfort on passive stretching, and detectable shortening of the affected muscle are other characteristic signs.

7 Neurological signs

Neurological assessment is essential when dealing with problems arising in any region of the spine, particularly when there is a suspicion of nerve root involvement. Limb pain which radiates below the elbow, or below the knee, is more likely to be radicular than referred. When such pain is accompanied by dysaesthesiae ('pins and needles', 'tingling' or 'burning') and numbness, root compression is very likely. Although it seems logical to confirm sensory impairment by performing light touch and pinprick tests, the mere existence of these symptoms in a dermatomal pattern is of equal significance to their objective confirmation. The assessment of motor function is of greater value; muscle power may be recorded 0–5 according to the MRC scale:

0 Nil
1 Detectable
2 Good
3 Against gravity
4 Strong, not normal
5 Normal

Appropriate assessment regimes for motor power in the upper and lower limbs are described in the succeeding chapters. Although girdle pain from thoracic spinal lesions may suggest nerve root compression, motor weakness of the intercostal muscles (should it exist) is not identifiable on clinical testing.

Four further points are worthy of note.

(1) Motor weakness which involves more than one nerve root, particularly if they are not adjacent roots, should arouse a suspicion of metastases. Only occasionally does spinal stenosis affect several nerve roots to the extent that diffuse motor loss is recorded.

(2) Very occasionally, a large thoracic disc prolapse is encountered which gives rise to spinal cord compression. When symptoms in the lower limbs are associated with thoracic spinal pain, a space-occupying lesion, for instance a disc herniation or tumour, should be suspected and a careful neurological assessment carried out.

(3) Cervical spinal stenosis may compress the long tracts as well as the emerging nerve roots. Any suspicion from the history should lead to a search for spasticity in the legs or other evidence of an upper motor neurone lesion.

(4) Neurological conditions which often give rise to spasticity of large muscle groups in the legs, such as multiple sclerosis, may present with leg pains. Tests of coordination are required and a careful appraisal of the motor system and reflexes should be made.

8 Shoulder and pelvic girdles

Biomechanically, the cervical and lumbar spines have close functional relationships with the pectoral and pelvic girdles respectively.

The shoulder joint and rotator cuff should be examined in neck disorders. Abnormal subacromial function may be present. The range of active abduction of the shoulders should be assessed in a patient with proximal thoracic spinal joint dysfunction too: full abduction is not possible in the presence of increased kyphosis of the thoracic spine.

The pelvis is a ring structure so that any disturbance at one point in the ring may provoke disturbance elsewhere. For example, loss of flexibility at the hip joints may give rise to lumbar spinal joint dysfunction. Similarly, sacroiliac dysfunction may be associated with stress at the pubic symphysis. Assessment of hip function, in addition to spinal and sacroiliac function, is thus imperative in lumbosacral and sacroiliac disorders.

MANAGEMENT

Management strategies may be constructed once a specific diagnosis has been made. Otherwise, treatment of symptoms, symptom complexes, or syndromes (for instance 'chronic low back pain', 'brachial neuralgia') either becomes randomized and speculative in respect of the available therapeutic modalities, or inflexible and dogmatic (which is worse). For instance, the practice of combining McKenzie's back extension exercises with mobilization for *all* patients with 'mechanical' low back pain is not only illogical (pre-supposing, as it does, that disc bulges which may be amenable to reduction by forced extension are always present), but it will inevitably aggravate certain conditions, such as degenerate facet joints.

Upon the establishment of a specific diagnosis, a management strategy may be constructed on sound scientific principles, for instance the use of spinal traction for intervertebral disc prolapse, or on an empirical basis, for instance manipulative and mobilization procedures for spinal joint dysfunction.

The prescription of analgesics (which may be helpful in very painful conditions) and non-steroidal anti-inflammatory drugs (which are often disappointing in their efficacy) should be considered as an adjunct to physical therapy; the thrust of this text, however, is towards an active 'physical' approach for specific 'mechanical' conditions.

Manipulation and mobilization

Manipulation is generally considered to be the use of techniques which utilize a low amplitude, high velocity thrust to the spine; controlled force is applied to a joint once the 'slack' of physiological movement has been taken up in one or more directions. **Mobilization** is the extension of those examination techniques which are used to assess joint play in one or several adjacent joints; in effect, the restrictive barrier to further movement is gently and repetitively put under pressure. Whatever the mechanism of apophyseal and sacroiliac joint dysfunction – whether mechanical (joint 'locking' or subluxation) or neurophysiological – manual techniques are often successful in their management. This certainly applies to episodes of acute spinal joint dysfunction which are probably self-resolving if sufficient time, often several weeks or months, is allowed to elapse, yet which may be treated, often with dramatic results, by mobilization or manipulation.

Wyke (1987) has stated that the experience of pain from the low back is inversely proportional to the discharge from mechanoreceptors located in the same or related tissue from which the pain is arising. Mechanoreceptor discharge, for instance as a result of spinal manipulation, depresses the centripetal flow of nociceptive activity.

When dysfunction is secondary to chronic ligamentous insufficiency, or is associated with symptomatic degenerative changes in the apophyseal joints, these manual techniques give negligible or temporary benefit only. A positive response may be expected in acute segmental dysfunction, involving disc prolapse as well as facet dysfunction, particularly if manipulation is combined with other techniques such as postisometric relaxation, a short course of traction, or an epidural injection.

Reassessment of the patient 2 or 3 days after spinal manipulation will determine the need for further treatments. For instance, when cervical spinal joint dysfunction results from whiplash, it is often necessary to mobilize the affected segment(s) on a number of occasions over several weeks.

Many studies have confirmed the early benefit from manipulation, though few trials have acceptable methodological standards (Koes *et al.*, 1991). Reviewers have often questioned the validity of this form of treatment because of the apparent lack of effect on the recurrence rate. The sensible approach, however, is to follow up the initial phase of restoration of normal function with rehabilitative measures to stabilize the affected segment, and thereby to reduce the likelihood of relapse.

The indication for manipulation is the diagnosis of spinal joint dysfunction. Contraindications include the presence of malignancy, infections and inflammatory disorders. In the neck, manipulation is contraindicated if widespread rheumatoid arthritis is present because of its predilection for the odontoid process and adjacent tissues; manipulation must be carried out with care (avoiding rotatory procedures) in the presence of vertebrobasilar insufficiency. In the lumbar spine, the cauda equina syndrome (in which acute retention of urine occurs) may be precipitated if manipulation is carried out for a central disc prolapse which compresses the sacral nerve roots; a history of paraesthesiae in the saddle area, or sphincter disturbance, indicates impending cauda equina entrapment for which a surgical opinion should be sought.

There are many mobilization and manipulative techniques, most of which are well documented and illustrated in texts such as Bourdillon (1992), Cyriax (1982), Grieve (1984), Lewit (1985), Maigne (1972), Maitland (1977), Mennell (1960), and Stoddard (1977). A synopsis of those techniques which are considered to be particularly useful is given in succeeding chapters.

Localized anti-inflammatory and muscle relaxant therapy

Various local applications are in common usage for symptomatic relief. Undoubtedly, heat increases local blood flow which helps to reduce muscle spasm. Since muscle spasm is secondary to an underlying disorder, however, any benefit will be temporary. There are pain relieving effects from the use of ice packs, ice-massage, and ultrasound; additionally, ultrasound may be used for facet dysfunction, and as an adjunct to mobilization, particularly if palpable tenderness is elicited over the affected joint(s). Ultrasound has no significant lasting effect when tenderness over the lumbosacral and sacroiliac ligaments is due to chronic ligamentous insufficiency; nor is it particularly helpful in symptomatic degenerative lesions of the apophyseal joints.

Massage is often more beneficial than other localized modalities, particularly when applied to trigger points. At the very least, it should be pleasurable and comforting. It may be used as an alternative, or as an adjunct, to cold application-and-stretch (a Travell technique which has replaced spray-and-stretch because of the latter's environmental unfriendliness). It is probable that all hands-on techniques involve some degree of placebo response, and it is logical, if time allows, to include massage in many therapeutic strategies. When tight muscles have been identified, commonly associated with TPs and areas of myotendinosis, stretching routines should be instituted as soon as the progress of the patient's articular condition allows.

Preferably, massage and stretching should be used as adjuncts to other treatments which have a 'mechanical' effect on the disturbed vertebral segment.

Traction

Since the time of Hippocrates, spinal traction in various guises has been used for the relief of spinal pain. Cyriax (1982) propounded the use of traction for a specific purpose – reduction of a prolapse of the nucleus pulposus in the cervical or lumbar spines. Logically, it should be sustained rather than intermittent, and given for between 15 and 30 minutes. The distraction force is gradually increased, and titrated against response, so that a force of 100–140 lb may be used on the lumbar spine in a well-built male. For the cervical spine forces of up to 30 lb may be used. Daily traction provides the best results, and treatment may need to be continued for up to 15 sessions. A positive response may not be identified until at least six sessions have been given, so that treatment should always be continued for at least this length of time, if tolerated.

Spinal traction, on an outpatient basis, is often successful for brachial neuralgia or for sciatica caused by an HNP; the prerequirements are a correct diagnosis, and an absence of neurological signs. Should neurological signs be present, caudal epidural injections (for sciatic root entrapment) or nerve block techniques (for either cervical or lumbar lesions) should be considered.

It has been postulated that gentle traction may help resolve joint dysfunction; certainly, it should provide mechanoreceptor stimulation and it is logical to contemplate a beneficial effect on the basis of reduction of muscle spasm. Unfortunately, this is not borne out by experience; little benefit is gained (apart from when joint dysfunction coexists with disc prolapse in segmental dysfunction), and discomfort may worsen. As a form of mobilization, intermittent traction may be considered if there is poor response to manual methods.

There are no contraindications to the use of traction so long as the tightness of the retaining harness is tolerated, and the condition does not worsen during the course of treatment.

Epidural Injections

Historically, Sicard in 1901 first described the technique of (caudal) epidural anaesthesia. Since then many practitioners, notably Cyriax (1982), have utilized and reviewed the effectiveness of this technique, with or without the addition of deposteroids to dilute local anaesthetics such as 0.5% procaine or lignocaine. Perhaps its principal use is for nerve root entrapment secondary to a protrusion of a nucleus pulposus in the lumbar spine. When neurological deficits are found on clinical examination, for instance diminished motor power, altered sensation or diminished reflexes, caudal epidural injections are the treatment of choice. The technique is safe, and is based on the premise that a reduction in the inflammatory reaction at the interface between disc and dural sheath of the nerve root occurs.

Injections are often repeated at intervals of one to two weeks, the number required being dependent upon patients' progress as determined by reduction of pain, diminishing dural tension signs, and improving neurological signs. A response rate of approximately 85% is found.

Other indications are 'hyperacute' lumbago, acute lumbar segmental dysfunction, and persistent low back pain due to dural irritation. Diagnostic epidurals may be used when doubts exist regarding the cause of sciatic pain (in particular). An analgesic response indicates a dural aetiology. The only contraindication is sensitivity to procaine or lignocaine.

Nerve block injections

The usefulness of local anaesthetics for management of chronic pain syndromes has been recognized for some time.

Sinuvertebral nerve block injections are used by orthopaedic physicians, pain relief specialists and anaesthetists for relief of pain associated with nerve root compression in the cervical and lumbar spines. A small amount of local anaesthetic, to which is often added a deposteroid, is injected as close to the intervertebral foramen as possible; the effectiveness of the local anaesthetic (which is used for its prolonged, rather than short-acting effect) is possibly due to the blocking of the nociceptive input at source or via its transmission along the sinuvertebral nerve. It is usually very effective in the cervical spine if nerve root entrapment is severe enough to give rise to neurological signs. It is given without X-ray screening, as a result of which localization of the correct segmental level may be inaccurate. Because of the plurisegmental connections of each sinuvertebral nerve, however, an injection at an adjacent foramen (but not, strictly speaking, at the 'correct' vertebral level) may still be beneficial.

A **paravertebral** nerve block (dorsal root ganglion block) is an injection into the nerve root dural sheath as it leaves the foramen; it is given under X-ray control as accurate localization is essential.

Spinal supports

Collars and corsets are commonly prescribed, but are often used inappropriately or as a substitute for more effective treatment. A collar restricts movement in the cervical spine, and is comforting in the first week or two after a whiplash injury (during which mobilization is contraindicated – unless the injury is relatively minor). Regrettably, it is often prescribed by physicians on the basis of the combination of a painful neck and the radiological changes of spondylosis; the majority of these patients would respond to mobilization should it be made available to them. The prolonged use of a cervical collar is often associated with delayed recovery from cervical whiplash.

Restriction of movement has been considered to be the principal contribution of a corset or lumbar support to the management of a painful back. However, it is probable that mobility at the lumbosacral joint is not restricted by a support, and possibly increased (as a result of restriction of the more proximal motion segments). If corsetry helps, which it seems to in some patients, it is probably due to the increase in intra-abdominal pressure.

Other injection treatments

Intra-articular injections of the apophyseal joints may be used for diagnostic and therapeutic purposes. In the investigation of thigh pain, for instance, diagnostic evaluation by intra-articular local anaesthetic under X-ray control may be helpful – reproduction of the patient's symptoms confirms facet joint pathology. The addition of steroid to the local anaesthetic creates a further therapeutic dimension.

When used to complement manipulation in the management of facet joint dysfunction, or to treat synovitis of the facet joint(s), the introduction of local anaesthetic and steroid to the posterior aspect of the relevant joint – a **facet block** – is often helpful. Intra-articular injection is unnecessary in these circumstances. Injection of the posterior capsule and capsular ligaments may be given in the clinic setting (without the need for X-ray screening); its efficacy may be due, in part, to the blocking effect on the medial articular branches of the posterior rami which supply the facet joints.

Local anaesthetic injections to trigger points may be helpful, particularly when joint mobility has been restored by mobilizing techniques yet one or two TPs remain. Dry needling (acupuncture) is stated by its exponents to be equally effective.

Sclerosant injections (of P2G – 25% dextrose, 2% phenol) to the spinal ligaments are used in the management of conditions associated with ligamentous insufficiency. They stimulate a proliferative fibroblastic reaction at the bony attachments of the ligaments, which is considered to be the basis for a subsequent strengthening effect. Most commonly, sclerosant injections are used for chronic sacroiliac and lumbar ligamentous insufficiency, including segmental instability. On occasions, they are beneficial in the dorsal spine.

To maximize stabilization they should be combined with an appropriate schedule of exercises and a fitness programme (see below).

Management of chronic pain

Consideration is given to the part played by socioeconomic and psychological factors in the perpetuation of spinal pain in Chapters 4 and 5. For patients with chronic pain which is refractory to the therapeutic regimes described in this text, behavioural therapy or inclusion in a back school programme may be useful.

TENS (transcutaneous electrical nerve stimulation) should also be considered. The gate control theory of pain (Melzack and Wall, 1965) suggests that the transmission of nociceptive stimuli to the brain via small myelinated and non-myelinated fibres may be suppressed by the excitation of large myelinated fibres. TENS selectively stimulates large fibres by virtue of its wave form, but patients may control current intensity, pulse frequency and, on some machines, the pulse width to achieve maximum pain relief. Production of endogenous opioids may be responsible for this analgesic effect. The effectiveness of TENS in chronic pain depends to some considerable degree upon the skill and patience of the therapist who, additionally, is required to combine an educational and counselling role with more traditional ministrations using hands-on techniques.

Acupuncture and **electroacupuncture** also have neurophysiological pain suppressing effects, and may be effective in musculoskeletal pain and neurogenic pain respectively. Either traditional Chinese acupuncture points or 'Western-type' points may be used for needle insertion; in the context of myofascial pain syndromes, the use of trigger points in muscles is logical.

REHABILITATION AND PROPHYLAXIS

Sufficient importance is attached to rehabilitation following a bout of back pain, and prevention of further spinal problems, to justify a chapter to be devoted to this topic. In brief, a spinal educational programme should contain the following elements:

1 Advice on posture.
2 Advice on dynamic lifting.
3 Instruction in ergonomics.
4 Muscle strengthening exercises, e.g. abdominals.
5 Flexibility exercises, when indicated.
6 Advice on overall fitness.

REFERENCES

Bourdillon, J.F. (1992) *Spinal Manipulation*, 5th edn, Butterworth-Heinemann, Oxford

Cyriax, J. (1982) *Textbook of Orthopaedic Medicine*, vol. 1, 8th edn, Baillière Tindall, London

DSS (Department of Social Security), Newcastle (1990) *Sickness and/or Invalidity Benefit: Spells of Certified Incapacity*, HMSO, London

Dwyer, A., Aprill, C. and Bogduk, N. (1990) Cervical zygoapophyseal joint pain patterns: a study in normal volunteers. *Spine*, **15**, 453–7

Feinstein, B., Langton, J.N.K., Jameson, R.M. *et al.* (1954) Experiments on pain referred from deep somatic tissues. *Journal of Bone and Joint Surgery*, **36A**, 981–97

Grieve, G.P. (1984) *Mobilization of the Spine*, 4th edn, Churchill Livingstone, Edinburgh

Hackett, G.S. (1956) *Joint Ligament Relaxation Treated by Fibro-osseous Proliferation*, Charles C. Thomas, Springfield, Ill.

Jayson, M.I.V. (1987) *Back Pain: the Facts*, 2nd edn, Oxford University Press, Oxford

Kellgren, J.H. (1939) On the distribution of pain arising from deep somatic structures with charts of segmental pain areas. *Clinical Science*, **4**, 35–46

Koes, B.W., Assendelft, W.J.J., van der Heijden, G.J.M.G. *et al.* (1991) Spinal manipulation and mobilisation for back and neck pain: a blinded review. *British Medical Journal*, **303**, 1298–303

Lewit, K. (1985) *Manipulative Therapy in Rehabilitation of the Motor System*, Butterworths, London

Maigne, R. (1972) *Douleurs d'origine vertébrale et traitements par manipulation*, 2nd edn, Expansion Scientifique, Paris

Maitland, G.D. (1986) *Vertebral Manipulation*, 5th edn, Butterworths, London
Melzack, R. and Wall, P.D. (1965) Pain mechanics: a new theory. *Science,* **150**, 971–9
Mennell, J.McM. (1960) *Back Pain: diagnosis amd treatment using manipulative techniques.* Little, Brown and Company, Boston, Mass.
Mooney, V. and Robertson, J. (1976) The facet syndrome. *Clinical Orthopaedics and Related Research,* **115**, 149–56
Nachemson, A.L. and Elfstrom, G. (1970) Intradiscal dynamic pressure measurements in lumbar discs. *Scandinavian Journal of Rehabilitation Medicine,* **Suppl 1**, 1–40
Porter, R.W. (1982) *Management of Back Pain,* Churchill Livingstone, Edinburgh
Stoddard, A. (1977) *Manual of Osteopathic Practice,* Hutchinson, London
Travell, J.G. and Simons, D.G. (1992) *Myofascial Pain and Dysfunction: the Trigger Point Manual,* vols 1 and 2, Williams and Wilkins, Baltimore, Md
Wyke, B.D. (1987) The neurology of low back pain. In *The Lumbar Spine and Back Pain* (ed. M.I.V. Jayson), Pitman Medical, London, pp.265–339

2
Cervical spine

The word 'orthodoxy' not only no longer means being right; it practically means being wrong.

G. K. Chesterton, *Heretics* (1905)

APPLIED ANATOMY

As the neck has to be a very mobile structure and, additionally, carry the weight of the head, its vertebral alignment and design is such that the vertebrae support each other. From both a functional and anatomical viewpoint, the craniocervical junction (C0-C2) – the occipito-atlantoid joint (C0/1) and the atlanto-axial joint (C1/2) – may be considered separately from the rest of the cervical spine.

Vertebrae

The **atlas** is a ring of bone which contains no vertebral body or spinous process, but has a lateral mass and a prominent transverse process on each side (Fig. 2.1). The concave superior facets are oval and articulate with the convex occipital condyles; the concave inferior facets articulate with the convex superior facets of the axis; and the posterior aspect of the anterior arch articulates with the odontoid peg

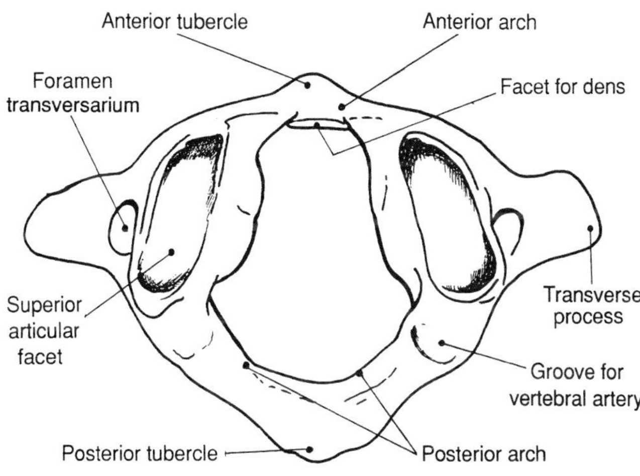

Fig. 2.1 The first cervical vertebra or atlas – superior aspect.

of the axis. The tip of each transverse process may be palpated between the mastoid process and the ramus of the mandible, and may be used as an anatomical landmark when assessing mobility in the upper cervical joints. The posterior tubercle, however, is not palpable clinically. The foramen transversarium lies close to the lateral mass and transmits the vertebral vessels and sympathetic nerves.

The **axis** has a body and more closely resembles the rest of the cervical vertebrae, except for the presence of the odontoid process (syn. dens) which projects superiorly and articulates with the atlas (Fig. 2.2). Anterior to the odontoid process is a facet on the back of the anterior arch of the atlas; posteriorly lies the thick transverse ligament of the atlas. The apical ligament (Fig. 2.3) attaches the apex of the odontoid process to the anterior margin of the foramen magnum. The alar ligaments (Fig. 2.4) are short, strong ligaments which pass upwards and laterally from the sides of the apex of the odontoid process to the medial aspects of the occipital condyles. The large spine of the axis may be palpated some 2 cm below the external occipital

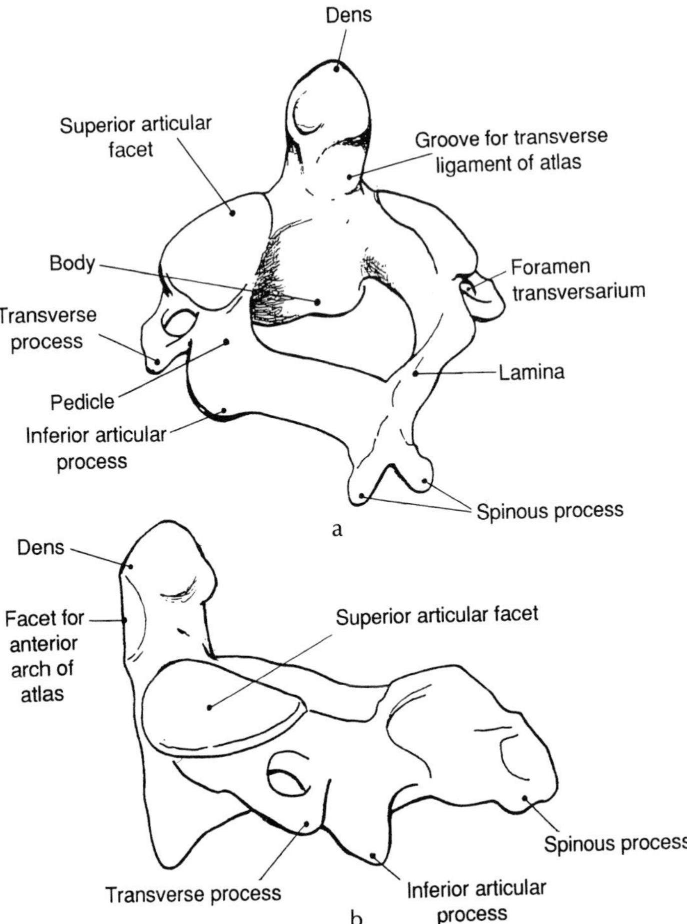

Fig. 2.2 The second cervical vertebra or axis – (a) superior and (b) lateral aspects.

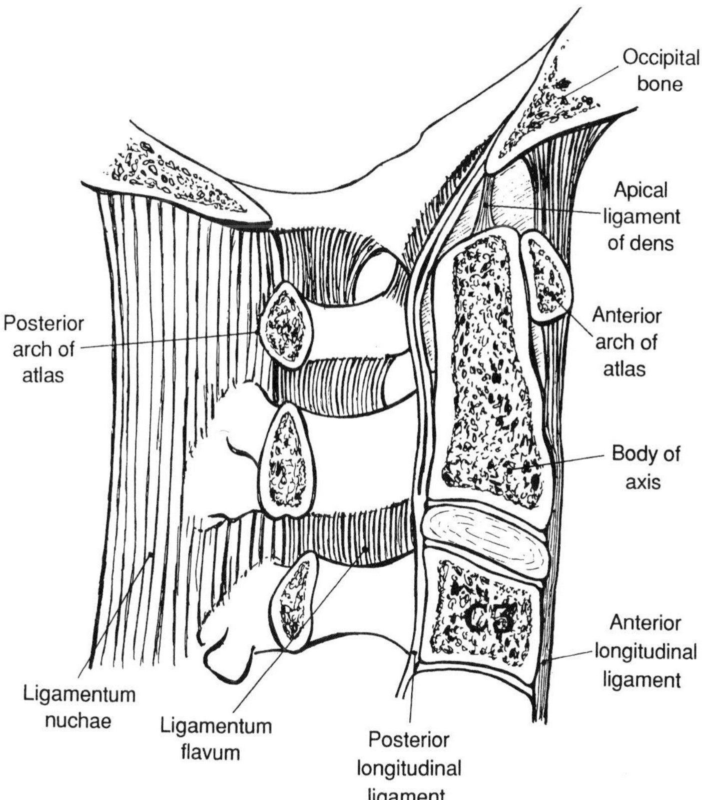

Fig. 2.3 Sagittal section of the cervical spine.

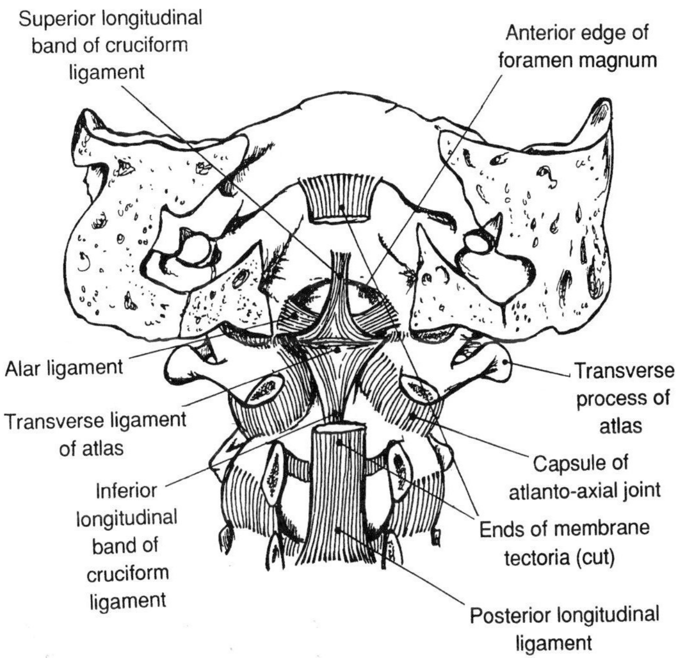

Fig. 2.4 Posterior aspect of atlanto-occipital and atlanto-axial joints. (From *Gray's Anatomy*, 1980, 36th edn, Churchill Livingstone, New York.)

protuberance. The articular facets transmit the weight of the head, allowing the odontoid process to rotate in respect to the atlas. The stability of the C1/2 joint is almost entirely dependent upon its ligaments – there are no intervertebral discs between C0 and C1 or between C1 and C2.

The **cervical vertebrae C2–C7** have characteristics which differ from the rest of the spine (Fig. 2.5). Each small transverse process

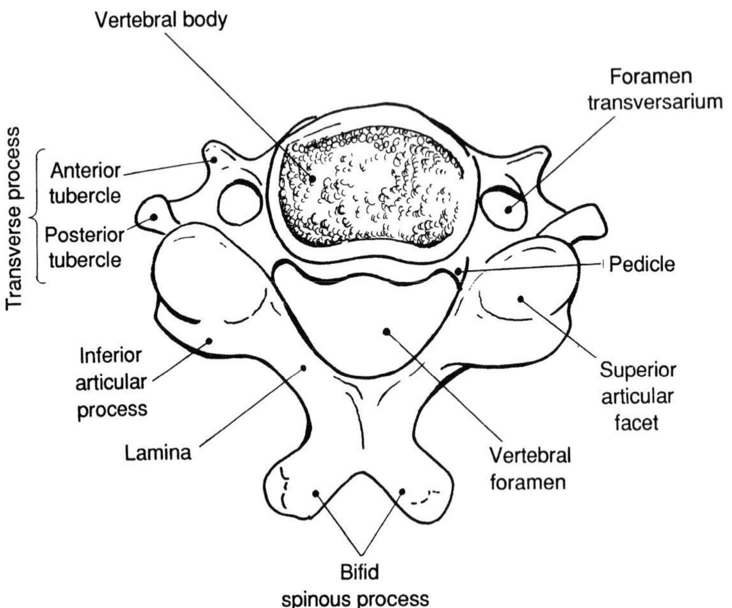

Fig. 2.5 A typical cervical vertebra – superior aspect.

contains a foramen transversarium which transmits a vertebral artery and vein (except at C7 at which the vertebral vein only is transmitted). The vertebral artery enters its bony canal at C6 and runs close to the articular processes, crossing the intervertebral canals, and ascending though the foramen magnum. The articular processes are approximately parallel on the two sides, inclined 45° to the transverse and coronal planes; on a lateral X-ray their orientation can be clearly seen, inclining from a postero-caudal aspect upwards and anteriorly towards the eyes. They are readily palpable posteriorly. The spines of C3–C5 are difficult to palpate because of the cervical lordosis.

The intervertebral discs do not extend the whole width of the vertebral bodies so that a further set of joints, the uncovertebral joints (of Luschka) also articulate between adjacent vertebral bodies (Fig. 2.6).

The **seventh cervical vertebra** is named the vertebra prominens because of its large spinous process. Care must be taken, however, during identification of the vertebral level by palpation of the spines,

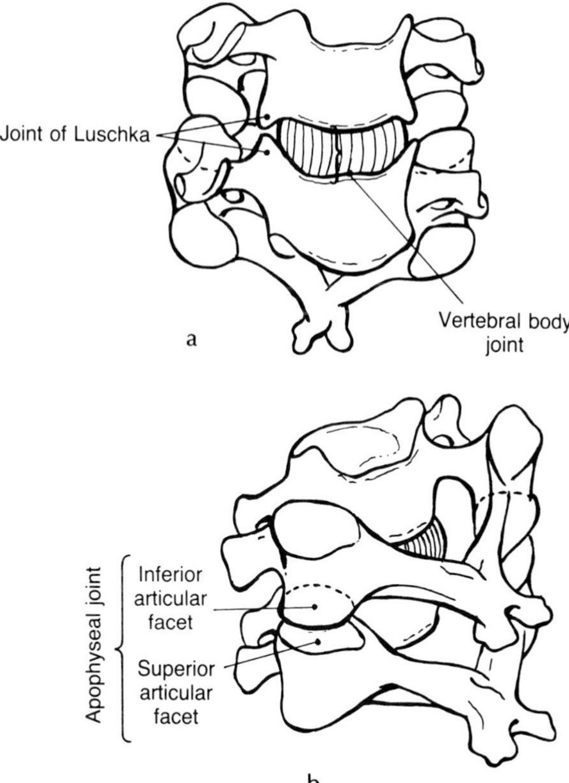

Fig. 2.6 (a) Anterolateral view of cervical spine demonstrating joints of Luschka. (b) Posterolateral view of cervical spine demonstrating apophyseal joints.

as both C6 and T1 may have prominent spines. Differentiation from C6 may be made by the fact that, when the neck is extended, the spine of C6 disappears from the palpating finger, while the spine of C7 remains prominent. The transverse processes of C7 may be elongated producing, in effect, rudimentary ribs and creating pressure on the adjacent nerve roots.

Muscles

Many muscles, small and large, act upon the head and neck, contributing substantially to the dissipation of forces as well as acting as prime movers. From a functional (and dysfunctional) point of view the following points are relevant.

- Weakness of these neck muscles is rarely seen – but weakness of the lower scapular fixators is common.
- Chronic fatigue (**myotendinosis**) in muscles such as trapezius and levator scapulae (Fig. 2.7) is probably very common. Sustained muscle contraction which is secondary to poor posture or tension causes painful ischaemia.
- Trigger points are particularly common: they are found predominantly in the levator scapulae (close to their inferior

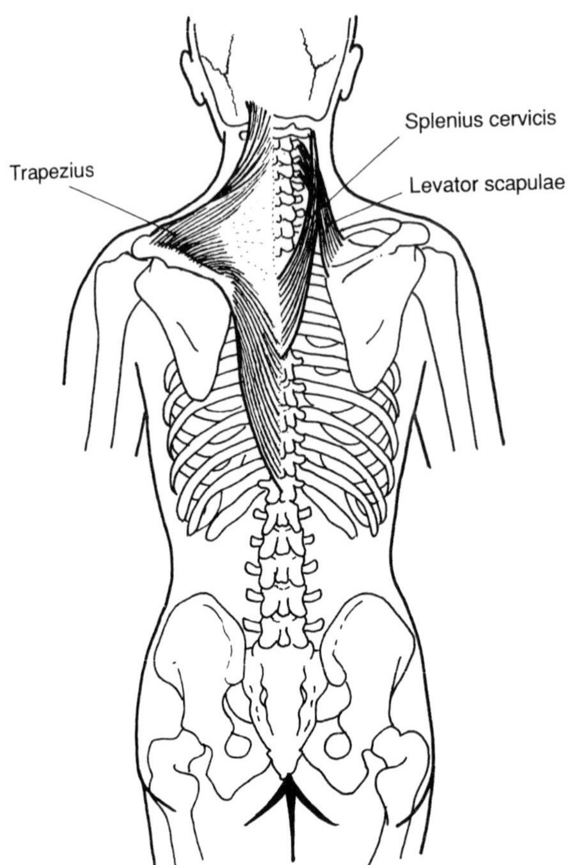

Fig. 2.7 Chronic fatigue in the upper trapezius and levator scapulae muscles is probably very common.

attachments at the superomedial border of the scapulae), in the upper and mid-points of the trapezii, and in the suboccipital muscles – rectus capitis posterior muscles and obliquus capitis muscles (Fig. 2.8). They have similarities to areas of myotendinosis, not least because of the characteristic of localized tenderness; trigger points, however, are usually secondary to joint dysfunction and may be treated by spinal manipulation.

Nerves

The spinal nerves are named by their relationship with the vertebra inferior to the intervertebral foramen through which they emerge (C1–C7); C8 emerges between C7 and T1 vertebrae (Fig. 4.9). During their course through an intervertebral canal (between C3 and C8) the dorsal and ventral nerve roots, united to form a common spinal nerve, are protected superiorly and inferiorly by the pedicles of adjacent vertebrae, medially by the body of the vertebra and the joints of Luschka, and laterally by the articular processes of the apophyseal joints (Fig. 2.9). Between C0 and C2, where there are no canals, the nerves emerge anteriorly in front of the articular masses and, consequently, rarely undergo true entrapment.

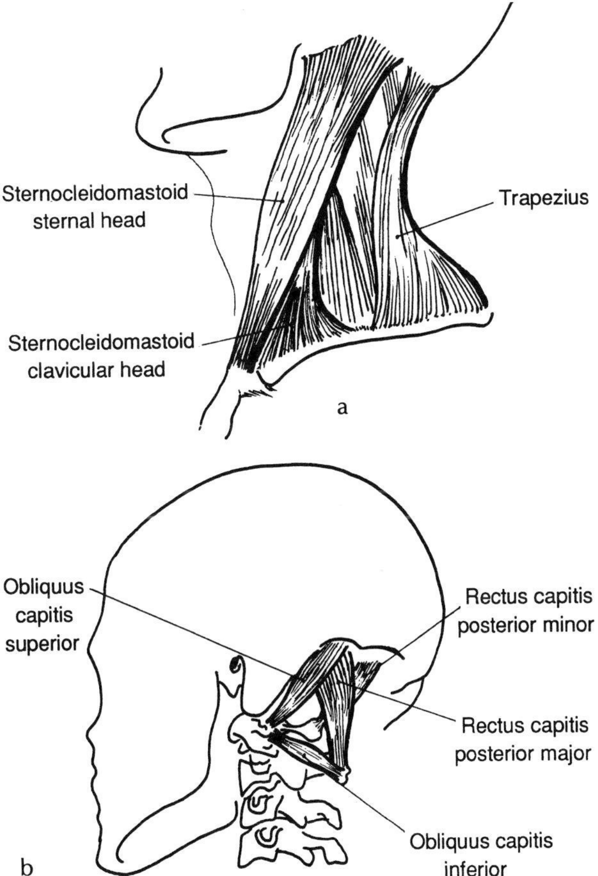

Fig. 2.8 The superficial neck muscles (a) and the suboccipital muscles (b) are demonstrated.

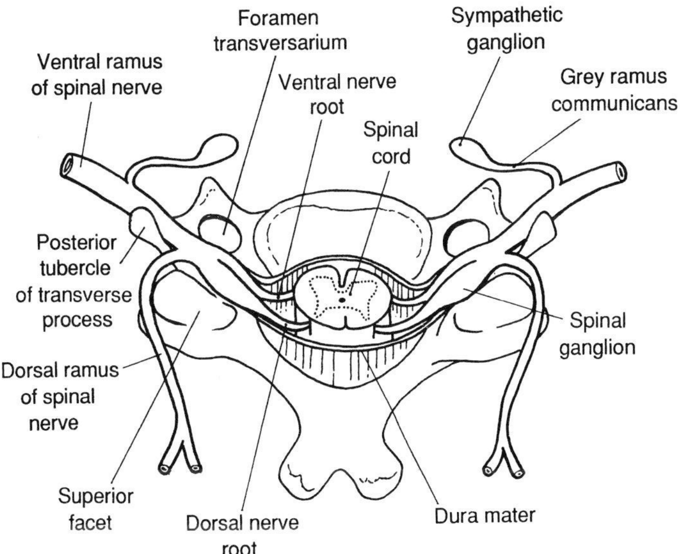

Fig. 2.9 The relationships of a spinal nerve in the cervical region are demonstrated. (From *Gray's Anatomy*, 1980.)

Upon emergence, each nerve divides into a dorsal ramus (supplying the posterior muscles and joint capsules) and a ventral ramus. The ventral rami C1–C4 form the cervical plexus and, via the occipital nerve, supply the larger neck and prevertebral muscles and the skin of the lower part of the scalp and neck. Afferent impulses from the posterior neck muscles, which are so important in the neck reflex and balance mechanisms, are transmitted via the C1–C3 dorsal rami; it is not surprising, therefore, that vertigo is a common symptom in proximal cervical joint dysfunction. The ventral rami C5–C8, together with T1, constitute the brachial plexus which supplies the musculature of the pectoral girdle and upper limb, and the skin of the upper limb. The trunks of the plexus lie in close relationship with the scalene muscles and, inferiorly, with the first rib. The plexus may be injured by traction on the nerve roots or on the ramifications within the plexus, and may be compressed by excessive tension (spasm) within the scalene muscles.

Postganglionic neurones of the sympathetic (autonomic) nervous system join the ventral rami via the grey rami communicantes. Ganglia in the cervical spine are situated proximally – the superior cervical ganglion – and inferiorly – the stellate ganglion; the middle cervical ganglion is found less consistently at the C6 level. From the superior cervical ganglion, postganglionic fibres reach their destination within the head via their plexiform association with the carotid arteries and their branches. Neurophysiological disturbance at the superior cervical ganglion is probably responsible for auditory and visual phenomena experienced by some patients following whiplash.

BIOMECHANICS

At the **craniocervical junction**, the movements between C0 and C1, and C1 and C2 may be considered separately. The principal movements between C0 and C1 are flexion and extension (nodding movements, otherwise referred to as inclination and reclination), approximating to a combined total of 25°. During flexion the occipital condyles glide backwards on the superior facets of C1; the reverse occurs during extension. Side flexion is limited to approximately 5° each side and results principally from axial rotation; when C1/2 rotation is locked by the examiner side flexion at C0/1 may be assessed clinically. Rotation is very limited and is also secondary to C1/2 rotation. Rotation, side flexion and anterior translation may be demonstrated during assessment of joint play.

The movements between C1 and C2 are complex. The principal movement is axial rotation which is limited by the joint capsules and the powerful alar ligaments. The combined atlas and head rotate around the odontoid process, and gliding movements take place between the articular processes. The extent of rotation is possibly up to 45° to each side in some individuals, comprising approximately

50% of total cervical rotation. When the neck is fully flexed, cervical rotation occurs predominantly at C1/2 and is restricted to 45°. As the neck extends, rotation is then possible at the distal cervical joints; in full extension, rotation is at its greatest, and is then augmented by movement at the proximal thoracic joints. The transverse ligament restricts flexion and extension at C1/2 to a few degrees only. Some side bending takes place during rotation.

Between C2 and C7, flexion and extension movements are fairly extensive. Essentially, flexion straightens out the normal cervical lordosis and amounts to some 25°. During flexion the proximal vertebral body tilts and slides on the one below. This forward translatory movement is often considerable in children (Fig. 2.10); it may also be identified clinically during joint play assessment. The spinal canal lengthens during flexion and the spinal cord elongates and becomes thinner. Kinesiological studies demonstrate that during cervical flexion, the initial movement is at C0/1, followed by flexion of the rest of the spine. Total cervical flexion amounts to approximately 40°.

Extension is of greater range, approximately 75°. The upper vertebra tilts and slides posteriorly, the ligamentum flavum buckles, and the intervertebral foramen is narrowed. In this position nerve roots may be compromised and the vertebral artery kinked. Rotation between C2 and C7 is associated with side flexion, and amounts to approximately 45° in each direction (Fig. 2.11). Rotation produces ipsilateral opening of the facets, resulting in narrowing of the intervertebral canal (Fig. 2.12). On the contralateral side compression of the articular facets occurs; in combination with tension in the joint capsules and torsion within the intervertebral disc, the approximation of these facets limits rotation. It can be seen that the nerve root is in danger of being compressed when the neck is extended and rotated to the painful side.

Kinesiological studies demonstrate that rotation is initiated at C1/2 and that with further movement in the upright position the C2–C7 levels undergo rotation. If the head is fully flexed, rotation is restricted and occurs primarily at C1/2. If the chin is tucked in, rotation occurs at C2/3. As the neck extends, rotational movements are recruited from the distal cervical spine.

Side flexion is coupled with rotation and is of the order of 35/40° to each side. Side flexion of the whole of the cervical spine is initiated at C0/2 where it is associated with axial rotation. The contralateral facet (and uncovertebral) joint spaces widen during side flexion.

PATHOANATOMY AND PATHOPHYSIOLOGY

Degenerative changes within the cervical spine are the inevitable consequence of man's upright posture. The changes of spondylosis – loss of disc height and hypertrophic osteophytosis – are maximal at

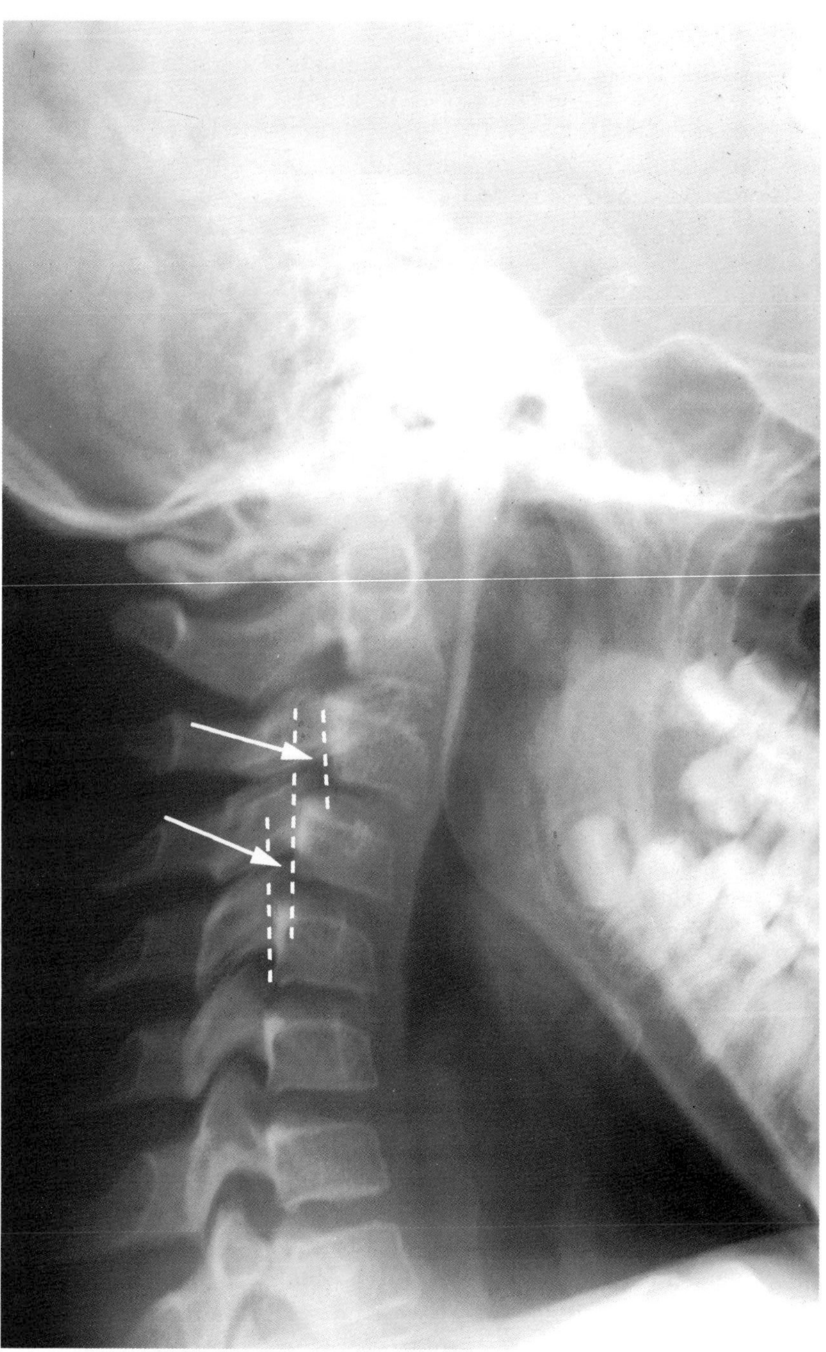

Fig. 2.10 Anterior translation of the proximal upon the distal cervical vertebra may be considerable in children. In this instance, anterior translation is well demonstrated at C3/4 and C4/5.

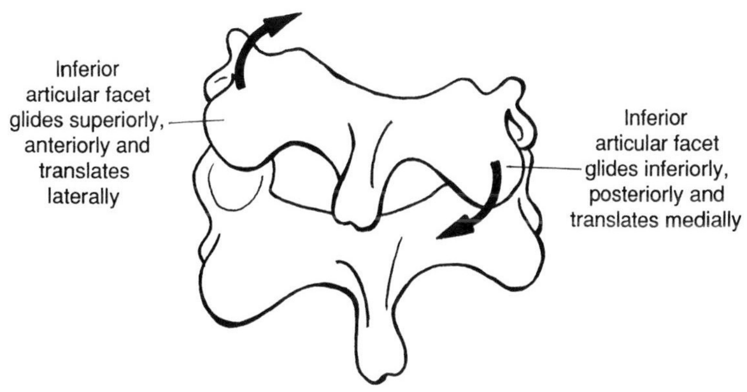

Fig. 2.11 Diagrams showing coupled movements of rotation and side flexion to the right in mid- and lower cervical regions.

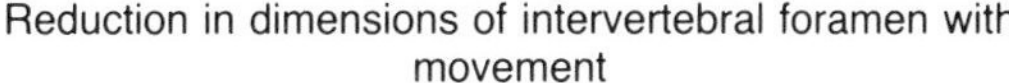

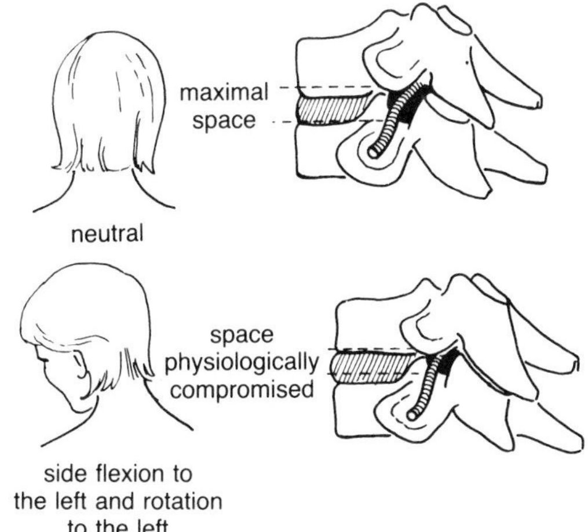

Fig. 2.12 Reduction in dimensions of intervertebral foramen with movement.

the site of maximal curvature, C4 to C6, presumably where maximal stress occurs. As recorded in Chapter 1, however, there is no correlation between the extent or site of degenerative changes on X-ray and the frequency or type of clinical condition responsible for a specific bout of neck pain. Undoubtedly, degenerative disc disease reduces its resilience to stress; in association with disturbed biomechanics of the posterior joints it provides an explanation as to why relatively minor stress, such as simply moving the neck sharply or in an unaccustomed fashion, may provoke the complaint of a 'ricked' or 'cricked' neck. Facetal dysfunction is the probable pathophysiological explanation for this common condition which is, in effect, the (reversible) response of a destabilized spine to various adverse factors.

The nucleus pulposus of the cervical intervertebral disc is sited in a relatively anterior position compared with the rest of the spine. This is one of several reasons proposed for the supposition that HNP (herniation of the nucleus pulposus) is an infrequent cause of root compression in the cervical spine. It is also postulated that the extra strength of the posterior longitudinal ligament and of the posterior annulus, and the interposition of the joints of Luschka exert a protective function in respect of the potential pressure from a disc bulge, or prolapse, upon the nerve roots in the intervertebral canal. However, the advent of soft tissue visualization techniques, in the form of CT scanning and MR imaging, has allowed the demonstration of nerve root compression by posterolateral herniation, particularly in the under 50–55 year age groups. In the 'middle years', that is late thirties to late fifties, root compression (which is often associated with loss of motor power and dysaesthesiae) is not uncommon, and is usually reversible. It is underdiagnosed as a result of a lack of adequate examination drills in common usage, and often inappropriately treated (nerve blocks are the only really effective conservative treatment if there are positive neurological signs). The natural history of the neurological consequences of root entrapment in this age group is complete resolution of the effects of motor denervation and disappearance of pain over the course of some months.

In common with the situation in the lumbar spine, an abnormal, bulging disc may give rise to symptoms which are probably mediated via nociceptive receptors in the posterior longitudinal ligament or dura mater and transmitted via the sinuvertebral nerve. Although the forceful injection of fluid into a normal cervical disc (in provocation discography) does not produce pain, its introduction into an abnormal disc gives rise to pain which is usually felt in the *interscapular* region; this may be abolished by the intradiscal introduction of local anaesthetic. Referred pain and referred tenderness in the interscapular area, usually just medial to the superomedial angle of one scapula, are common in lesions of the cervical spine; when pain in this region is reproduced by neck movements the likelihood of a discogenic cause is high.

Degenerative changes, in the form of osteophytes from the angles of the vertebral bodies lifting up the longitudinal ligaments, are thought to be protective (of the discs) in nature. Osteophytes on the posterior surfaces of the vertebral bodies, and osteophytes from the apophyseal joints, however, may give rise to spinal cord compression. The diameter of the spinal canal may become considerably reduced in neutral sagittal rotation. In cervical flexion, when the cord is elongated, its normal contour may be indented by posterior bulging of one or more disc(s) and by adjacent osteophytes. In extension, buckling of the ligamentum flavum may also indent the cord from its posterior aspect. This is of particular relevance in the elderly in whom disc thickness diminishes throughout the spine and cervical spondylosis is common; the thoracic kyphosis is often increased, the head is pushed forward, and a secondary exaggeration of the cervical lordosis occurs. Myelopathy, when secondary to cervical spondylosis, often presents insidiously with altered sensation or loss of coordination in the legs; it is often asymptomatic, yet may be detected if the Babinski responses are included in the routine examination of those patients whose problems are centred on the cervical spine.

At each segmental level in the normal spine, there is usually plenty of room for the common spinal nerve, its sheaths and the epidural contents within the intervertebral canal. The nerve is fixed immediately outside the foramen, though it is free to move within the canal; indeed, its position changes in response to movements of the cervical spine. The diameter of the foramen may be influenced by degenerative changes such as osteoarthritis of the apophyseal joints. Osteophytic intrusions into the foramen may be clearly visualized on oblique X-rays of the spine, yet are often asymptomatic (Fig. 2.13). Symptomatic nerve root compression may occur if the foraminal diameter is further compromised by a bulging disc or by

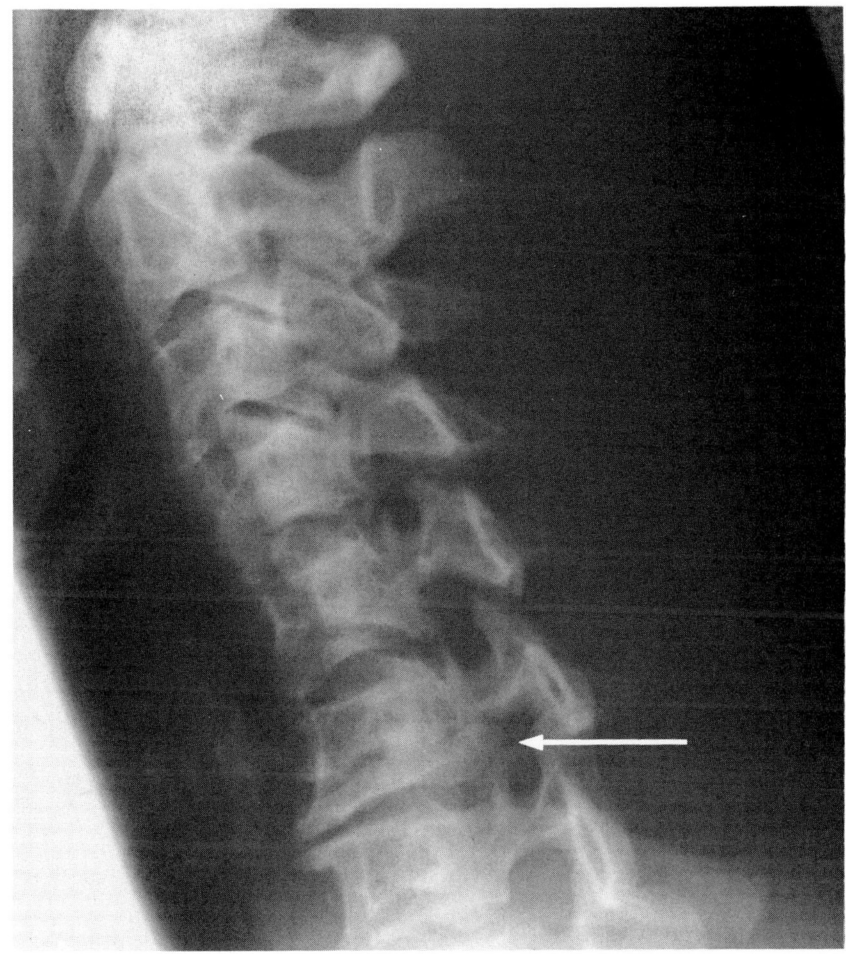

Fig. 2.13 Oblique X-ray of the cervical spine revealing osteophytic intrusions into the intervertebral foramina

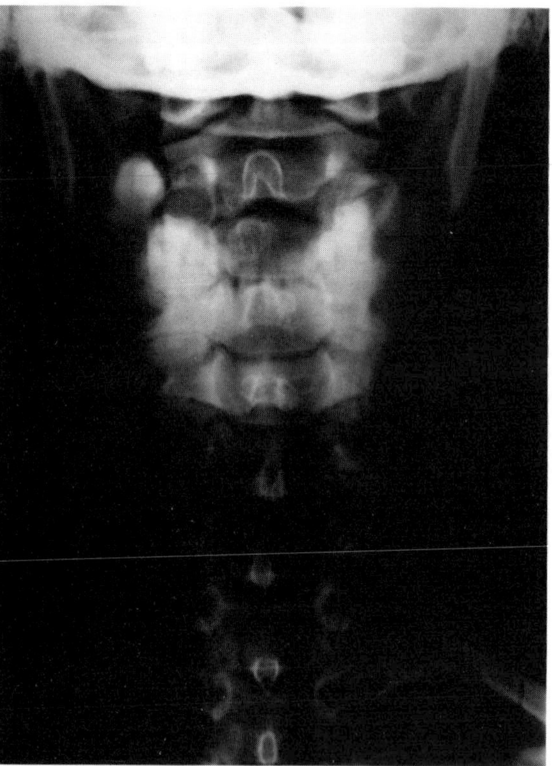

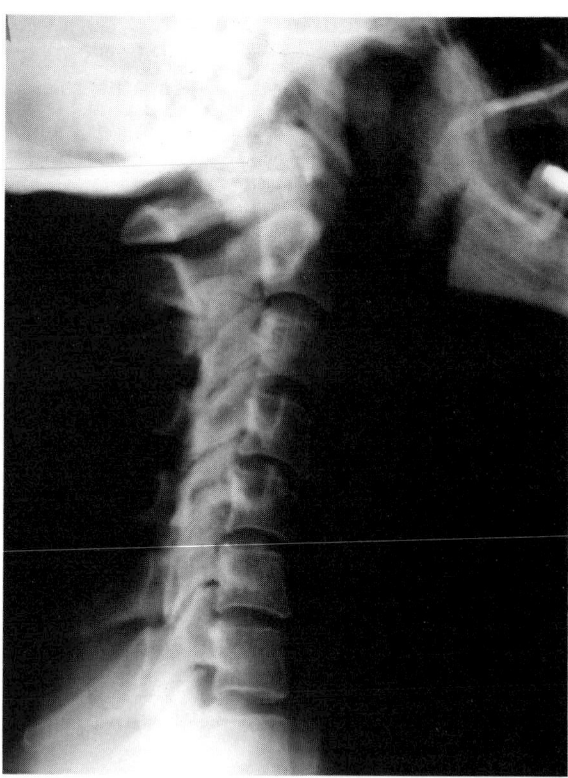

Fig. 2.14 Anteroposterior and lateral X-rays of the cervical spine revealing osteoarthritis of the apophyseal joints between C2 and C6.

inflammatory oedema. Extension and rotation of the spine to the affected side close the foramen and precipitate radicular symptoms. The clinical situation, as reflected by the complaint of radicular symptoms and corresponding signs on examination, may be reversible, despite radiological evidence of substantial osteophytic outgrowths, if the pathophysiological changes in the soft tissues resolve. If symptoms persist for between 3 and 6 months, and particularly if neurological signs are persistent or progressive, decompressive surgery may be required.

Osteoarthritis of the apophyseal joints may be observed on X-ray as subchondral sclerosis and narrowing of the joint margins (Fig. 2.14). Clinically, it gives rise to stiffness of the neck, that is, reduction of the mobility of the neck in the typical capsular pattern – all movements painlessly reduced in range other than flexion, which is spared for the most part. The condition behaves in a similar way to osteoarthritis elsewhere; often, stiffness is the principal and characteristic feature but discomfort, possibly due to synovitis, supervenes if the neck is subjected to too much stress.

Occasionally, synovitis is persistent – usually in the proximal spine, for instance C2/3. It is often well localized, and characterized by a prolonged period of painful restriction in mobility which is not helped (and may be made worse) by manipulation or even gentle mobilization. It is often helped by steroid injections around the affected joint(s). Very occasionally, it is associated with polymyalgia rheumatica or with diffuse idiopathic skeletal hyperostosis (DISH) (Fig. 2.15). In younger patients a stiff cervical spine is more likely to be due to ankylosing spondylitis.

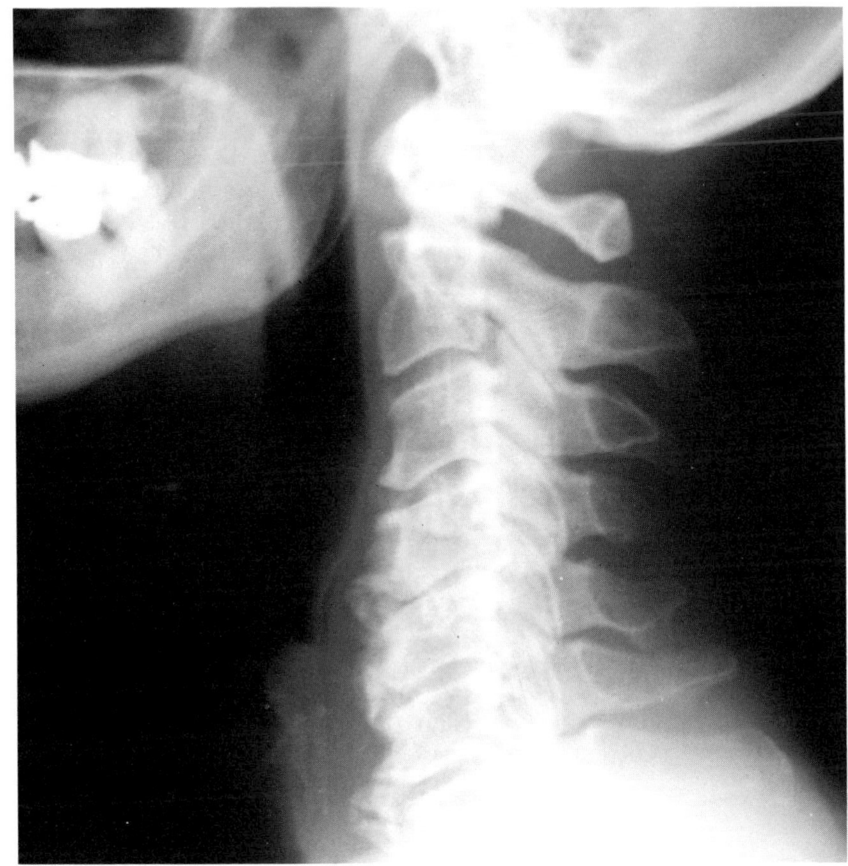

Fig. 2.15 The typical changes of diffuse idiopathic skeletal hyperostosis (DISH) are demonstrated.

Dysfunction

The pathological changes so far described in this chapter have a primary aetiological role in the *minority* of patients who seek help for cervical spinal conditions. Nevertheless, abnormal biomechanics and neurophysiological disturbances, which account for the majority of neck-related complaints, for instance spinal joint dysfunction and myotendinosis ('myofasciitis'), may, in some cases, be secondary to structural destabilization. Disturbed function may be diagnosed on the basis of painful hypomobility in a vertebral segment, when the presence of radiologically detectable degenerative changes is largely irrelevant. As explained in Chapter 1, it is this author's contention that spinal joint dysfunction may be considered to be a neurophysiological disturbance centred upon the apophyseal joints. Confirmation that the apophyseal joints may be a source of (chronic) neckache and headache was provided by Bogduk, who demonstrated complete, though temporary, relief from pain in a number of patients following cervical medial branch nerve blocks or apophyseal joint blocks (Bogduk and Marsland, 1988).

Joint dysfunction provides a nociceptive stimulus which results in ancillary signs via reflex neural pathways – local muscle hypertonicity and skin changes, and trigger points some distance from the primary disorder. Disturbance of the autonomic nervous system, in addition to somatic dysfunction, may be apparent: the complaints of dizziness, tinnitus, headache and visual disturbance are commonly associated with spinal dysfunction at the craniocervical junction. Dysfunction at C5/C6 may give rise to reflex disturbances at the shoulder joint or subacromial joint.

Myotendinosis, the characteristic feature of which is the presence of myofascial TPs – commonly in the levator scapulae and trapezii, but which, according to Travell and Simons (1983), may arise in *any* muscle – is due to muscle overload. In the neck, shoulder, and proximal thoracic regions, common precipitating or aggravating factors are situations in which the involved muscle becomes fatigued by constant use in its shortened position – for instance, reading, typing and long car journeys. Sudden, excessive stretching (as in whiplash – see below) is another common precipitant.

Over recent years the phenomenon of RSI (repetitive strain injury) has emerged. In this condition, which affects office and factory workers who use their hands and arms repetitively, symptoms are experienced in the neck, shoulder, arm or hand. By convention, the term RSI excludes specific conditions such as tenosynovitis in the forearm, carpal tunnel syndrome and nerve root entrapment in the neck. In fact, it is characterized by the absence of 'detectable' clinical signs. In the author's experience, *careful* examination of these patients often reveals signs of cervical spinal joint dysfunction or areas of myotendinosis; joint mobilizing techniques or treatment to localized myofascial TPs may then help the cervical symptoms, and sometimes the referred symptoms in the arm. However, there is a substantial group of patients with RSI, usually due to repetitive typing or keyboard operation, in whom no established pathological or functional changes can be elicited. The relevance of ergonomics to RSI is examined in greater detail in Chapter 5.

Acute wry neck (or torticollis)

This is the equivalent condition in the neck to lumbago in the lumbar spine. In the young adult (usually under 30) it very probably reflects an acute disc prolapse, in which the neck is held in fixed rotation and side flexion as a result of gross protective muscle spasm. The absence of root pain does not preclude the diagnosis of disc herniation: root pain is unusual under the age of 35 unless recurrent severe strain is applied to the neck as happens in some sports such as (scrummaging in) rugby football. In the child, protective muscle spasm may be secondary to adenitis in the neck. In the newborn, a sternomastoid injury is the most probable cause.

Spasmodic torticollis

Although the patient inexplicably, and apparently uncontrollably, twists his head in a particular direction, control may be exercised by manual pressure by the patient or the examiner on the head. It is thought to result from a disorder of the extrapyramidal nervous system.

Hysterical torticollis

This is characterized by voluntary elevation of the scapula in association with neck flexion towards the painful side.

WHIPLASH

Definition

The term **whiplash injury** was coined in 1928 by Harold Crowe to describe the mechanism of injury to the neck when the head was moved suddenly, initially into hyperextension, then into flexion (Breck and Van Norman, 1971). The common cause is a rear-end vehicle collision, although it is not uncommon for other types of accident, for instance head-on collisions, side-on collisions and roll-overs to give rise to neck injuries too. The reasons why rear-end (acceleration) collisions are the most common cause are, first, the biomechanical strain associated with hyperextension pushes the neck beyond its physiological range of movements, and secondly, the often unexpected nature of the collision occurs without preceding voluntary bracing of the spine. When used in a general sense, 'whiplash injury' includes all types of bony, discal or other soft tissue pathology. In its narrow sense, all conditions are excluded apart from what may be described as 'sprain' of the posterior elements (or, more specifically, as spinal joint dysfunction), which is often associated with myofascial trigger points in the base of the neck.

Epidemiology

Whiplash injury after road traffic accidents is common. It is estimated that approximately 30% of those involved in rear-end collisions complain of neck-related symptoms when attending hospital Accident and Emergency Departments; a further group of 35% experience delayed symptoms which not uncommonly arise within the next 12 to

24 hours (Deans *et al.*, 1987). There has been an increase in whiplash injuries in the UK since the wearing of seat belts became compulsory in 1983 for front seat passengers and drivers. The occupants of the front seats suffer more than rear seat passengers. The benefit from the use of head restraints is contentious (see below). Although considered to be a twentieth-century phenomenon, it had been identified by J. E. Erichsen in 1886 under the diagnostic label 'railway spine' as a result of railway accidents (Teasell and McCain, 1991).

Biomechanics

Kinematic and experimental studies reveal that the initial effect on the spine following forward acceleration of the vehicle is forward propulsion of the trunk and shoulders (Fig. 2.16). As a result of the inertia of the head, the cervical spine is (hyper)extended in relation to the shoulders; once the inertia is overcome, the neck rapidly flexes.

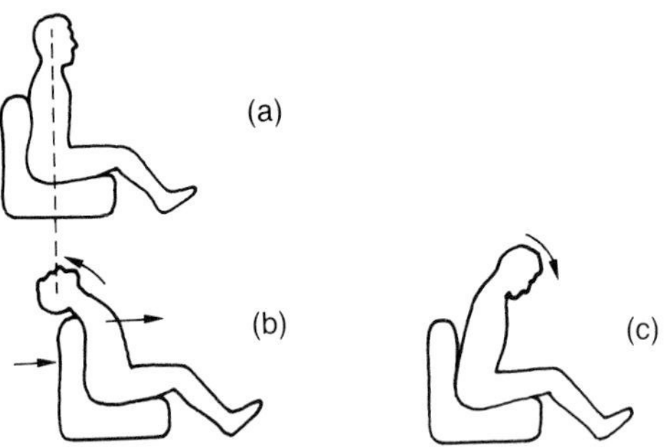

Fig. 2.16 Diagram of the movements of the upper body during whiplash showing: the position of the body at impact (a); the position of the shoulders have accelerated forwards (b); and the position once the head flexes (c). The arrows indicate the direction of movement of various parts of the body. (From Bogduk, N., 1986, Anatomy and pathophysiology of whiplash. *Clinical Biomechanics,* **1**, 92–101.)

Appreciation of this initial forward movement of the trunk (leaving the head behind) facilitates an understanding of the relationship between the incidence of whiplash injury and the use of head restraints. Unless the occiput is resting very close to the restraint (the recommended distance is less than 25 mm) at the time of impact, hyperextension of the neck will occur since the head remains virtually stationary in respect to the front of the restraint; even when resting on the restraint, some degree of extension is probable.

Pathophysiology and pathoanatomy

During the hyperextension phase the anterior spinal structures (anterior longitudinal ligament, intervertebral discs and prevertebral muscles) are strained, and the oesophagus and sternomastoid muscles are stretched. Posteriorly, the apophyseal joints and the spinous processes are compressed.

During the flexion phase the degree of damage is limited by the chin impinging against the chest. The odontoid process abuts the anterior arch of the atlas, and forward motion of the atlas transmits the strain to the atlanto-occipital joints. The posterior ligaments are subject to strain and the vertebral bodies and intervertebral discs subject to compression.

Associated injuries are sprain of the temporomandibular joint, brain damage or dysfunction, and cord 'concussion'. Fractures are relatively uncommon; nevertheless *X-rays should be taken* (other than in minor cases) to exclude odontoid peg, apophyseal and vertebral body fractures. Other radiological features which may be observed are reversal of the cervical lordosis, presumably due to muscle spasm; increased prevertebral soft tissue shadowing, which is more likely to be due to bleeding from the prevertebral muscles than from a vertebral body fracture; and angular deformity of the cervical vertebrae, possibly representing injury to the posterior ligaments. MRI has not proved to be a useful investigatory tool to date as the images are usually negative in respect of soft tissue pathology.

The presence of degenerative changes should be noted: although there is a poor correlation between these changes and the incidence of symptoms following whiplash, their presence is generally considered to be associated with more prolonged symptoms. More severe structural abnormalities, such as facet joint dislocation (which is inevitably associated with a fracture) and step deformities of one vertebra on another, require assessment by an appropriate specialist.

Whiplash symptoms often persist for several months, during which the two consistently found pathophysiological features are cervicothoracic **spinal joint dysfunction** and **myofascial trigger points**. While it is probable that TPs are secondary to joint dysfunction in most patients with neck problems, the biomechanical stresses involved in whiplash are perhaps more likely to give rise to primary trigger points (myotendinoses). The presence of a TP in the levator scapulae muscle, for instance, could explain the frequently experienced reference of pain to the medial border of the scapula and to the ulnar border of the arm (Travell and Simons 1983).

Symptoms

Most patients with whiplash injury complain of neck discomfort and stiffness; discomfort often radiates proximally to the occiput (indicating a C0/1 or C1/2 joint disturbance) and distally to the interscapular region (indicating mid/distal cervical joint disturbance). Headache is particularly common. Blurred vision, dizziness and other complaints which are probably due to sympathetic nervous discharge are not infrequent. Temporary paraesthesiae and numbness in the arms may be due to compression of the brachial plexus secondary to scalene muscle spasm, or to root irritation secondary to synovitis of the facet joints, but more prolonged symptoms are likely to be associated with spinal joint dysfunction and myofascial TPS, or occasionally with nerve root irritation caused by a disc prolapse. Dysphagia is also a common complaint during the first few days, probably due to bleeding from the pharynx, oesophagus, or prevertebral muscles.

Diagnosis

Clinically, the establishment of a specific diagnosis following whiplash requires an identical examination regime to that for any other patient presenting with similar symptoms, irrespective of the source. Usually, precautionary X-rays have been performed at Accident and Emergency departments, so that the principal decision for the therapist to make is whether there is any evidence of disc prolapse which, although relatively unusual in these circumstances, would call for specific therapeutic measures. The most common problem is cervical spinal joint dysfunction, which often proves to be particularly indolent at the proximal cervical joints and at the cervicothoracic junction. TPs, in the levator scapulae and trapezius for instance, are almost invariably present and often very persistent. Temporomandibular joint dysfunction, thoracic joint dysfunction, and sacroiliac dysfunction often coexist.

In the first week after whiplash, during which there is often considerable pain and stiffness in the neck, it is probable that contributions to the overall symptomatology are made by strains of most of the soft tissue structures within the neck, not least by capsular and ligament strain and synovitis of the apophyseal joints. During this time it is reasonable to offer palliative therapy only, for instance local cold applications and the use of a soft cervical collar.

Management

After one week a further evaluation is made, followed by gentle mobilization procedures for joint dysfunction if the acute phase is beginning to settle. The most useful regime for the majority of patients is the combination of gentle mobilization, muscle energy techniques, massage (for TPs predominantly), and a programme of graded stretching exercises. Patients should be weaned from the regular diurnal use of cervical collars after 1–2 weeks for fear of muscle atrophy, muscle shortening and dependency; nocturnal use may be helpful for a longer period of time. After the first few weeks regular reassessment should identify the need for continuing treatment or, should a pattern of disc prolapse become established, for additional therapy such as cervical traction. Usually, however, patients tend to be worse with traction, and the main thrust of treatment should be towards the resolution of joint dysfunction and TPs.

Prognosis

Much retrospective analysis, often on selected groups of patients, has been undertaken to determine the prognosis from whiplash; these statistical conclusions vary considerably. It is probable that poor prognostic indicators in patients in their forties and beyond are pre-existing degenerative changes, and prolonged immobilization in a collar. Other factors indicating a poorer prognosis following whiplash are persisting sleep disturbance, depressive diatheses, lower socioeconomic groups and personality traits which contribute to reduced 'coping' skills.

The use of early mobilization techniques has been shown to be effective in shortening the length of disability; also, a home mobilization programme following instruction by a physiotherapist may be helpful. However, most statistical surveys do not evaluate the benefit of adequate mobilization treatment, and it is probable that the recorded incidence of 25% or more of patients who continue to be symptomatic one year after injury (Deans *et al.*, 1987; Hohl, 1974; McNab, 1964) may be reduced significantly with appropriate treatment.

Neurosis

A comment in respect of neurosis associated with whiplash is necessary. Henry Miller (1961) wrote extensively and influentially of accident neurosis (or 'compensation' or 'litigation' neurosis) which may complicate progress in a small percentage of patients, although this situation is not usually difficult to recognize.

There is often a latent period of a few weeks or even months during which time the patient's anxiety may be considered to be a natural reaction to the fright of the accident. Thereafter, gross dramatization of symptoms associated with a somewhat hystrionic reaction to examination are cardinal features of accident neurosis. Miller's description of the patient's behaviour at the initial medical consultation for the assessment of his condition is particularly apt:

> If he is being examined at the request of the insurance company he frequently arrives late. He is invariably accompanied, often by a member of his family, who does not wait to be invited into the consulting room but who resolutely enters with him, and more often than not takes an active part in the consultation, speaking for him, prompting him, and reminding him of symptoms that may for the moment have slipped his memory. The patient's attitude is one of martyred gloom, but he is also very much on the defensive, and exudes hostility, especially at any suggestion that his condition may be improving . . . the most consistent clinical feature is the subject's unshakeable conviction of unfitness for work.

Perhaps under these circumstances, thankfully the minority, the therapist's counselling role should be positive, to complement Dr Miller's further observation that doctors should 'encourage a robust attitude to minor injury'.

Regrettably, the other side of the coin is seen more frequently – **iatrogenic** anxiety, associated with the persistence of symptoms and resulting from insensitive or inadequate management, or associated with the dreaded diagnosis of 'arthritis' (based on the presence of degenerative changes on X-ray). This situation is exacerbated by poor rapport with the physician or therapist (usually the former) who is frustrated by lack of therapeutic response, and is suspicious either of unconscious deception by the patient ('hysteria') or conscious deception ('malingering'). The worst scenario is the prolonged use of cervical collars after injury, often based upon the mistaken supposition that any active treatment such as mobilization, should it have ever been considered, is contraindicated in the presence of 'arthritis' or 'spondylosis', and which leads to persistence of somatic symptoms and anxiety, and to the risk of established chronic pain and illness behaviour. Once such chronic illness behaviour has become established, the role of compensation may be relatively minor, and the experienced therapist recognizes the need for behaviour modification therapy.

HISTORY

Apart from young adults who present for the first time with an acute wry neck and have no relevant past history, most patients with neck pain give a history of recurrent bouts of pain in the past. These are usually explained as resulting from sitting in a draught, for instance by an open window. Possibly a new characteristic, such as referred pain, or anxiety regarding the nature of and reason for the recent recurrence, persuades the patient to seek attention. The circumstances in which pain has been experienced in the past, its location, speed of onset and longevity, should all be established. The susceptibility of the patient to spinal derangement may be gauged; this could be of assistance during the subsequent assessment, and particularly in respect to advice regarding prevention of further injury.

The characteristics of the presenting symptoms should be clearly established. A common situation, as in the thoracic and lumbar spines, is for a sudden pain to be felt in the paraspinal region during an unguarded moment, such as turning quickly or awkwardly. Both an overall feeling of neck stiffness and restriction in mobility in specific directions progress over the next 24 hours. If the cervical spine has become destabilized by degenerative disc disease, or by recent disc prolapse or whiplash injury, relatively minor stresses may give rise to joint dysfunction.

Alternatively, the history may be insidious, in which case no association has been made with any particular event or incident, and the patient has gradually become aware of increasing discomfort and stiffness; these symptoms may have been ignored for a while yet their persistence prompts attendance for advice. This is particularly evident if brachial symptoms supervene.

The location of the symptoms gives a useful guide to the nature of the lesion. Headache (whether occipital, vertical, or frontal), dizziness, tinnitus and aching in the temporal and facial regions suggest craniocervical dysfunction. Pain felt unilaterally in the mid-point of the neck, radiating to the 'shawl' area (usually the supraspinous area of the scapula), is often due to joint dysfunction in the mid/distal cervical spine. Feinstein *et al.* (1954) demonstrated **referred pain** patterns following noxious stimulation of interspinous musculotendinous tissue innervated by the posterior rami of the cervical spinal nerves; interestingly, referred pain to the ulnar side of the arm was consistently produced by stimulation of the 7th and 8th cervical segments, though referral to the radial side of the arm occurred in none of their subjects. Dwyer *et al.* (1990) outlined referred pain patterns in normal volunteers following intra-articular injection of the cervical apophyseal joints with contrast medium under fluoroscopic screening (Fig. 1.30); in a further group of patients with suspected apophyseal joint pain, diagnostic predictions from established pain patterns were confirmed by local anaesthetic blocks of the medial branches of the posterior rami.

Pain felt diffusely in the neck, and more specifically along the medial border of the scapula when the neck is moved in certain directions, suggests (but is not pathognomonic of) a disc prolapse. Brachial discomfort, felt diffusely in the shoulder and upper arm, is a common complaint and should not be considered to be true radicular pain unless other characteristics are present. Patients' dermatomal localization of **radicular pain** in the arm (due to root compression) is often less exact than in the lumbar spine; paraesthesiae, and particularly numbness, are rather better localized. Paraesthesiae are only felt in the arm from lesions involving the C6, C7 and C8 roots (that is, excluding C5). The most commonly affected is the C7 root, when symptoms are experienced in the index, long and ring fingers. Small areas of hypoaesthesia (or, paradoxically, areas of exquisite hyperaesthesia) may be present paravertebrally at the segmental level of spinal joint dysfunction.

The temporal relationship between radicular symptoms and neck symptoms should be established: it is not unusual for patients to fail to recall preceding neck pain and stiffness when their present complaints are localized to the arm. Pain felt in the pectoral region and axilla is not uncommon in a C7 root palsy.

Further enquiry may need to be made in respect of paraesthesiae; their relationship to posture, and their diurnal or noctural predominance, for instance, are often important factors when considering the differential diagnosis. Noctural discomfort may be very troublesome, particularly when caused by a cervical disc prolapse or whiplash. Turning over in bed, or raising the head from the pillow, may be extremely painful, prompting patients to describe their neck as weak, as well as stiff and painful.

EXAMINATION

Demeanour

In clinical practice there are two sets of circumstances in which very abnormal behavioural characteristics may be apparent at the initial interview. In the first, gross exaggeration of the normal responses to examination is combined with dramatization of symptoms in 'accident neurosis'. The second circumstance is 'hysterical torticollis', in which a youngster, usually a teenaged girl, presents with a neck held determinedly in a fixed position and with responses to questioning which vary from resentment to frank hysteria.

Disturbances of affect, otherwise, are secondary to persistence of pain and/or the inability of doctors (to a much greater extent than therapists) to understand the problem or develop a rapport with the patient. All too frequently, symptoms such as headaches and dizziness tend to be dismissed as expressions of tension or anxiety, when a spinal cause may be detected by careful examination. Patients with strong neurotic traits are as liable as the rest of the population to develop musculoskeletal problems!

Appearance

A torticollis is unmistakable. Spinal posture in the sitting position at interview, and in the standing position during examination, are noted. In particular, a rounded upper back signifies a likely propensity to ligamentous strain and myotendinosis. In these patients, the exaggerated thoracic kyphosis is associated with forward projection of the head and hyperextension of the neck (Figs 3.5, 3.12). Often, further rounding of the back, by drooping of the shoulders and protraction of the pectoral girdle, increases the likelihood of cervicothoracic and shoulder symptoms considerably.

In advanced ankylosing spondylitis, a fully extended neck fails to compensate for the kyphotic trunk, and the patient loses his ability to look upwards.

Standing (or sitting): articular examination

Global articular signs are recorded as active, then passive, movements of the neck in six directions: flexion, extension, rotations to right and left, and side flexions to right and left. The examiner observes:

1 Reproduction of pain.
2 Range of movement.
3 End-feel.

Pain and range of movement may be recorded using the chart demonstrated in Fig. 2.17. Resisted muscle contraction tests may also be employed, although they have little discriminant value. If metastases invade muscle attachments to a vertebra, pain on contraction may be detected; and, in acute torticollis and whiplash, discomfort and apparent weakness may be demonstrated for a few days in the acute phase.

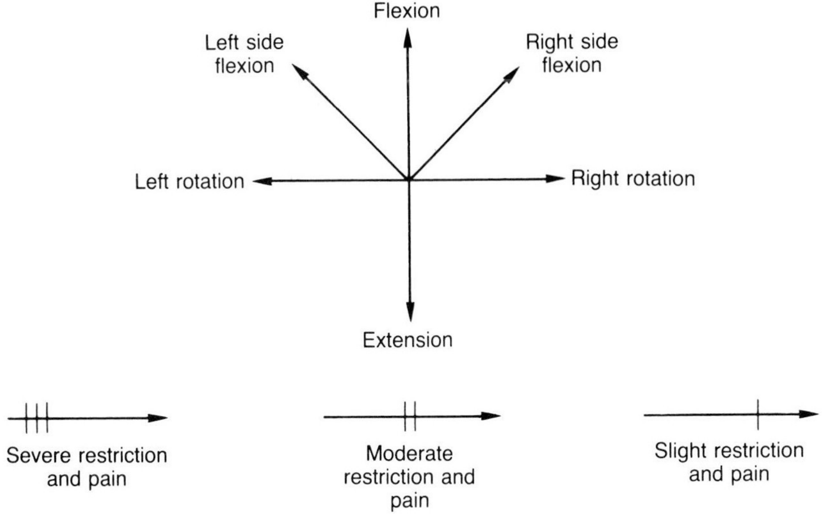

Fig. 2.17 A method of recording range of movement at the cervical spine.

The assessment of active movements informs the examiner which movements are painful, and which movements are apparently restricted. The end-feel on passive movements yields further information on the reason for restricted movement in specific directions. A hard end-feel on rotation indicates the limit of a normal range of movements; a restricted, possibly asymmetrical, range of rotations with a hard end-feel is associated with advancing years. A feeling of muscle tension at the end of range is typical of spinal joint dysfunction; it is not possible to differentiate this from a nuclear disc prolapse on end-feel alone. The muscle spasm, accompanied by the look of pain and apprehension on the face of a patient with spinal malignant deposits, is very characteristic.

The pattern of global mobility restriction is recorded. The capsular pattern in the cervical spine (for instance in ankylosing spondylitis and rheumatoid arthritis) is a restricted range of all movements, except flexion which is often only minimally affected. Other conditions – spinal joint dysfunction, cervical disc prolapse and nerve root entrapment – give rise to a non-capsular (partial articular) pattern. Nerve root entrapment in the elderly, due to a combination of osteophytosis and disc bulge, is aggravated by extension and ipsilateral rotation, both of which reduce the intervertebral foraminal diameter. The passive range of coupled extension and ipsilateral rotation may be found useful as a provocative test for radicular pain in relatively minor degrees of root entrapment.

Standing (or sitting) neurological examination

When dealing with 'mechanical' lesions of the cervical spine, the objective confirmation of sensory loss in the upper limbs is often unrewarding and, thankfully, unnecessary; the patient's *complaint* of localized numbness, particularly when associated with the other radicular symptoms of pain and paraesthesiae in a dermatomal pattern, is highly predictive of nerve compression. Clinical assessment of motor function in the upper limbs is much more useful, and should be included in the examination of all patients with neck pain, irrespective of the presence of radicular symptoms. Muscle power may be assessed by manually resisting its contraction, and recorded according to the MRC scale (see 'Neurological signs', Chapter 1); this is helpful when assessing and reassessing relatively gross loss of power, though less useful in the more subtle degrees of weakness at the MRC4 ('strong, not normal') level. A suitable schedule should include the muscles associated with the following movements (which are listed with their root innervations):

Rotation of neck (sternomastoid) C1.
Shrugging of shoulders (trapezius) C2,3,4.
Abduction of shoulder (deltoid and supraspinatus) C5.
External rotation of shoulder (infraspinatus) C5.
Flexion of elbow (biceps brachii) C5,6.
Extension of wrist (extensor carpi) C6.
Flexion of wrist (flexor carpi) C7.
Extension of elbow (triceps) C7.
Ulnar deviation of wrist (flexor and extensor carpi ulnaris) C8.
Extension of thumb (extensor pollicis) C8.
Adduction of thumb (adductor pollicis) C8.
Extension of fingers (extensor digitorum) C8.
Approximation of fourth/fifth fingers (interossei) T1.

The tendon jerks may be elicited, though their sensitivity is not as high as a careful appraisal of muscle function:

Biceps C5,6.
Brachioradialis C5,6.
Triceps C7.

Dural stretch tests (syn. abnormal brachial plexus tension tests; neural tension tests) should be performed if there is doubt concerning

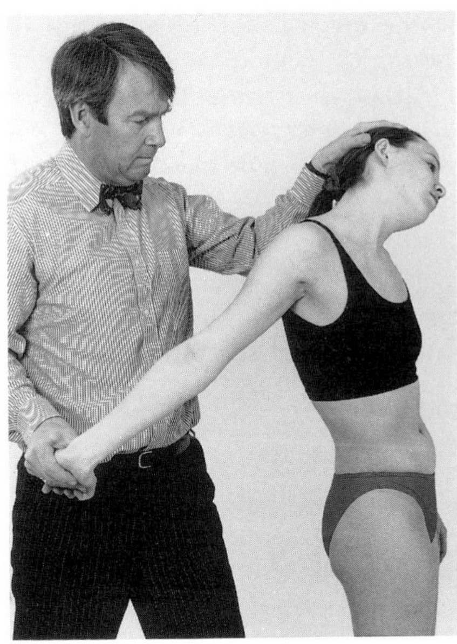

Fig. 2.18 Demonstration of neural tension in the mid- and distal cervical spine.

the cause of pain in the shoulder and arm, particularly if the distribution is along the C5 dermatome. The test, developed by Elvey (1986) in Perth, Australia, stretches the nerve roots and their dural sheaths at the C5, C6 and C7 levels by applying tension to the brachial plexus and the peripheral nerves in the upper limb (Fig. 2.18). The position of the patient in which maximal tension is applied is:

Contralateral side flexion of the neck.
Abduction (to 90°) and extension of the shoulder.
Depression of the shoulder girdle.
Extension of the elbow.
Supination of the forearm.
Dorsiflexion of the wrist.

Tension (and, therefore, the sensitivity of the test) is controlled by the degree of side flexion of the neck and/or extension of the elbow. Reproduction of shoulder or arm pain indicates excessive nerve or nerve root tension which, in the context of disorders of the cervical spine, is most likely to arise at the C5/6 and C6/7 intervertebral levels.

Functional examination of the glenohumeral, subacromial and acromioclavicular joints by active, passive and stress (provocation) tests, in addition to resisted movements, should be performed. A minimum requirement is an assessment of active abduction followed by resisted abduction of each shoulder, which collectively act as a screening test for abnormal shoulder biomechanics (as well as for C5 nerve root paresis). If abnormalities are detected, these may be due to dual pathology; alternatively, the common neural pathway of C5 may be the mechanism for apparent disorders at both the neck and the shoulder.

Although neurological assessment in the lower limbs is performed, for the most part, with the patient in the supine position, an assessment of gait may be helpful at this stage.

Supine

In this position, joint play assessment in the cervical spine may be carried out. Additionally, localized muscle hypertonus and segmental tenderness over the spinous processes and the articular processes may be detected.

Joint play assessment

This is a most useful part of the examination. It provides further information on segmental mobility that is not available from the global neck tests so far described; on the other hand, it may be impossible to perform these tests with any degree of sensitivity in the early stages of acute disc prolapse in young adults or in severe whiplash, because of the intense muscle spasm. Under most other circumstances, however, segmental differentiation is possible during joint play assessment. Joint play also serves as a sound starting point for mobilization of the neck, which is, essentially, an extension of the examining technique (Mennell, 1960).

Long axis traction

This gives the examiner an indication of the degree of play along the long axis of the spine, although it is non-specific in respect of segmental localization (Fig. 2.19). Muscle relaxation occurs after

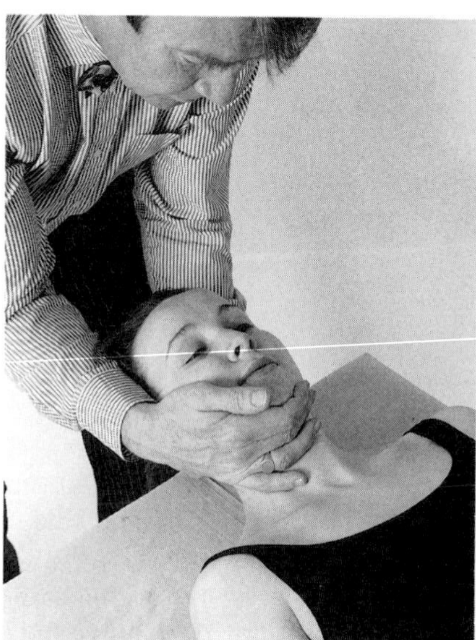

Fig. 2.19 Joint play and mobilization of the cervical spine – long axis traction.

5–10 seconds of manual distraction of the joints of the neck (applied to a level at which the patient starts to slide along the couch). It should be performed with the chin tucked in to straighten the cervical lordosis.

Side gliding

Most patients are able to relax during this procedure, although one or two visits are necessary sometimes for confidence to be gained by the anxious. Side gliding is produced by the examiner's hands cupping the occipital bone bilaterally (Fig. 2.20); segmental specificity is achieved by pressure from the radial margins of the examiner's index fingers on each side of the neck. Tenderness over the articular masses and transverse processes is sought, and hypomobility noted.

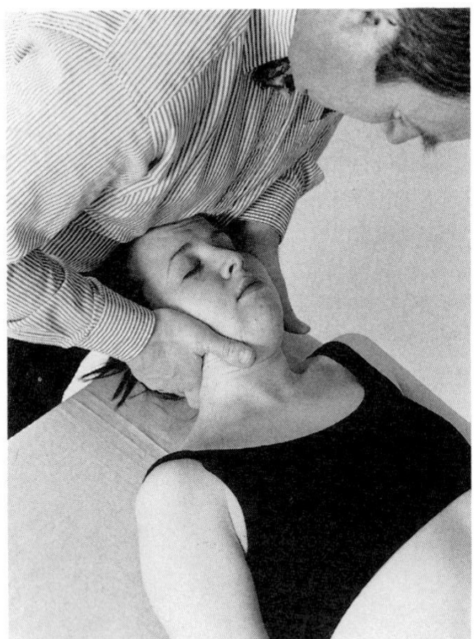

Fig. 2.20 Joint play and mobilization of the cervical spine – side gliding.

Side bending

Segmental localization is again achieved by the use of the index finger of one hand to fix a vertebra, and the complementary use of the other hand to provide a side bending force to the head and proximal cervical spine (Fig. 2.21).

Anteroposterior glide

The index finger of one hand directs the application of anterior translation pressure at a vertebral segment (Fig. 2.22a); subsequently, posterior translation is produced by backwards pressure applied

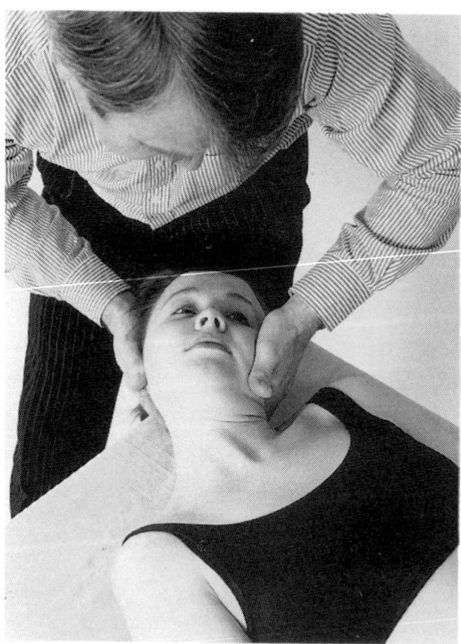

Fig. 2.21 Joint play and mobilization of the cervical spine – side bending.

through the web between the thumb and index finger of the other hand on the patient's chin (Fig. 2.22b). Anteroposterior glide is particularly helpful in the mid- and proximal cervical spine, less so distally.

Coupled rotation and side bending

Overpressure may be exerted when a comfortable passive range of rotation to right, then to left, has been reached, Further joint play is

a

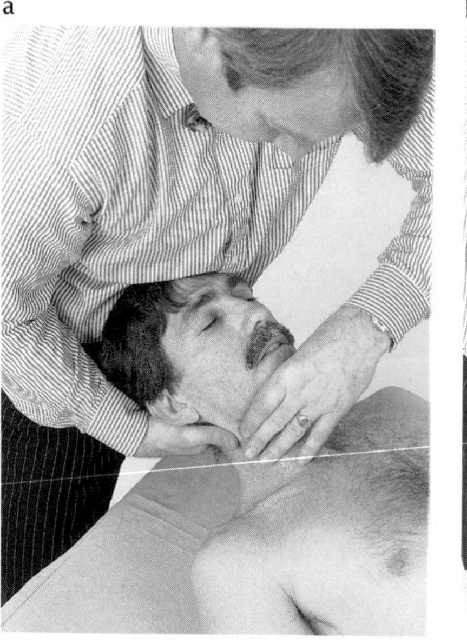

b

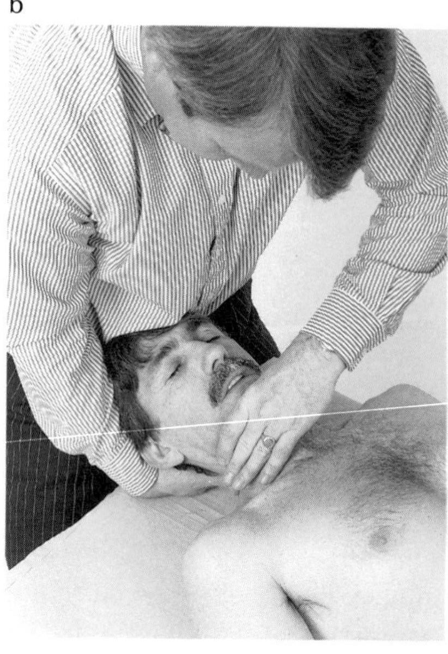

Fig. 2.22 Joint play and mobilization of the cervical spine – anteroposterior glide.

produced, and discomfort noted. Of greater usefulness in the proximal cervical spine, however, is the addition by the examiner of side bending to the fully rotated neck (Fig. 2.23a). Once C1/2 rotation has been maximized, a rocking movement into side flexion of the head on the rotated neck procures movement at the C0/1 joint (Fig. 2.23b). In elderly patients, in whom vertebrobasilar insufficiency is suspected, moderate rotation only is employed, to a degree which does not provoke symptoms of dizziness.

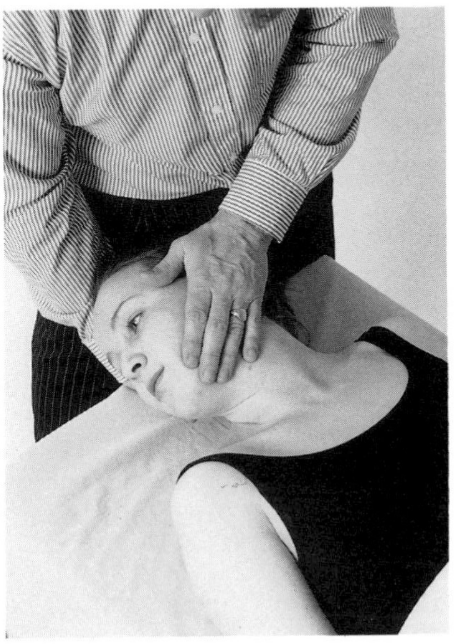

a

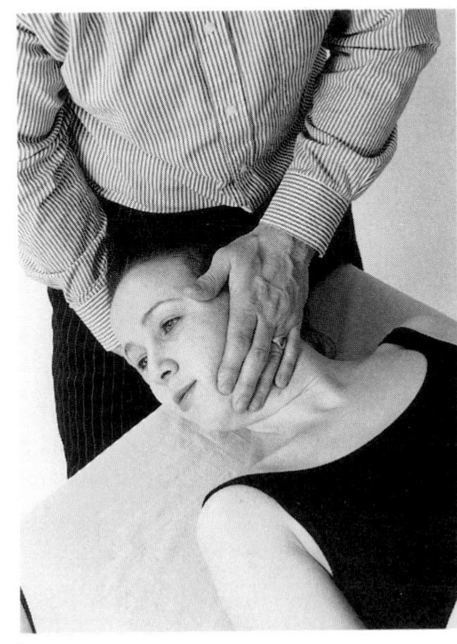

b

Fig. 2.23 Occipito-atlantoid (C0/1) joint play and manipulation.

Muscle hypertonus

Palpation yields further information on the segmental level of joint dysfunction by the identification of trigger points (localized muscle hypertonus). Tenderness and tension in the suboccipital muscles indicate a lesion at the craniocervical junction (C0–C2). Paraspinal muscle hypertonicity is a consistent finding in dysfunction between C2 and C5. A trigger point is commonly found in the mid-point of the trapezius in dysfunction in the mid-cervical spine; and in the levator scapulae, near its distal attachment, in dysfunction in the distal cervical spine. Trigger points in the trapezius and levator scapulae are more easily identified when the patient assumes the prone or sitting position.

Spinous process tenderness

Light pressure over the spinous process at the affected level commonly causes discomfort. This may be confirmed by palpation with the patient in the prone position, though the latter examination is superfluous unless the therapist prefers this position for Maitland-type mobilization (Maitland, 1977), and for identification of trigger points.

INTERPRETATION

Cervical disc prolapse

Intervertebral disc prolapses give rise to different clinical syndromes, depending upon their size and location in respect to the spinal canal into which they protrude. The capacity of the spinal canal and the presence of degenerative changes at the intervertebral foramina are additional factors which may influence the course of the clinical condition.

Acute wry neck (torticollis)

This condition in a young adult is usually unmistakable: the combination of a very short history and gross articular signs, characterized by fixed side flexion, offers little room for differential diagnosis. Spontaneous resolution usually takes place within 10 days. Effective relief of symptoms may be procured by muscle energy techniques in the first 24–48 hours, followed by (joint play) mobilizing techniques.

Acute central (posterior) prolapse

Posterior neck pain, radiating to the shoulders, is associated with reversal of the cervical lordosis (manifesting clinically as a fixed flexion posture). This is the least common presentation of a cervical disc prolapse; progression from a central to a posterolateral protrusion is the usual outcome.

Posterolateral prolapse

Unilateral (posterior) neck pain is often associated with scapular pain. A common complaint is of stiffness and discomfort in the neck, and pain along the medial border of the scapula. A partial articular pattern is found; although some active movements remain unrestricted, rotation towards the painful side is usually painful. Joint play assessment is characterized by substantial hypomobility which is associated with muscle spasm. Areas of referred tenderness (trigger points) are usually found in the distal levator scapulae. Manipulation and mobilization procedures have a good but temporary effect, symptoms tending to recur after 24 hours. Resolution may occur following repeated manipulations although progress is often slow.

Daily cervical traction is more reliable, and is positively indicated if symptoms have been present for two weeks or longer.

If brachial pain (felt in the shoulder and upper arm) is experienced in addition to neck pain, this may be due to nerve root pressure; confirmation by dural tension tests should be attempted. If neck movements do not give rise to arm pain, mobilization is often successful.

If pain is felt predominantly in the arm, and particularly if the radicular pain is provoked by some neck movements, traction is the treatment of choice.

Root entrapment

Pressure on the C5, C6, C7 or C8 nerve roots produces radicular symptoms – namely, root pain, dysaesthesiae and numbness.

C5 root entrapment

The muscles affected are the supraspinatus, infraspinatus, deltoid and biceps brachii. The biceps jerk and/or the brachioradialis jerk may be absent. A C4/5 disc prolapse is responsible. Difficulty with diagnosis may be experienced for the following reasons:

1 C5 dermatomal pain, which is felt predominantly in the lateral aspect of the upper arm, is a common presenting symptom of primary disorders of the shoulder joint and the rotator cuff, which are themselves particularly common in the middle aged.
2 Weakness of abduction of the shoulder is common to both a supraspinatus tear and a C5 root paresis.
3 Disordered biomechanics of the glenohumeral and/or subacromial joints may be secondary to cervical spinal disorders in which there is no true nerve root compression.
4 Paraesthesiae, which are normally a distinguishing characteristic of nerve compression, are absent at this level.

Clearly, the history should be taken carefully to identify preceding neck pain and stiffness. This is particularly important once the nerve palsy has become well established, and the neck signs on examination are minimal or 'negative'. Some salient features on examination are:

1 Muscle weakness often involves the deltoid and biceps brachii as well as the spinati: demonstrable weakness on resisted forward flexion of the dependent arm indicates denervation of the anterior fibres of the deltoid.
2 Painless weakness is demonstrated on resisted contraction (suggesting nerve compression rather than muscle tear).

The differential diagnosis includes:

1 Other causes of muscle denervation, e.g. brachial plexus traction injury, suprascapular nerve palsy (affecting the spinati), circumflex nerve injury secondary to anterior dislocation of the shoulder (affecting the deltoid). There is a history of trauma in these instances.
2 Other causes of myopathy or tendinopathy, e.g. neuralgic amyotrophy (involving the shoulder girdle muscles); rotator cuff rupture (usually involving the spinati).

C6 nerve root entrapment

Pain is felt in the anterolateral upper arm, and radial aspect of the forearm and hand. Paraesthesiae are felt in the thumb and index finger, and are often accompanied by numbness. Weakness of biceps brachii, brachioradialis and extensor carpi radialis may be found, but is often not gross. The entrapment is caused by a C5/6 disc protrusion.

In the differential diagnosis, carpal tunnel syndrome, which gives rise to more extensive paraesthesiae affecting the radial three and a half digits, may need to be considered. Intrinsic disorders (ruptures and tendinitis) of the biceps give rise to discomfort within the C6 dermatome, but paraesthesiae are absent and contraction of the biceps (which is tested by resisting flexion of the elbow and supination of the forearm) gives rise to discomfort in addition to weakness.

C7 nerve root entrapment

This is by far the most common root affected; prolapse of the C6/7 disc gives rise to C7 root palsy. Pain is felt along the extensor aspect of the arm; paraesthesiae are felt in the index, long and ring fingers, and may be accompanied by numbness at the tip of one or more fingers. Muscle weakness is common, particularly of the triceps. Weakness of the wrist flexors and pectoralis major may be substantial too. Occasionally, marked wasting of the pectoralis major may be observed. The triceps jerk may be depressed or absent, but is an unreliable sign. Patients often find relief from nocturnal symptoms by sleeping with the hand of the affected arm behind the back of their neck.

When there is a typical story of neck pain, radicular pain, and paraesthesiae within the C7 dermatome, and weakness of the triceps is demonstrated, the diagnosis is obvious enough. In sports injury practice, weakness of the triceps may be encountered as a result of intrinsic injury at, or close to, its insertion onto the olecranon.

C8 nerve root entrapment

Symptoms are felt along the inner border of the arm as far as the ulnar border of the hand. Paraesthesiae are felt in the long, ring and little fingers. Numbness is commonly experienced at the tip of the little finger. C8 root palsy is due to a C7/T1 disc prolapse.

Weakness of the ulnar deviators of the wrist and the small muscles of the hand is noted. In particular, weakness of extension and adduction of the thumb, and extension of the fingers may be profound.

As the dysaesthesiae commonly affect the little finger, or little and ring fingers only, the differential diagnoses include those conditions which affect the lower trunks of the brachial plexus, and those conditions which affect the ulnar nerve. In the **thoracic outlet syndrome** the lower trunk of the brachial plexus is compressed against the first rib as a result of drooping of the shoulder girdle. A cervical rib may have the same effect, that is, the production of paraesthesiae, often affecting all the fingers, when pressure is released – either during the evening when the elbows rest on the wings of an armchair, or during the night. The brachial plexus is the neural element of a neurovascular bundle, all the elements of which may be compressed at the thoracic outlet. Additional symptoms may be caused by pressure on the subclavian artery or vein, for instance swelling and stiffness in the hand.

The ulnar nerve may be compressed in the groove behind the medial epicondyle of the elbow (when it is either secondary to trauma or to osteoarthritis), or in Guyon's canal in the wrist (for instance, 'handlebar palsy' in cyclists).

Reversible or non-reversible?

In the elderly, root entrapment at any level may be the result of progressive osteophytosis. Oblique X-rays may demonstrate substantial narrowing of the relevant intervertebral foramina. Discomfort in the neck and arm may be minimal, and the principle finding is (uni- or multisegmental) weakness. Commonly, however, there is a discogenic element to the root entrapment, and a conservative management strategy is often indicated in the first instance. Adverse radiographic findings are not a contraindication to treatment by traction or sinuvertebral nerve block injections. When faced with a worsening neurological situation, however, particularly if progressive weakness suggests the involvement of more than one root, procrastination is best avoided and referral for a neurosurgical opinion is indicated.

For younger patients, that is the 35–55 year age group, in whom a disc herniation is responsible for positive neurological signs, manipulation of the cervical spine is contraindicated; it does not improve the condition, and the patient may blame the therapist for worsening symptoms. Traction may provide some relief. The only effective treatment, however, is the use of nerve block injections which, when given by physicians experienced in this technique, often foreshorten the painful phase considerably. Root pain, otherwise, resolves spontaneously within 3 months; a further few months is often required for recovery of muscle function.

Cervical spinal joint dysfunction

Joint dysfunction may occur at any level within the cervical spine, and gives rise to varying degrees of disability. In its least severe form, from the examiner's point of view, the 'global' movements of the cervical spine, in the standing or sitting position, may be unimpaired; recognition then depends on joint play assessment – a search for hypomobility, and on palpatory techniques – a search for localized muscle hypertonus. In mid-cervical and distal cervical lesions, trigger points may be palpated some distance away from the primary source of dysfunction, for instance in the trapezius or levator scapulae.

In relatively severe cases, there are more obvious global articular signs, including limitation of rotation and/or flexion and extension. The extent of restriction of mobility is variable, however, and the examiner is dependent upon joint play assessment and muscle hypertonicity for segmental localization. Localized muscle spasm and tenderness may be intense, particularly overlying the articular masses between C2 and C4.

Joint dysfunction associated with hypomobility at the craniocervical junction or at C2/3 is a common cause of neckache, headache (occipital, vertical and frontal), dizziness, facial pain, tinnitus and vertigo. Reflex sympathetic (nervous system) irritation is the probable neural explanation for these symptoms which were initially described by Barré as the 'posterior cervical syndrome' (1926). In some patients, nervous tension may play a significant role in the aetiology of, or persistence of, muscle tension. Dysfunction of the proximal cervical joints, when associated with marked muscle hypertonus, may be responsive to physical treatment such as the combination of massage to the suboccipital muscles and gentle mobilization. The response is often temporary, however, and the therapist is required to adopt a strong counselling role, to help reduce mental stress, in order to establish prolonged relief.

If headaches are a prominent feature intracranial pathology may need to be excluded. The characteristics of headaches which are caused by joint dysfunction are their variation with posture and activity, and the existence of localized signs in the neck. Deep massage to the suboccipital muscles is often helpful. Occasionally, frankly migrainous headaches have an association with joint dysfunction, which is probably one of several aetiological factors in this distressing condition. Some patients find that their attacks may be aborted, or reduced in frequency, by cervical manipulation.

A search for other causes of temporal and facial pain may be necessary – for instance TMJ (temporomandibular joint) dysfunction, which is often secondary to whiplash and is sometimes referred to as 'jaw-lash', or temporal arteritis, which may be associated with polymyalgia rheumatica. Other features of **TMJ dysfunction**, in which damage to the intra-articular disc commonly occurs, are limited jaw opening, clicking and tinnitus. A disc tear may be detected by palpation of the TMJ through the external auditory meatus, using the tip of the little finger, when a 'clonk' is felt on opening or closing the jaw. Localized muscle spasm may be palpated.

Joint dysfunction in the mid- and distal cervical spine may give rise to referred pain in the 'shawl' or interscapular areas. Examination of the thoracic spine, in addition to the cervical spine, should always be undertaken as proximal thoracic joint dysfunction clearly enters into the differential diagnosis. It is not unusual for cervical and thoracic lesions to coexist.

If cervical rotation is found to be substantially restricted in the presence of muscle spasm and hyperaesthesiae, particularly in the proximal or mid-cervical spine, synovitis of the underlying joint(s) should be suspected. This is either secondary to acute injury such as whiplash, or due to osteoarthritis. Mobilization is then ineffective, and treatment by ultrasound, shortwave, or injection of steroid and local anaesthetic should be commenced. When due to osteoarthritis, the symptoms may be prolonged for years, but partial relief may be expected following treatment nevertheless.

For the majority of patients with joint dysfunction, mobilization or manipulation is effective. Gentle mobilization procedures are the treatment of first choice – for instance, an extension of the techniques used in joint play assessment. If necessary, more vigorous techniques with a greater degree of thrust may be employed.

Myotendinosis

On occasions trigger points persist, despite adequate resolution of spinal joint dysfunction. These may be associated with inadequate posture, poor working conditions or excessive nervous tension, any one or all of which may need to be addressed. The head-forward, round-shouldered posture is particularly common, and is associated with tight pectoral muscles, and overload of the trapezii and the levator scapulae.

Myotendinoses in the region of the neck and shoulder may be associated with overuse symptoms in the forearms and hands, and contribute to one of the myriad forms of RSI (repetitive strain injury). Appropriate advice on ergonomics and workload must be given to prevent the development of a chronic unrelenting condition.

Individual trigger points may be helped by massage, cold applications-and-stretch (after Travell), subcutaneous sodium salicylate injections and intramuscular injections of local anaesthetic.

TREATMENT

Mobilization, manipulation and post-contraction relaxation

Joint mobilization is the principal treatment for cervical spinal joint dysfunction. When successful, it restores normal segmental mobility, reduces muscle hypertonicity, and abolishes the reflex changes which are manifested via the autonomic nervous system. Mobilization, manipulation and post-contraction relaxation ('muscle energy') techniques may be employed. Although purists take care to distinguish between mobilization and manipulation on the basis of the presence, or otherwise, of a thrust element, the two terms are used interchangeably in this text – the more so as some of the techniques for the cervical spine which are often described as mobilization have a thrust element to them.

Post-contraction relaxation

Post-contraction relaxation (syn. post-isometric muscle relaxation; muscle energy techniques of Mitchell) is a useful technique when there is gross muscle spasm, such as in acute torticollis. Resisted (isometric) contraction of the tight muscle(s) is followed by relaxation during which an increased range of movement is noted. Augmentation of the contraction and the relaxation phases may be produced by respiration, and by eye movements, as described by Lewit (1985). During contraction, the patient breathes in deeply and looks upwards or towards the direction of attempted movement; relaxation is then combined with exhalation and looking downwards or looking towards the direction of relaxation. The examiner may provide the resistance to contraction; alternatively, gravity may be used as a resistance, followed by gravity-assisted relaxation. Once a patient has received adequate instruction, gravity-assisted exercises may be used at home. In acute torticollis, other mobilizing techniques may be utilized once a significant improvement in range of movement has been achieved.

Post-contraction relaxation is also useful in joint dysfunction, particularly when patients find difficulty in relaxing during other manual treatments. It may also be used in the management of resistant trigger points in muscles as an alternative to cold applications-and-stretch, or to injections of local anaesthetic.

Mobilization and manipulation

The therapist chooses the most comfortable position for spinal mobilization by giving due regard to the patient's size and the height of the couch. Although some manipulations of the cervical spine may be accomplished with the patient in the sitting position, the conclusion of the examination will have taken place with the patient in the supine position; conveniently, this is the most appropriate position in which to commence gentle mobilization.

Initially, mobilization should be an extension of the procedures adopted for joint play assessment – particularly side bending, side gliding, and anteroposterior glide. Once the patient's cooperation has been establised, a small amplitude thrust may be added to (a) long axis traction, (b) side flexion, (c) C0/1 rock in rotation. These manoeuvres are particularly helpful in patients suffering from residual dysfunction in the proximal cervical spine following whiplash. Twenty minutes treatment (once the acute phase has settled), given once or twice a week for 2 or 3 weeks, may make the difference between 6 weeks of whiplash discomfort on the one hand, and 6–12 months on the other.

Joint dysfunction in the mid-cervical spine may benefit from an 'unlocking' procedure in the Stoddard (osteopathic) mould (Stoddard, 1977). A standard manipulation is to lock the cervical spine into rotation and then into side flexion to the other side, followed by a thrust using the radial border of the index finger for segmental localization (Fig. 2.24). Although it is normally a safe practice to manipulate in the direction of relative comfort, a critical review of the examination signs by the manipulative therapist is necessary after each procedure involving thrust. A revision of the technique, or one performed in the opposite direction, may be required. Two to three days, at least, should elapse prior to reassessment. Once weekly, or twice weekly, treatments may be necessary, depending upon the responsiveness of the lesion.

An alternative strategy is to manipulate with manual traction, which has the advantage of opening up the facet joints and reducing the risk of vertebral artery kinking. Although Cyriax (1982) advocated the use of very strong traction, using the combined

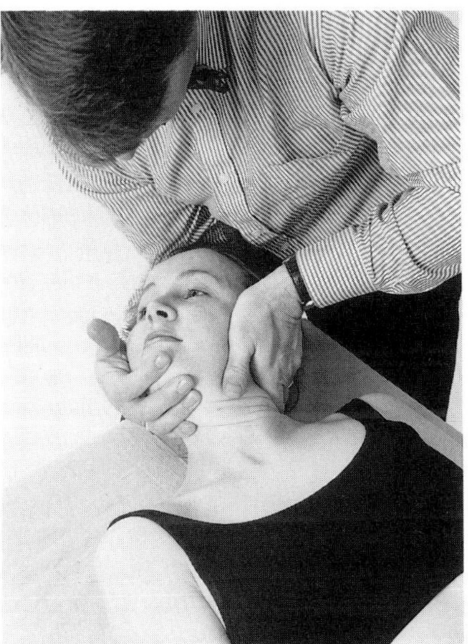

Fig. 2.24 A standard manipulation for cervical spinal joint dysfunction – the spine is locked into rotation and then into side flexion in the other direction prior to the application of thrust.

distracting force of the manipulator at the neck and his assistant at the ankles, manipulation is often successful without such strong force (which, in any case, is not tolerated by every patient). Manual traction may be applied to the neck with the chin partially tucked in, to flatten the cervical lordosis, until the therapist feels the patient's body starting to move on the couch; this point may be delayed by the use of couch coverings which increase friction. Manipulations may then be performed as previously described; for maximum benefit, and for safety, the slack should be taken up first with straight axial distraction, then in rotation and/or side flexion, prior to a high velocity, low amplitude thrust being applied.

As the indication for manipulation is joint hypomobility associated with dysfunction, it follows that the contraindications include all other conditions. Some conditions such as metastases, and rheumatoid arthritis affecting the cervical spine, should be suspected from the history and examination, and the patient referred to an appropriate specialist; in these circumstances, manipulation is specifically contraindicated. Other conditions, such as disc herniations which give rise to nerve root compression, are unresponsive, and, if the condition worsens and a root palsy supervenes, the therapist may be blamed. Manipulation must be performed with care in the presence of vertebrobasilar insufficiency, giving rise to positional vertigo or dizziness (usually in neck extension); techniques involving a significant degree of rotation and extension should be strictly avoided.

Sustained traction (using a harness)

Daily cervical traction, for instance using 30 lb sustained pull for 20 minutes, is undoubtedly of considerable value for an established disc prolapse, particularly when root compression has not given rise to positive neurological signs. The most comfortable, and effective, position is for the patient to recline with the neck flexed by some 20°/30°. An average of ten treatments is required. In the presence of neurological signs indicating nerve root entrapment, traction is not effective in ameliorating root pain, but it may reduce residual discomfort felt in the neck.

A number of neck suspension devices are available for home use; they appear to be less effective, possibly because they do not achieve a satisfactory reduction of cervical lordosis.

Sinuvertebral nerve block

The direction of the cervical nerve root canals is downwards and forwards, medial to lateral. Should a direct route to the intervertebral foramen be required (to procure a dorsal root ganglion block), an anterolateral approach under X-ray screening is required. Happily, a sinuvertebral nerve block, using a posterior approach and without screening, is usually equally effective. Two per cent lignocaine 2 ml and 10 mg triamcinolone hexacetonide are introduced at the appropriate level to the superior margin of the posterior articular masses, some 3 cm from the midline. Diffusion of the solution occurs anteriorly, and relief is often gained immediately or within a few hours. Two or three treatments, at intervals of one to two weeks, are often effective when root pain is secondary to a disc prolapse producing a root palsy, in which case spontaneous resolution of the symptoms would be anticipated over a period of 3–4 months. Should root pain be secondary to foraminal osteophytosis, temporary improvement only is found, and surgical decompression is required.

REHABILITATION AND PREVENTION OF INJURY

Exercises

The use of exercises and postural correction, and aspects of rehabilitation and prevention of further symptomatology by attention to ergonomics, are considered further in Chapter 5. While patients are undergoing treatment for joint dysfunction a useful self-mobilization exercise for them to do at home, or elsewhere, is 'double-chinning': in the standing position, the chin is repeatedly retracted to give a 'double chin' and then protracted (Fig. 5.13). Additionally, the shoulders are braced somewhat, thereby reducing the proximal thoracic kyphosis and, secondarily, further reducing the cervical lordosis.

Patients with a C7 root palsy should be advised to attempt to sleep with their affected arm behind their head or neck; they may already have discovered for themselves that this manoeuvre often gives relief. Supportive pillows of different types are available – the principal requirement is for support to the mid- and distal cervical spine to prevent sagging while asleep.

Prevention of injury in sport

Aspects of hyperflexion and hyperextension injuries to the cervical spine as a result of road traffic accidents have been considered in the section on 'whiplash'. Regrettably, head restraints have been found to be of little prophylactic benefit following rear-end vehicular collisions because the initial forward propulsion of the trunk is primarily responsible for the consequent hyperextension of the neck.

Until relatively recently, it had been thought that hyperflexion and hyperextension were also the predominant mechanisms responsible for severe cervical spinal injuries (for instance compression fractures, fracture-dislocations, and cord injuries) seen occasionally during sports such as rugby football, American football, ice-hockey, trampolining and diving. However, more detailed analysis suggests that *axial loading* is the primary mechanism involved, particularly when the neck is slightly flexed, thereby straightening out the usual lordosis and reducing the ability of the neck muscles to assist the vertebral bodies and intervertebral discs in the absorption of compressive forces.

In the context of prevention of injury it is worth stressing that restricted flexibility of the cervical spine (as elsewhere in the spine as a whole) from whatever cause, for instance degenerative changes, or previous fusion, or muscular tightness, results in *impaired dissipation of forces*. Thus rugby players are at increased risk of serious cervical injuries if returning to sport after injuries which seriously compromise the flexibility of the cervical spine.

REFERENCES

Barré, J.A. (1926) Sur un syndrome sympathique cervical postérieure et sa cause fréquente: l'arthrite cervicale. *Revue Neurologique,* **33**, 1246

Bogduk, N. and Marsland, A. (1988) The cervical zygapophyseal joints as a source of neck pain. *Spine,* **13**, 610–17

Crowe, H., cited in Breck, L.W. and Van Norman, R.W. (1971) Medicolegal aspects of cervical spine strains. *Clinical Orthopaedics and Related Research,* **74**, 124–8

Cyriax, J. (1982) *Textbook of Orthopaedic Medicine*, 8th edn, Baillière Tindall, London

Deans, G.T., Magalliard, J.N., Kerr, M. *et al.* (1987) Neck sprains – a major cause of disability following car accidents. *Injury,* **18**, 10–12

Dwyer, A., Aprill, C. and Bogduk, N. (1990) Cervical zygapophyseal joint pain patterns 1 and 2. *Spine,* **15**, 453–61

Elvey, R.L. (1986) Treatment of arm pain associated with abnormal brachial plexus tension. *Australian Journal of Physiotherapy,* **32** (4), 225–30

Feinstein, B., Langton, J.N.K., Jameson, R.M. *et al.* (1954) Experiments on pain referred from deep somatic tissues. *Journal of Bone and Joint Surgery,* **36A**, 981–97

Hohl, M. (1974) Soft-tissue injuries of the neck in automobile accidents: factors influencing prognosis. *Journal of Bone and Joint Surgery,* **56A**, 1675–82

Lewit, K. (1985) *Manipulative Therapy in Rehabilitation of the Motor System,* Butterworths, London

McNab, I. (1964) Acceleration injuries of the cervical spine. *Journal of Bone and Joint Surgery,* **46A**, 1797–9

Maitland, G.D. (1977) *Vertebral Manipulation,* 4th edn, Butterworths, London

Mennell, J.McM. (1960) *Back Pain; Diagnosis and Treatment Using Manipulative Techniques*, Little, Brown and Company, Boston, Mass.

Miller, H. (1961) Accident neurosis. *British Medical Journal*, 919–25; 992–8

Stoddard, A. (1977) *Manual of osteopathic practice*, Hutchinson, London

Teasell, R.W. and McCain, G.A. (1991) Clinical spectrum and management of whiplash injuries. *In Painful Cervical Trauma* (eds D. Tollison and J. Satterthwaite), Williams and Wilkins, Baltimore, Md, pp. 292–318

Travell, J. and Simons, D.G. (1983) *Myofascial Pain and Dysfunction: the Trigger Point Manual*, vol. 1, Williams and Wilkins, Baltimore, Md

3
Thoracic spine

We read every day, with astonishment,
things which we see every day, without
surprise.

Earl of Chesterfield *Letters*

APPLIED ANATOMY

Vertebrae

The 12 thoracic vertebrae have slightly wedge-shaped bodies which contribute to the permanent kyphosis of the thoracic spine. In comparison with the cervical and lumbar discs, the thoracic intervertebral discs are relatively thin, being 7 mm thick on average and approximately one-quarter of the height of the vertebral body (Fig. 1.14). The thoracic vertebrae have other characteristic features to accommodate the articulations with the ribs (Fig. 3.1). The positions of the articular facets vary somewhat throughout the thoracic spine. The heart-shaped bodies T1–T9 have an oval facet on their side to articulate with the head of the corresponding rib, and a small demi-facet inferiorly to accommodate the head of the more caudal rib. The bodies of T10–T12 have single facets.

The spinous processes slope downwards, maximally in the middle of the thoracic spine; that of T12 is almost horizontal. Identification of vertebral level by palpation of the spinous processes may be difficult; the most reliable method is to count downwards from T1 when the spine is flexed (and the spinous processes are separated from each other). The transverse processes (except at T11 and T12) contain a facet at their tip for the tubercle of the corresponding rib. There are no facets on the transverse processes of T11 and T12; indeed, the transverse processes of T12 are short, and the general characteristics of this vertebra, including the plane of the inferior articular processes, resemble the lumbar vertebrae. The articular processes (Fig. 3.2), which form the apophyseal joints between T1 and T11, lie at an angle of 60° or more to the transverse plane; they also form a 20° angle to the coronal plane such that, at each vertebral level, they form the arc of a circle whose centre lies within the vertebral body (Fig. 3.3). This orientation allows rotation as well as flexion and extension.

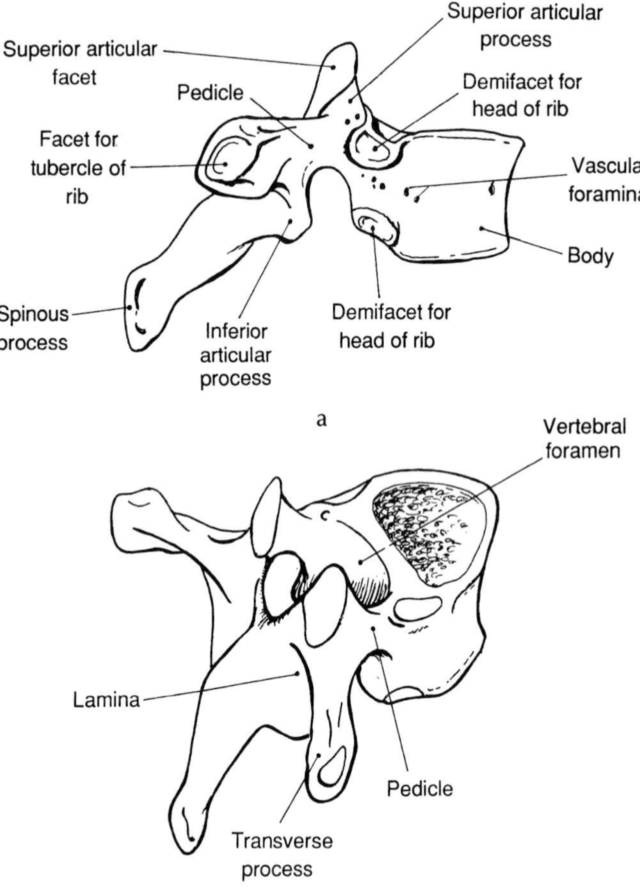

Fig. 3.1 A typical thoracic vertebra – lateral (a) and posterolateral (b) views.

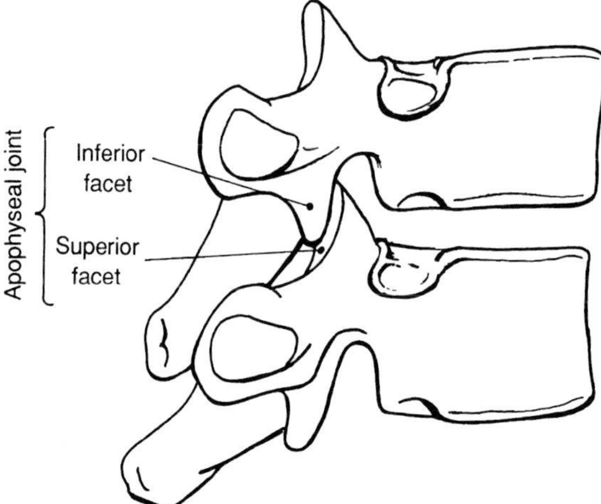

Fig. 3.2 A typical thoracic apophyseal articulation (lateral view).

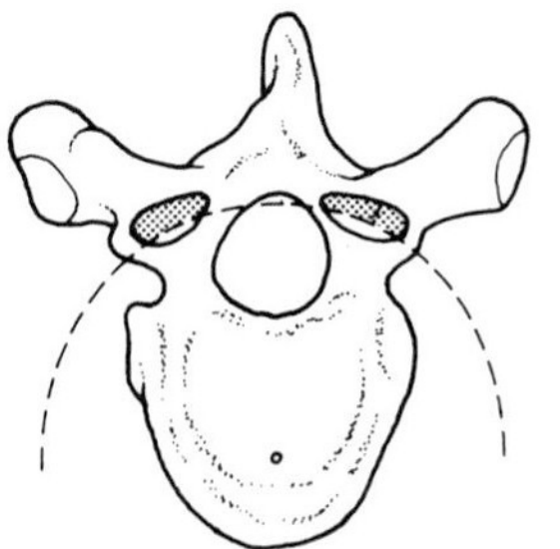

Fig. 3.3 The superior articular surfaces of the thoracic facet joints face backwards, upwards and laterally, such that they form the arc of a circle whose centre lies within the vertebral body. (From Palastanga, N., Field, D. and Soames, R., 1990, *Anatomy and Human Movement*, Butterworth-Heinemann, Oxford.)

Thoracic cage

The thoracic spine is the posterior margin of the thoracic cage, the other bony structures being the ribs and the sternum. The upper seven ribs articulate with the sternum via their costal cartilages (at the sternocostal joints). The costal cartilages of the 8th, 9th and 10th ribs articulate with the costal cartilage above (at the interchondral

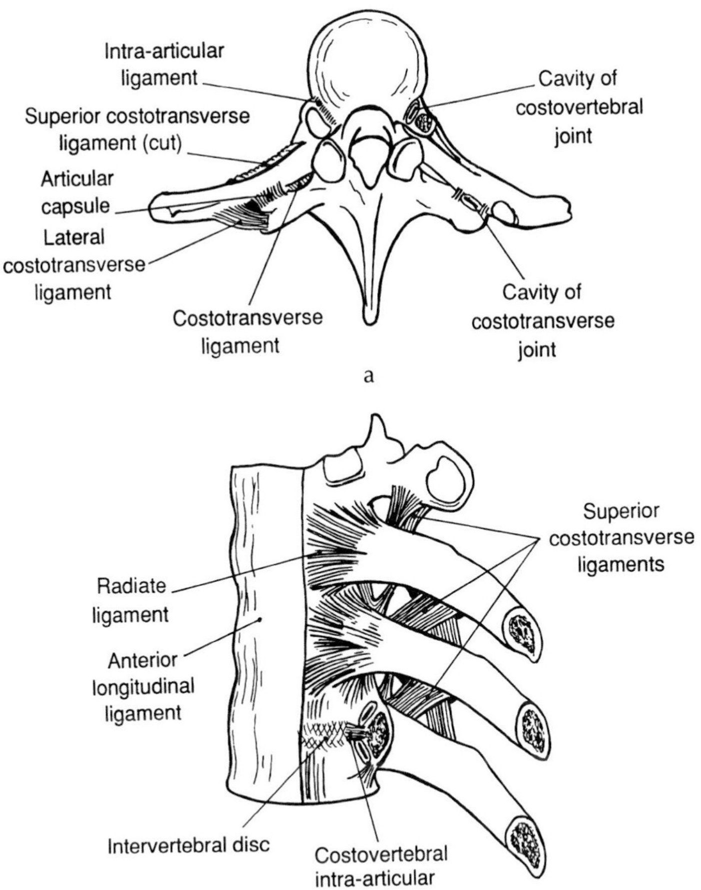

Fig. 3.4 Costovertebral and costotransverse joints – superior (a) and lateral (b) views. (From *Gray's Anatomy*, 1980, 36th edn, Churchill Livingstone, New York.)

joints). Posteriorly, the heads of ribs 2–10 articulate with the bodies of the corresponding vertebrae and that of the vertebra above (at the costovertebral joints), and the tubercles articulate with the corresponding transverse processes (at the costotransverse joints). The first rib articulates only with T1; similarly, rib 10 articulates only with T10. Ribs 11 and 12 are 'floating', having no costotransverse joints and no articulation anteriorly. The costovertebral joints (Fig. 3.4) are synovial joints and have well-developed ligaments – the radiate ligament of the head of the rib and an intra-articular ligament (except at T1, 10, 11 and 12).

Muscles

The 'round-shouldered' posture, with which is associated a variety of symptoms arising from the region of the cervicothoracic junction (for instance neckache, backache, and thoracic outlet syndrome), is characterized by increased thoracic kyphosis, protraction of the pectoral girdle and compensatory hyperextension of the cervical spine (Fig. 3.5). The muscles which elevate and retract the scapula, such as the trapezius and levator scapulae, may suffer from fatigue and exhibit areas of myotendinosis. The pectoralis major, which adducts and medially rotates the humerus, tends to shorten. Correction of these muscle imbalances is necessary for the re-establishment of a good spinal posture.

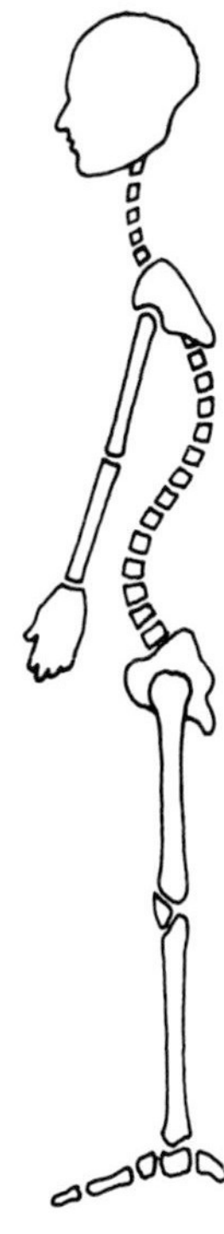

Fig. 3.5 The 'round-shouldered' posture – increased thoracic kyphosis and protraction of the pectoral girdle and compensatory hyperextension of the cervical spine. (From Hutson, M.A., 1990, *Sports Injuries: Recognition and Management*, Oxford University Press, Oxford by permission of Oxford University Press.)

Movements of the thoracic spine are controlled by the same groups of muscles which act on the lumbar spine – the trunk flexors (abdominals and psoas), rotators, side flexors and extensors. They are considered in some detail in Chapters 1 and 4.

Nerves

The posterior rami of the spinal nerves divide into medial branches which supply the muscles of the back, the posterior joints, and their ligaments; and lateral branches which terminate as cutaneous nerves supplying the back of the shoulder, the posterior and inner aspects of the arm, the posterior thoracic region, and, distally, as far down as the iliac crest and lateral buttock (T12). Frequent anastomoses between the posterior rami and their branches are common, creating a plurisegmental system of innervation of the skin and soft tissues. The ventral rami form the intercostal nerves; unlike the situation in the cervical and lumbar regions, root entrapment is an uncommon event in the thoracic spine and, in any case, is not detectable by signs of motor weakness.

BIOMECHANICS

The orientation of the articular processes of the apophyseal joints favours **axial rotation**. Overall, this amounts to some 35° in each direction, and is brought about by the action of the abdominal oblique muscles. Tension in the annuli fibrosi and the posterior ligaments is created, but the principal restraint to further movement is the bony thoracic cage. Rotation is accompanied by distortion of the ribs and shearing forces to the sternocostal and costochondral joints. There is no such restraint to rotation in the distal thoracic spine where the lower two ribs have no anterior attachment. Mobility at the thoracolumbar junction (T12/L1), however, is limited by the lumbarization of the 12th thoracic vertebra.

Interestingly, during walking, rotation of the upper thoracic spine is in the opposite direction to rotation in the lower thoracic and lumbar spines; maximal intervertebral rotation occurs at T7/8. Clinically, mid-thoracic joint dysfunction is common.

Side flexion amounts to some 20–25° on each side and is coupled with rotation. Relatively greater movement is possible in the distal thoracic spine.

There is a considerably greater range of **flexion** than **extension**; in total there is approximately 50–70°. According to some authorities most movement occurs in the lower half of the thoracic spine as a result of the greater elasticity of the longer lower ribs, and particularly between T11 and T12, and between T12 and L1. As in the lumbar spine, flexion from the upright position is controlled by the eccentric contraction of the paraspinal muscles, and from the supine position by the abdominal muscles. Extension from the upright position is controlled by eccentric contraction of the abdominals, and from the prone position by isotonic contraction of the paraspinals. In extension, the degree of rotation and lateral flexion is considerably reduced.

Joint play in the direction of extension or side flexion/rotation may be demonstrated in the thoracic spine by various examining techniques which involve pressure on the spinous processes; accessory movements at the rib articulations may be demonstrated by localized pressure on the transverse processes.

Rib movement is either active (during respiration) or passive (secondary to movements of the thoracic spine). The axis for movements of the upper ribs is along their necks, creating rotation and a 'pump handle' action. The axis for the lower ribs is anteroposterior, allowing a gliding motion at the costotransverse joints (which are flatter in this region) as well as rotation, resulting in a 'bucket handle' movement. It is possible that subluxation of a costotransverse joint in the T6–T9 region is a cause of sudden thoracic and intercostal pain during vigorous, repetitive activities involving thoracic rotation and protraction of the shoulder girdle, such as rowing and punching. By their attachments to the ribs anterior to the scapula, the scapular protractors, serratus anterior and pectoralis minor, may create excessive strain on the ribs and cause disruption at these costotransverse joints.

PATHOANATOMY AND PATHOPHYSIOLOGY

The pathoanatomical changes which occur in the cervical and lumbar spines, namely disc degeneration and apophyseal joint destabilization, undoubtedly occur also in the thoracic spine. Bruckner *et al.* (1989) have demonstrated *disc degeneration* on MR imaging, particularly at T7/8, in young women with interscapular pain. Radiographic evidence of disc narrowing and marginal osteophytosis of the vertebral bodies (usually anterior and lateral) reflects more established age-related changes. Sometimes these x-ray changes too are present in the younger age groups, for instance in the third and fourth decades, possibly caused by excessive strain on the thoracic vertebrae in sports such as rowing. However, in clinical practice, the incidence of *disc prolapse* of sufficient severity to present as nerve root entrapment, or spinal cord compression, is extremely low. The relative stability of the region, provided by the elasticity of the thoracic cage, and the fact that weakness of the annulus tends to occur on the concavity of the sagittal spinal curves, presumably accounts for this.

The vast majority of conditions of acute onset are due to **joint dysfunction**, and are often easily managed by joint manipulation.

Although the most common site for dysfunction is probably the mid-thoracic spine, lesions may occur throughout this region. Maigne (1980) has emphasized the relatively high incidence of dysfunction at the thoracolumbar junction which gives rise to pain radiating to the iliac crest and buttock. Dysfunction at the cervicothoracic junction, and between T1 and T3 is also common, e.g. after whiplash. Fraser (1990) identified a specific T3 syndrome in which upper back pain is associated with autonomic nervous system changes in the upper limb which may include paraesthesiae, muscle weakness and vasomotor responses in a non-dermatomal pattern. Radiographic degenerative changes usually indicate a reduced range of rotation and extension, and appear to increase the likelihood of subsequent joint dysfunction.

The nature of thoracic spinal joint dysfunction is conjectural; it would seem logical that the apophyseal joint is the site of spinal joint dysfunction, as elsewhere in the spine. Disturbances at the rib articulations should be considered, however, and descriptions of the various types of *rib dysfunction* may be found elsewhere (Bourdillon, 1992, for instance). Confirmatory tests for rib dysfunction include identification of asymmetry of the rib angles and of the anterior ends of the ribs, and specific tissue texture changes. In practice it would seem likely that the majority of, if not all, examining and manipulative techniques for joint dysfunction provide a mechanical, or mechanoreceptor, stimulus to both the spinal joints and the rib articulations, and their differentiation may be obscure.

Scheuermann's disease (vertebral osteochondrosis)

Although this condition may affect the mid-thoracic spine it is usually found in the distal thoracic and lumbar spines. It is a disorder of growth in teenagers, particularly in 15–16-year-old boys. Vertical protrusions of the nucleus pulposus occur through defects in the cartilaginous end-plates of adjacent vertebrae, forming Schmorl's nodes (Fig. 1.23). Additionally, growth at the epiphyseal ring is disturbed anteriorly, giving rise to irregular appearances on X-rays (Fig. 3.6). These changes occur over several segments and are associated with degenerative changes in the intervertebral discs. The marked feature is anterior wedging of several vertebrae, resulting in *increased kyphosis*. Clinically, there is restricted mobility in the distal thoracic spine, but compensatory hypermobility (and increased stress) occurs at the lumbar and cervical lordoses.

Scheuermann's disease may be asymptomatic, being found as a painless kyphosis on routine examination. In active children, however, particularly boys who play sports such as cricket and rugby, localized discomfort may be a presenting symptom. In such instances, it is sensible to restrict activities to a level at which discomfort disappears. This active phase of osteochondritis is self-limiting; swimming should be encouraged in the meantime, and heavy lifting or weight-training eschewed. Subsequently, mobilization may help

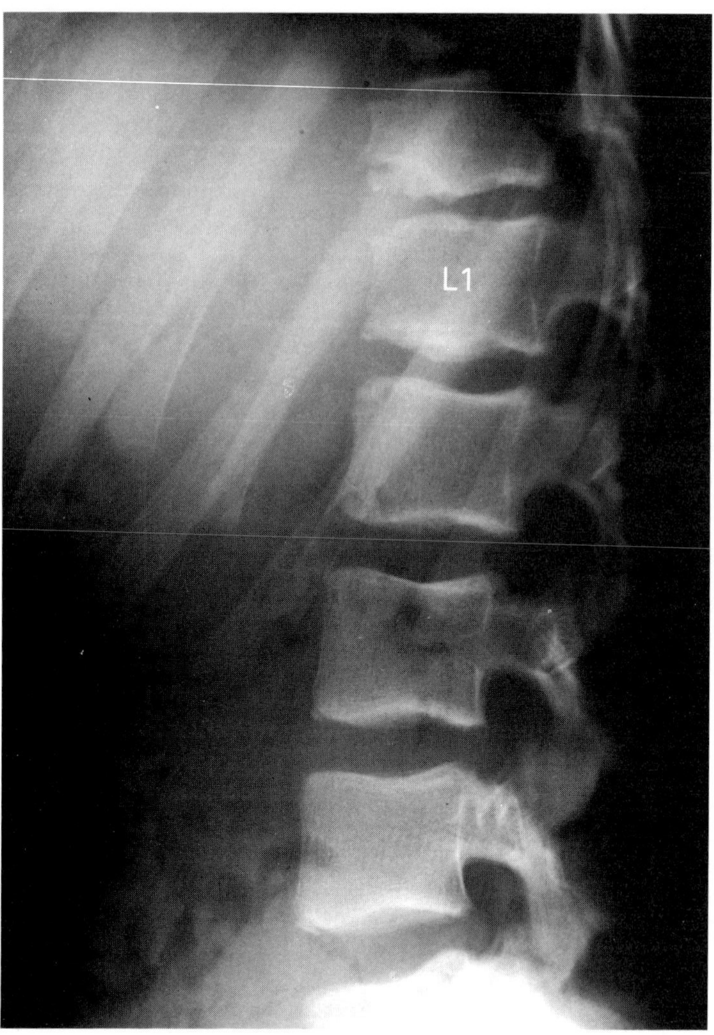

Fig. 3.6 Scheuermann's disease – anterior erosions at L1/2 and L2/3 are demonstrated.

restore a little mobility in the affected segments. The kyphosis is permanent, however, and gives rise to an increased incidence of low back (and cervical) pain in future years (Stoddard, 1977).

Senile kyphosis

The degenerative changes associated with spondylosis in the thoracic spine – principally narrowing of the anterior portions of the discs, sclerosis of the adjacent borders of the vertebral bodies and anterior

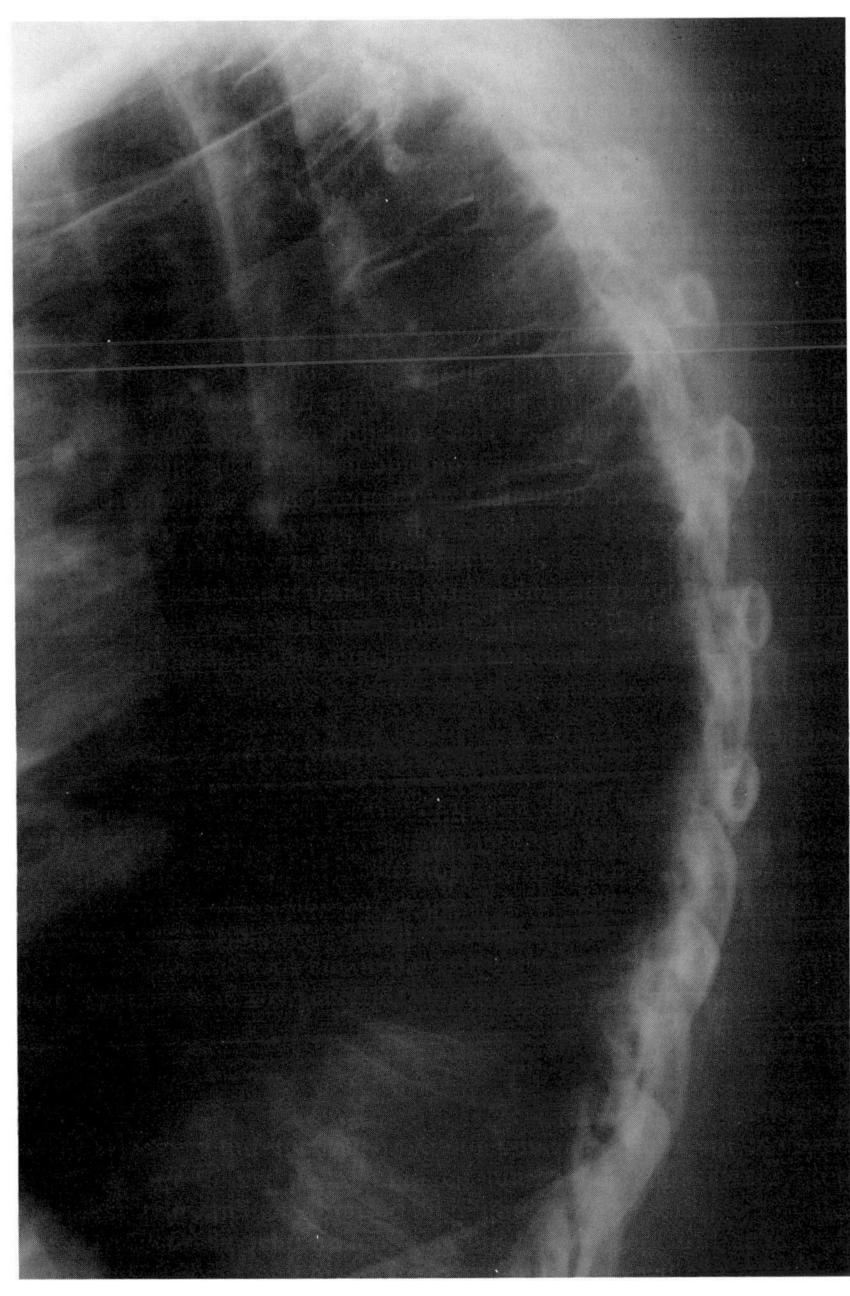

Fig. 3.7 Senile kyphosis – degenerative changes associated with increased kyphosis of the thoracic spine.

osteophytosis – give rise to wedging and considerable restriction in spinal mobility (Fig. 3.7). If the resultant exaggerated kyphosis is found predominantly in the proximal thoracic spine it is often covered by thickened subcutaneous tissue, the combined prominence being referred to as a 'dowager's hump'. Mobilization, particularly in extension, may be helpful.

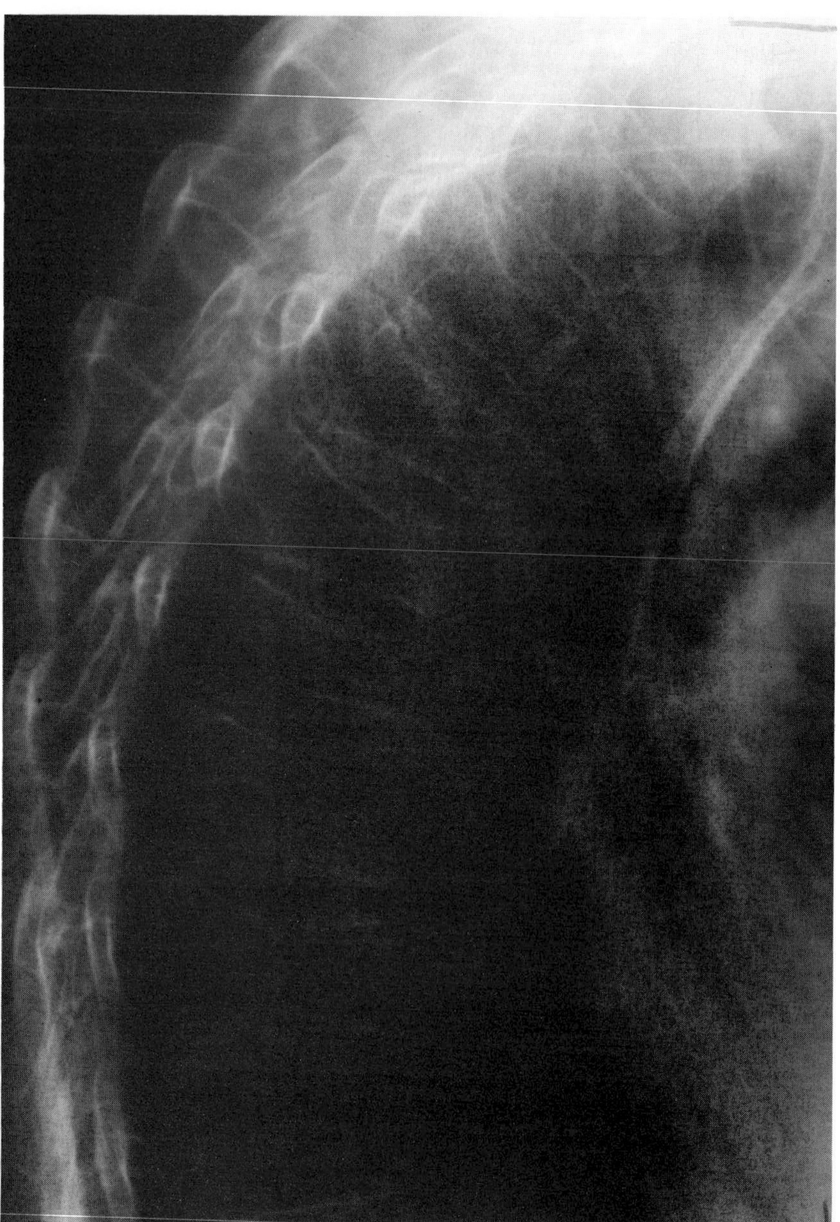

Fig. 3.8 Osteoporotic wedge compression fractures are seen in the thoracic spine on this lateral X-ray.

Spinal osteoporosis

This is seen principally in postmenopausal women, though the possibility of other diseases affecting the thoracic spine, particularly multiple myeloma, must be considered. Activities which jar the spine provoke discomfort, which is due to at least minor collapse of one or more vertebrae, and a thoracic kyphosis is found on examination. The condition is characterized, however, by the incidence of pathological compression fractures which often give rise to girdle pain, and sometimes to a localized kyphus (Fig. 3.8). Multiple episodes of vertebral body collapse, which are identifiable on X-ray, may have occurred, each incident having been accompanied by varying degrees of pain or discomfort. The worst of the pain settles in 2–3 months as the fracture heals.

Osteoporosis that is severe enough to cause danger of vertebral fracture is an exaggeration of age-related change, which itself results from hormonal changes. In women, the incidence of postmenopausal osteoporosis may be reduced by regular participation in sports or recreational activities, which increase bone density, prior to the menopause. After the menopause, physical activity continues to give a degree of protection. If prophylaxis is deemed to be required, for example after hysterectomy with oophorectomy, this can be achieved by hormone replacement therapy. Once significant osteoporosis has occurred, the only proven method of improving bone stock is by cyclical etidronate and calcium therapy.

Thoracic scoliosis

Compensatory

A mild degree of scoliosis may result from unequal leg length – either real or associated with sacroiliac locking – and is considered to be compensatory (or functional). No rotational deformity is present, and the scoliosis disappears on sitting (Fig. 3.9). A further type of secondary (compensatory) scoliosis occurs in the thoracic spine as a response to a 'sciatic scoliosis' in the lumbar spine. This disappears, of course, as the primary cause, a lumbar disc protrusion, resolves. Occasionally, a scoliosis is secondary to poliomyelitis or to spinal neurofibromata.

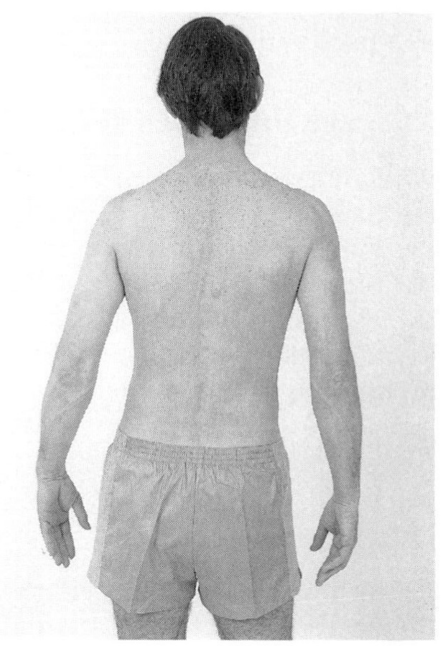

Fig. 3.9 A compensatory scoliosis of the thoracolumbar spine is usually secondary to leg length inequality or to a sciatic scoliosis in the lumbar spine.

Structural

Congenital scoliosis is secondary to other abnormalities such as hemivertebra, and is variable in its severity.

Adolescent idiopathic scoliosis (AIS) is a fixed lateral curvature of the spine, and is particularly common in girls from the age of 10–12 onwards; it usually affects the thoracolumbar spine. The degree of scoliosis ceases on termination of bone growth, usually between the ages of 16 and 18. It is often a benign painless condition, though radiographic measurement of the angle of the scoliosis may be necessary in severe cases, and referral to a scoliosis clinic for further assessment is then indicated.

The mechanics of the development of lateral curvature in a rod such as the spine have been studied and confirm the clinical observation that an accompanying axial rotation is inevitable (Fig. 3.10). Burwell and co-workers in Nottingham have used morphological data to interpret how the deformity may be brought about through a developmental anomaly of locomotor control in the central nervous system causing asymmetry of trunk muscle function (Burwell and Dangerfield, 1992). This asymmetry involves mainly rotators attached to ribs during cyclical activities such as walking which leads to a failure of rotation control in the spine. Breakdown of rotation occurs in association with a lateral spinal curvature and with a short-segment lordosis to create the deformity of AIS: the vertebral bodies rotate to a greater degree than the spinous processes in the direction of the convexity of the curve, resulting in prominence of the posterior ribs on that side. This 'rib-hump' may be identified in relatively minor degrees of AIS on forward bending of the trunk.

Spinal pain is uncommon until middle age is reached when, in the more severe forms, disc erosion at the site of maximum curvature of the scoliosis gives rise to painful compression of one vertebral body against another.

Thoracic ankylosing spondylitis

Although ankylosing spondylitis affects the sacroiliac joint initially and, subsequently, the rest of the spine, cases are met in which the predominant symptoms are from the thoracic spine (Fig. 3.11). The costotransverse joints are affected too, and gradually become fixed, thereby substantially affecting respiratory excursion. A distinctive feature is discomfort around the chest which is independent of posture or other activities. Indeed, the dorsal and ribcage stiffness is often eased by physical activity; there is usually night pain and the patient is worst when waking.

Other pathology

In the middle-aged and elderly, malignancy should be suspected if there is a history of persistent or increasing pain, which is unaffected by posture and is present at night. The thoracic spine is a not uncommon site for myelomatosis. Carcinoma of the oesophagus usually gives rise to dysphagia, though it may present with persistent discomfort in the posterior thoracic region. The examiner's suspicions are aroused by the absence of localized signs on examination of the spine.

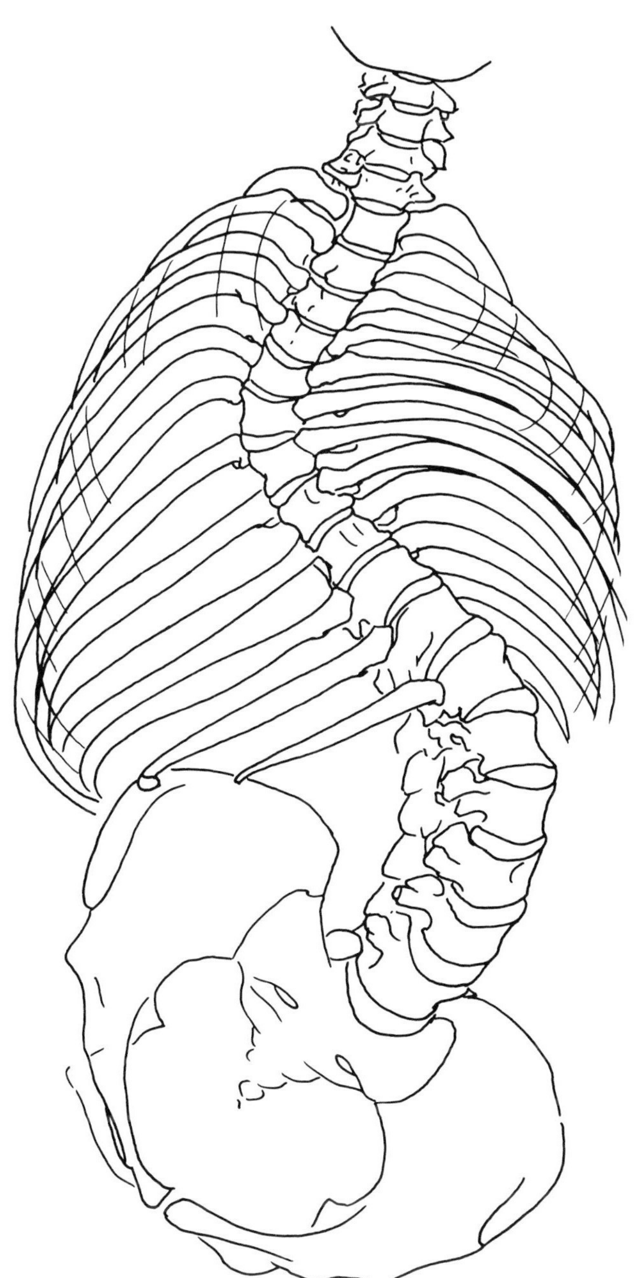

Fig. 3.10 Axial rotation accompanies lateral curvature in adolescent idiopathic scoliosis (AIS). (From Palastanga *et al.*, 1990.)

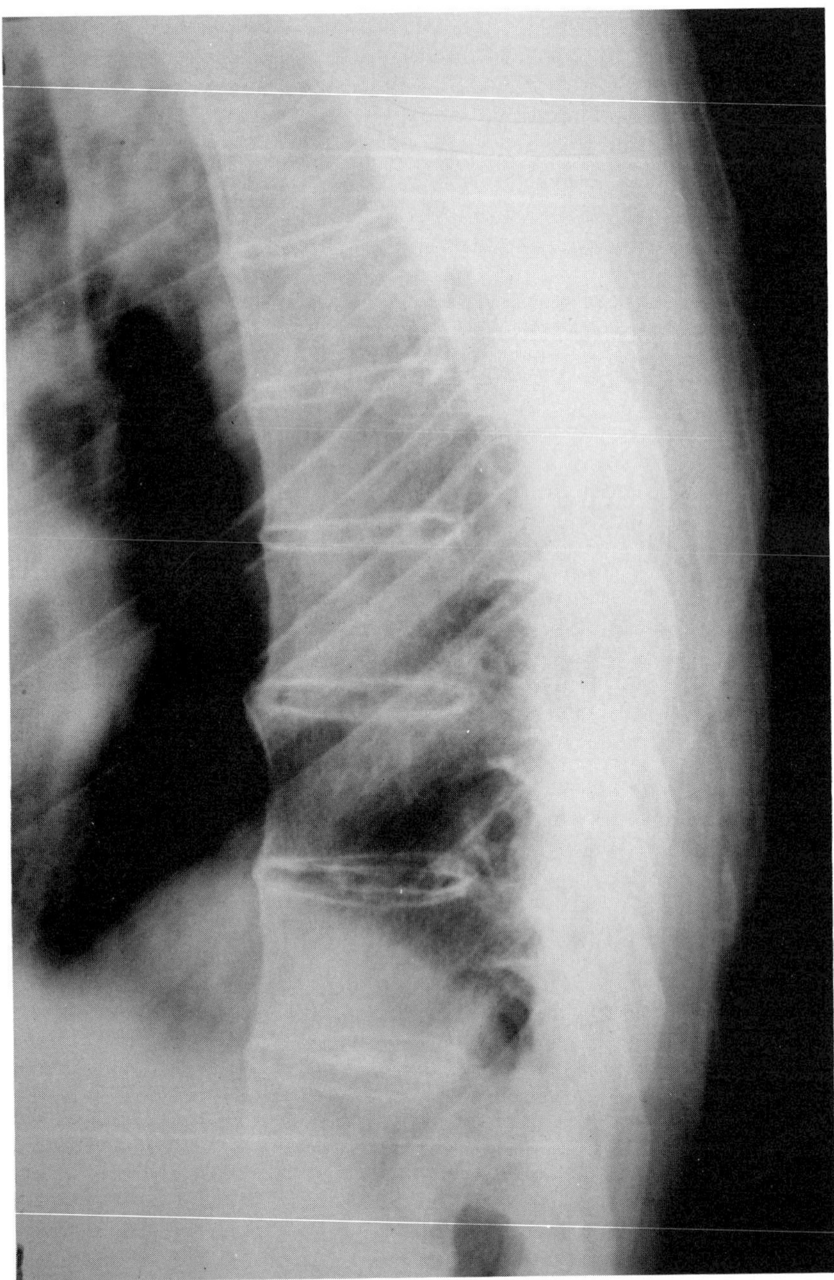

Fig. 3.11 Squaring of the bodies of the thoracic vertebrae and the formation of syndesmophytes are typical features of a 'bamboo spine' due to ankylosing spondylitis.

HISTORY

Site of pain

Discomfort that is felt in the 'shawl' area, particularly when associated with trigger points within the trapezius, is more likely to be associated with dysfunction in the mid- or distal cervical spine than with lesions in the proximal thoracic spine. Similarly, medial scapular discomfort may be a manifestation of cervical disc prolapse, necessitating a full examination of the cervical spine. Proximal thoracic lesions too may give rise to localized posterior thoracic discomfort and, to add to diagnostic difficulties, it is not unusual for conditions in the cervical and thoracic spines to coexist. This is a particularly frequent occurrence after whiplash injury. T3/4 lesions may give rise to discomfort in one or both arms.

Mid-thoracic joint dysfunction usually gives rise to well-localized discomfort which is felt at the level of the back of the bra in females, either in the midline or in the paraspinal region unilaterally. Radiation of discomfort around the posterolateral chest wall may occur, even as far as the anterior chest. Nerve root compression should then be suspected. Referred pain from the distal thoracic spine may be felt in the loin, and as far as the iliac crest and the iliac fossa.

If bilateral girdle pain is experienced, particularly with an acute onset, vertebral collapse, for instance an osteoporotic compression fracture, should be suspected. Occasionally, degenerative changes (thoracic spondylosis) in an elderly patient may be responsible for a similar picture.

Onset

Pain that is felt in the mid-thoracic spine may have an acute onset, when it is often associated with a twisting or bending movement. Alternatively, extension and rotation of the spine may have occurred, as in twisting to reach for a briefcase in the back seat of a car. In these situations, acute joint dysfunction is suspected.

More commonly, discomfort has a subacute onset, being felt, for instance, the morning after a session of gardening, or a game of squash rackets or other vigorous sports. An insidious onset *per se* should not necessarily lead one to suspect more serious pathology, as many patients do not recall any particularly strenuous activity that preceded the onset of their symptoms. In these circumstances, adverse postural characteristics, such as prolonged car driving or extensive hours spent operating a VDU, may be the primary aetiological factors in the development of thoracic pain.

Characteristics

Proximal thoracic spinal lesions often interfere with a patient's capacity to lift and carry heavy items, for instance shopping bags. Twisting and turning are painful, usually to a greater degree to one side than the other. Racket sports and golf tend to be provocative.

Pain on deep inspiration, and on coughing and sneezing, may convince the patient, or sometimes the examiner, that a lesion exists in the lungs or pleura. Activities that involve reaching out with the arms, particularly if this results in grasping, are usually painful.

Many household chores are painful. It is common for sleep to be interfered with; the patient usually finds that some positions are comfortable, others not. Morning stiffness is common, whatever the pathology.

Associated symptoms

Referred pain from the proximal thoracic spine may be felt anteriorly in the chest or in the arms; from the distal thoracic spine, symptoms may be referred to the abdomen, loins, or iliac fossae. The presence of visceral symptoms, particularly the complaint of dysphagia, should lead the examiner to consider further relevant investigations. If necessary, referral to an appropriate specialist should be arranged for this purpose. The absence of localizing signs in the thoracic spine should always stimulate a search for an alternative diagnosis.

Not uncommonly, pain may be experienced contemporaneously in the neck, in the thoracic spine, and in the lower back. Such plurality of symptoms is particularly likely after whiplash injuries to the spine arising from road traffic accidents. A specific search for additional spinal lesions, such as sacroiliac dysfunction, must be made, and appropriate corrective treatment instituted.

The complaint of heaviness and/or numbness in the legs raises the possibility of cord compression.

EXAMINATION

The whole of the spine should be assessed; appropriate exposure of the patient by undressing to the underclothes is necessary.

Posture

The overall posture of the patient should be observed. A marked thoracic kyphosis is a common finding, and may be associated with drooping of, and protraction of, the shoulders (Figs 3.5, 3.12). This postural trait is not just confined to adolescent girls and women with heavy breasts. The middle-aged of both sexes are inclined to reveal their sagging connective tissues and their mid-life crises in their posture. Signs of stress in the male business executive may be manifested in the attitude of the spine, particularly the thoracic spine, as well as in a harassed countenance.

On the other hand, there may be a structural cause. An active young man with an exaggerated thoracic kyphosis and back pain may have Scheuermann's disease of the thoracolumbar spine, or ankylosing spondylitis. An elderly patient is more likely to have developed chronic degenerative changes in the thoracic spine, or osteoporotic compression fractures, giving rise to wedging and the appearance of a 'dowager's hump'.

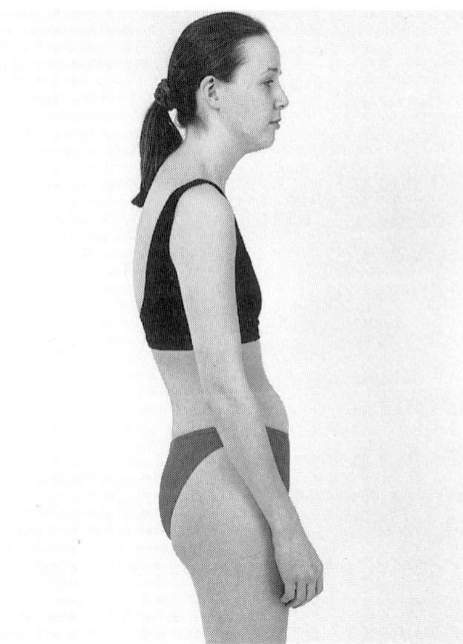

Fig. 3.12 Poor spinal posture gives rise to round shoulders, thoracic kyphosis and compensatory cervical hyperextension.

Standing

A more angular and localized kyphus is usually due to vertebral collapse.

A scoliosis may be detected: a prominent rib hump indicates a structural scoliosis. Asymmetry of the dimples overlying the posterior superior iliac spines suggests that the compensatory thoracolumbar scoliosis is secondary to leg length inequality or sacroiliac dysfunction.

Asymmetry of the height of the shoulders and unilateral prominence of the anterior margins of the ribs are particularly common findings, and their relevance to thoracic spinal pathology should be assessed following completion of the examination. Shoulder height asymmetry is often postural and of little relevance.

Of greater importance is a preliminary assessment of the mobility of the cervical spine as cervical lesions may be a source of interscapular pain. Active abduction of the shoulders should also be assessed; a restricted range is found in the presence of restricted mobility of the proximal thoracic spine, and in association with a marked thoracic kyphosis. Forward flexion of the arms, as in reaching forwards, may also be uncomfortable in these circumstances.

Standing: dural signs

Pain on neck flexion, either active or passive, is believed to indicate dural irritation. It is a common finding in mechanical lesions of moderate severity and is difficult to explain other than by the presence of a disc bulge or prolapse pressing against the adjacent dura mater. Pain on protraction or approximation (active or passive) of the shoulders indicates dural irritation at D1 or D2.

Standing: trunk movements

The active movements of trunk flexion, extension and side flexions to right and left are assessed for pain and restriction in range. The rib hump of structural scoliosis becomes more prominent when viewed tangentially during forward flexion. A 'flattened' section, that is a lordotic segment or two in the thoracic spine, indicating a relatively severe degree of dysfunction, may be observed on trunk flexion. Stiffness of the lumbar spine too may be noted during this part of the examination.

Sitting

Passive rotation of the thoracic spine is best examined with the patient sitting to fix the pelvis. The patient clasps her hands behind her head and abducts the upper arms to separate the elbows; the examiner assists rotation to first one side and then the other by placing one hand on the nearest elbow and, if preferred, the other hand on the scapula of the other side (Fig. 3.13). It is easier to detect unilateral restriction, by comparison with rotation in the other direction, if the patient sits on the edge of a low couch. Pain towards the end of normal range, or painful restriction of rotation in one direction, are frequent findings in thoracic spinal joint dysfunction.

With the patient leaning forwards, a thump to the thoracic spine, at successive segmental levels, may be given using the hypothenar muscle mass and the crook of the little finger with the fist clenched. This is performed gently at first, then more vigorously if tolerated. Surprisingly, this is not at all painful unless bony pathology such as a compression fracture is present.

a

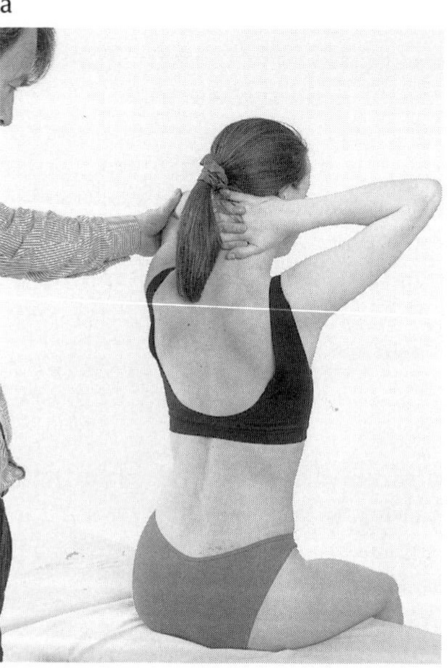

b

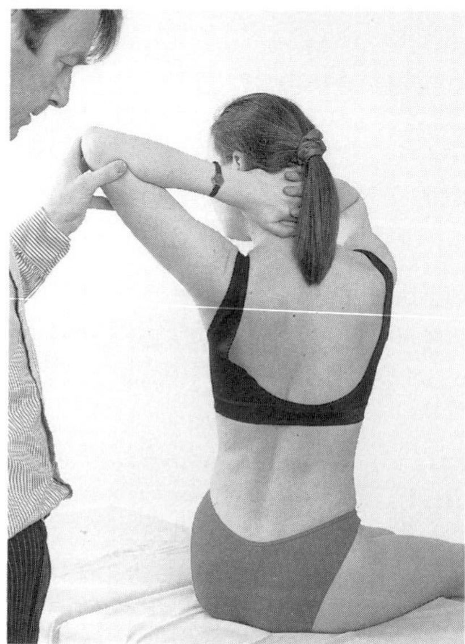

Fig. 3.13 Passive thoracic rotation should be assessed with the patient sitting.

In the sitting position compensatory scoliosis due to leg length inequality will be seen to disappear.

The thoracic cage is examined. Prominence of one or more ribs, anteriorly or posteriorly, may be noted. The swelling of a 'sprung' costochondral joint may be observed, and tenderness confirmed by palpation. The joint may click when the trunk is rotated.

The ribs and intercostal spaces are palpated: localized tenderness is sought in a suspected rib fracture or intercostal muscle strain, both of which may enter into the differential diagnosis of girdle pain, or coexist (for instance following trauma) with thoracic spinal joint dysfunction.

During inspiration and expiration, the degree of movement during, and any discomfort associated with, the excursion of the thoracic cage are identified. Compression of the chest, first anteroposteriorly, then bilaterally, is used to detect fractures (e.g. of the sternum or the ribs).

Prone lying

Skin rolling (Fig. 3.14) is performed throughout the length of the thoracic spine, and extended distally as far as the iliac crest and upper buttock (to identify lesions arising from the thoracolumbar junction). Patches of increased turgor and tenderness may be found paravertebrally at the site of a segmental lesion; they are more frequent on the painful side though are often present on the painless side too. Extremely tender patches, which accompany the equally tender but deeper trigger points, are found in fibromyalgia; they are multiple and favour the upper half of the back of the chest.

Tenderness to light pressure or stroking over the spinous processes in the proximal thoracic spine indicates a hyperaesthetic state caused

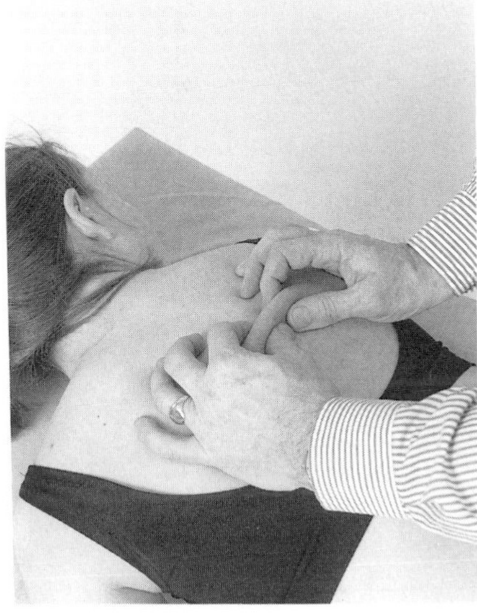

Fig. 3.14 Skin rolling is demonstrated.

by involvement of the autonomic system in dysfunction of the cervicothoracic junction. Areas of hyperaesthesia, or sometimes of hypoaesthesia, may occur at other segmental levels too.

Trigger points, particularly common in the levator scapulae when associated with lesions of the distal cervical spine, but sometimes found in other muscle groups, should be sought.

The segmental compression test

This is a most useful screening test for dysfunction. The ulnar border of the hand (effectively, the 5th metacarpal) is used to produce localized hyperextension at each vertebral level. Alternatively, compression may be applied using the thumb and the index finger of the examining hand. Segmental mobility and patient discomfort are recorded. In the proximal thoracic spine, it is usually easier to stand ahead of the patient and to apply compression to the spinous processes of T1–T4 using the 1st metacarpal (or both thumbs). When using the 1st or 5th metacarpal of an examining hand it is helpful to reinforce compression with the other hand (as demonstrated in Fig. 3.15). The examination couch should be sufficiently low to allow the examiner to lock his arms straight at the elbows.

Lateral springing

Lateral springing is performed by applying pressure to first one side, and then the other side, of each spinous process using the tips of both thumbs (Fig. 3.16). Once more, the degree of movement and any associated discomfort are noted.

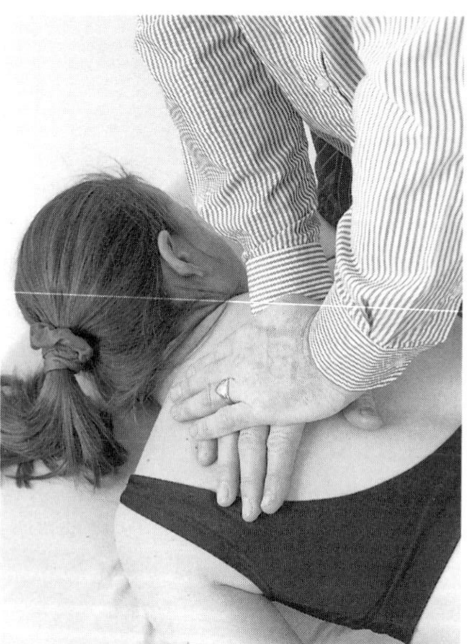

Fig. 3.15 Thoracic spine – segmental compression test.

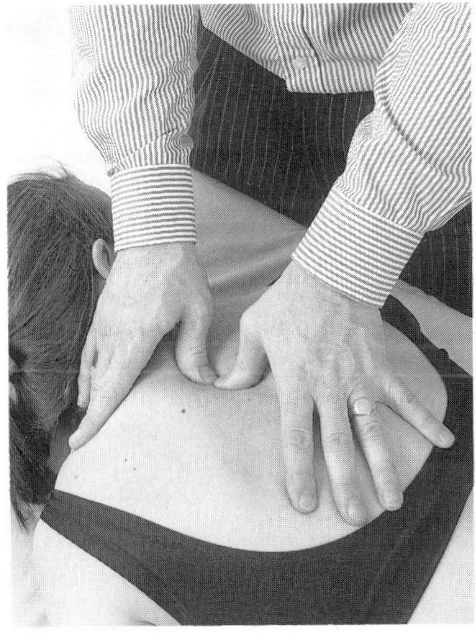

Fig. 3.16 Thoracic spine – lateral springing.

Both the segmental compression test and lateral springing test are examples of joint play assessment and should be performed throughout the thoracic spine (to avoid missing multiple lesions).

Costovertebral stress tests

Posteroanterior compression is applied to each rib, 3–4 cm from the midline. Pressure is applied with the thumb, or the pisiform bone, or the base of the thenar eminence; reinforcement with the other hand is desirable (Fig. 3.17). Discomfort should be recorded.

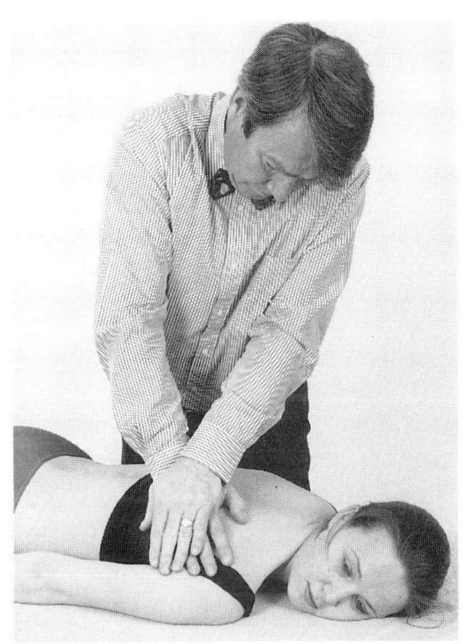

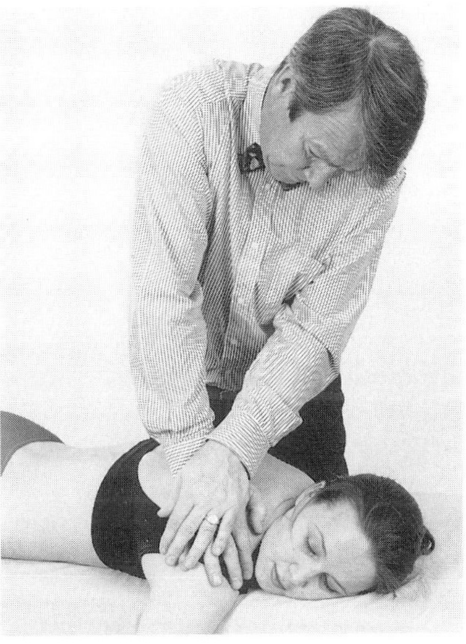

Fig. 3.17 Thoracic spine – costovertebral stress.

Neurological assessment

This is particularly valid if spinal cord compression is suspected from the history (for instance paraesthesiae in the feet), or following the detection of a spastic gait or incoordination of the legs. The subsequent examination should then include a full appraisal of the sensory and motor systems, reflex changes and Babinski responses.

INTERPRETATION

Thoracic disc prolapse

Very occasionally, a prolapse of the nucleus pulposus in the thoracic spine is sufficiently large to give rise to spinal cord compression. The combination of thoracic symptoms and articular signs, and upper motor neurone signs in the lower limbs, suggests a space-occupying lesion within the spinal canal. Further investigations should be undertaken by an appropriate specialist. Scanning techniques, particularly MRI, have largely overtaken the invasive technique of myelography in the assessment of disc prolapse. Straight X-rays are unrevealing.

When posterior thoracic and unilateral chest pain are accompanied by pain on neck flexion, indicating dural irritation, a posterior (or posterolateral) disc prolapse is probably present. One or more adjacent lordotic segments may be seen on trunk flexion. Rotation in one direction is almost invariably restricted; rotation in the other direction may be uncomfortable but not restricted to the same degree. Overall, some of the movements of the thoracic spine are of full painless range, indicating a partial articular pattern. If acute, the patient is very apprehensive about any sudden movements; getting in or out of a car, and applying a seatbelt, for instance, involve twisting movements and are particularly painful. Deep inspiration is usually painful.

Manipulative reduction is nearly always successful; several sessions of treatment may be required over several weeks.

Spinal joint dysfunction

Apophyseal joint dysfunction is particularly common, though rarely severe, in the thoracic spine. Referred pain may be felt in the chest or the abdomen (from mid- and distal thoracic lesions). Although discomfort may be felt on rotation of the thoracic spine in one direction, and possibly on other movements, the overall restriction in range, in the partial articular pattern, is not as substantial as that associated with a disc prolapse. Indeed, in a relatively minor joint dysfunction, there may be no obvious restriction of global movements, or discomfort at the end of range, in the standing or sitting positions. Localized superficial tenderness, segmental provocation pain and hypomobility on joint play assessment are the cardinal indicators of joint dysfunction.

Trigger points in the trapezius, rhomboids and levator scapulae muscles are more commonly associated with distal cervical spinal lesions. Positive skin rolling, however, is a better localizing sign for thoracic joint dysfunction. Segmental hypomobility, discomfort on compression and lateral springing in the proximal thoracic spine, and an exaggerated thoracic kyphosis are particularly common in the middle-aged. When faulty posture is apparent, corrective exercises play an important part in treatment.

Mobilization (without impulse) and manipulation (with impulse) are used in combination with appropriate exercises, e.g. flexibility exercises for the spine and shoulders, strengthening exercises for the lower scapular fixators, and postural and ergonomic assessment.

Costovertebral joint dysfunction ('rib lesions')

The osteopathic concept of ribs fixed in inspiration or expiration and the corroborative signs of asymmetry, tissue texture change and tenderness (Bourdillon, 1992) are not considered in any detail here. For the inexperienced, if pressure pain is identified over the angle of a rib, manipulative correction should be attempted.

Ankylosing spondylitis

The history of backache in a young adult, which is not aggravated by daily activities but may be painful at night and may be accompanied by morning stiffness, raises the possibility of a spondyloarthropathy. The typical examination findings in a moderately advanced case are a flat lumbar spine and a markedly kyphotic thoracic spine. Thoracic excursion on deep inspiration is restricted. Trunk movements are generally of poor range; in particular, side flexions and rotations are very limited bilaterally. There are no localizing signs on joint play assessment. In the earlier stages, X-rays may reveal typical changes of sacroiliitis; as the condition advances, squaring of the vertebrae and syndesmophytes are seen, leading eventually to a 'bamboo spine' (Fig. 3.11).

Lesions of the thoracic cage

As a result of vigorous or repetitive sporting activity, stress fractures of the ribs, intercostal muscle strains and disturbances of the costochondral joints may occur. These conditions are not usually accompanied by backache, but, nevertheless, may enter into the differential diagnosis of unilateral chest pain. Although pain is felt on deep breathing and spinal rotation, examination of the thoracic spine is otherwise negative. Localized chest wall tenderness is present; when a costochondral joint is 'sprung', that is subluxated, a localized swelling of the joint may be seen and felt.

As a result of head-on vehicle collisions, a fractured sternum is commonplace. Tenderness and bruising over the anterior chest, and pain on chest compression are found, but healing is normally uneventful. The same deceleration forces may also give rise to thoracic spinal injuries which are usually symptomatic for a much longer period of time.

Vertebral crush fracture

An osteoporotic spine is liable to (multiple) vertebral body collapse. Girdle pain is often present. In the early stages after the onset of pain, trunk movements are uniformly painful, particularly rotations, and the patient moves from the sitting position with considerable discomfort. There is segmental compression pain at the site of the collapse.

After some weeks, mobility improves and any persisting pain is often due to a disturbance of an apophyseal or costovertebral joint – the signs often become unilateral, and tenderness is then elicited on compression of the affected joint.

TREATMENT

Mobilization/manipulation

Manipulative techniques (involving thrust) are usually very effective in spinal joint dysfunction: the results are often dramatic. Therapists should become familiar with a variety of suitable techniques and use them as required. Occasionally, and unexpectedly, a joint dysfunction may be refractory to one particular manipulative procedure; unless a contraindication exists, such as worsening pain, other techniques should be attempted. The following techniques are 'tried and tested' and are commended.

Springing (into forced extension)

This is an extension of the segmental compression test, using the hypothenar eminence of one hand, reinforced by the other hand (Fig. 3.15). The patient lies prone on a low couch and the low amplitude, high velocity thrust should be applied with the therapist's elbows locked into extension, thereby transmitting some body weight.

Crossed hands technique

This also forces the spine into extension but with a rotational element in addition. The base of the thenar eminence (effectively, the tubercle of the scaphoid) of one hand, and the base of the hypothenar eminence (the pisiform bone) of the other hand, are used to effect

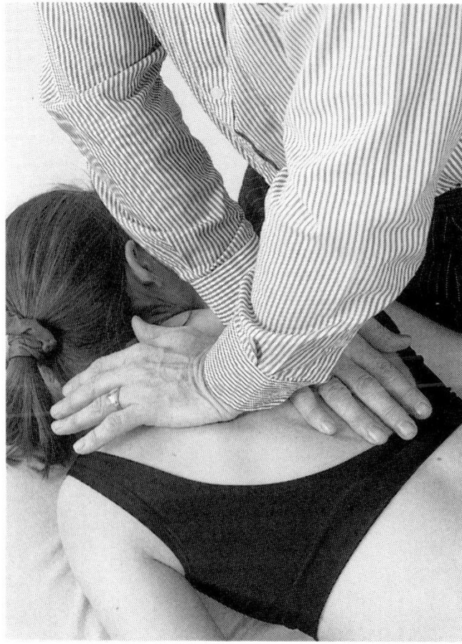

Fig. 3.18 Thoracic spine – crossed hands manipulation.

pressure on the transverse processes of a vertebra (Fig. 3.18). A high velocity thrust is imparted by the hands in opposite directions (one caudally, one cranially). Both this and the previous technique should be used after the patient breathes out. Undoubtedly, a significant mobilizing force is administered simultaneously to the costovertebral joints.

Roll-over technique

The disadvantage of the prone lying techniques described is that the chest is compressed against the couch, which is not to every patient's liking. This may be avoided by using a manipulative technique which involves rolling the patient over from a side lying position into a supine position so that an extension thrust may be made against the examiner's hand which is positioned posteriorly at the appropriate vertebral level (Fig. 3.19). The patient should either fold his arms across his chest or, preferably, clasp his fingers behind his neck and approximate his elbows, to facilitate leverage of the thoracic spine into extension. The hand adjacent to the spine is positioned so that either the thenar eminence, or the combination of the thumb and index finger, takes up the slack and then resists the backwards thrust of the chest.

'Lift off' or 'knee in back'

The author's preference is to link arms with the patient in the manner shown, and to ask the patient to flex, then extend, his trunk (Fig. 3.20). As the trunk nears the upright position, the examiner uses his

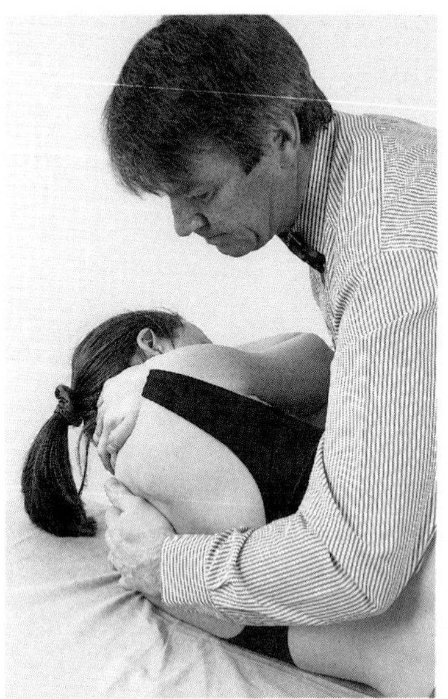
a

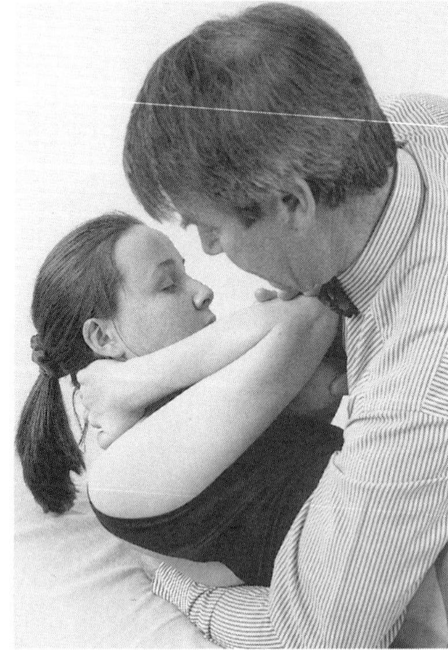
b

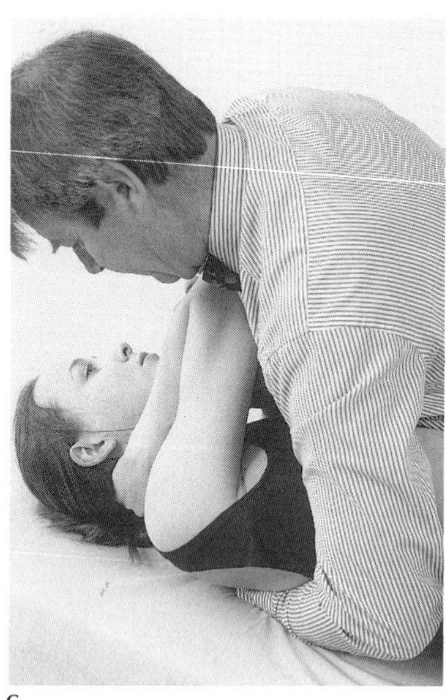
c

Fig. 3.19 Thoracic spine – roll-over manipulation sequences.

a

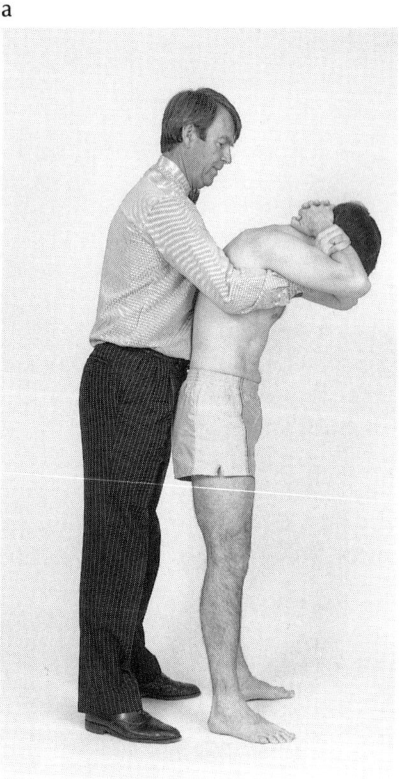

b

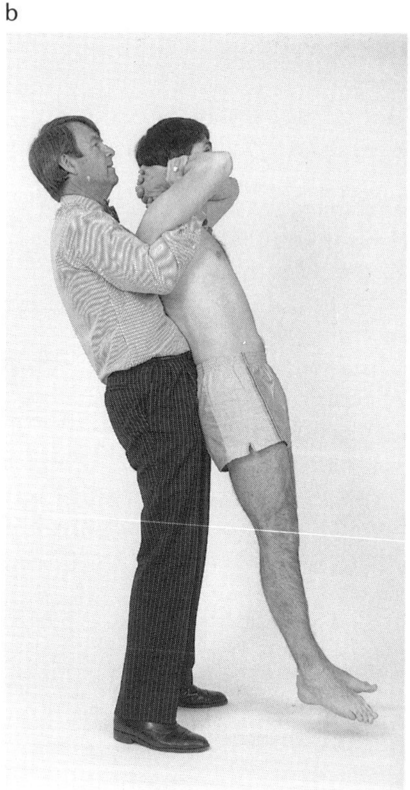

Fig. 3.20 Thoracic spine – lift-off manipulation.

own chest (abutting against the dorsal spine of the patient) and his body strength to lift the patient off the ground, and in the process to extend the thoracic spine. Although a relatively crude manoeuvre, it may, nevertheless, be quite effective. An alternative technique, which is more suitable for a therapist of more diminutive stature, is to press a knee (using a small cushion) against the back of the (sitting) patient to produce the same effect.

Proximal thoracic spine (and cervicothoracic junction)

A thrust technique which is usually effective is to use the tip of the thumb or the thenar eminence, to produce a side bending/rotational stress upon a vertebra via its spinous process. This is similar to, but more forceful than, the lateral springing examination procedure, and requires stabilization of the proximal spine with the other hand and arm. With the patient in a side lying position facing the therapist, and the thumb or thenar eminence of the manipulating hand producing the desired lateral springing force, the therapist's other hand laterally flexes the neck towards and rotates the neck away from his own body (Fig. 3.21). In the mid- and distal thoracic spines, a similar technique may be used, using the thumb to fix the relevant vertebra via its spinous process, and the other hand to procure side flexion and rotation of the spine proximal to the lesion.

Thoracolumbar junction

A rotational manipulation of the type used for the lumbar spine is employed. Rotation is controlled by the examiner's arms and

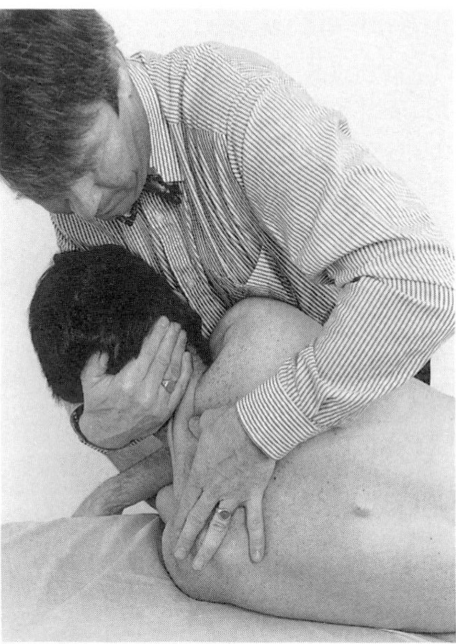

Fig. 3.21 Thoracic spine – a suitable manipulation technique for the proximal thoracic spine is demonstrated.

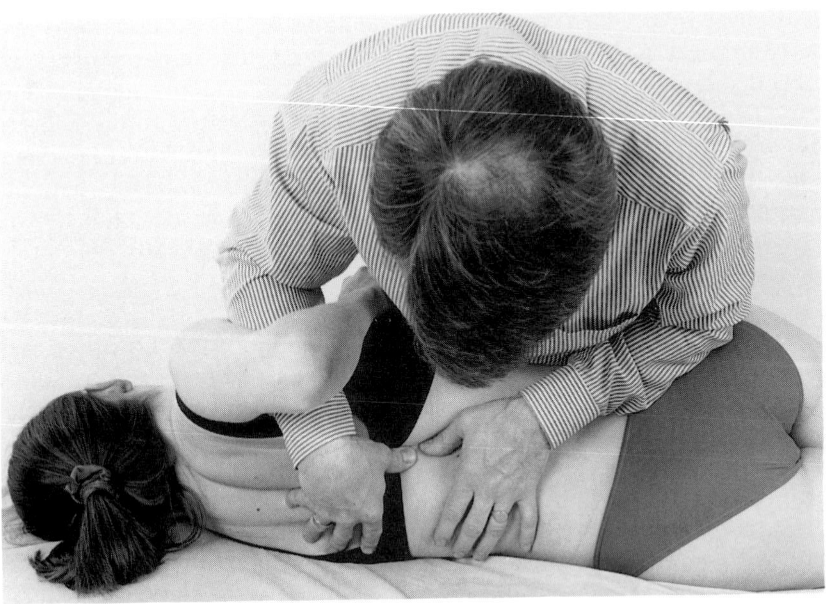

Fig. 3.22 Thoracic spine – a suitable manipulation technique for the distal thoracic spine is demonstrated.

segmental overpressure produced using the thumb against a spinous process (Fig. 3.22). This technique may be used also for the distal thoracic spinal joints as far up as T9.

Mobilization

Mobilization, using an oscillatory technique of the (Maitland) type used for lateral springing (Fig. 3.16), but without any thrust element, may be very effective for the proximal thoracic spine in particular.

Costovertebral springing

The thenar eminence, which is placed on the angle of the appropriate rib on the side of the patient furthest from the examiner, may be used to procure springing of a costovertebral joint (Fig. 3.17a). For the proximal rib articulations, the patient may abduct her scapula by hanging her arm over the side of the couch (Fig. 3.17b). Alternatively, the hypothenar eminence may be used to spring the angle of the rib on the side of the patient adjacent to the examiner.

Injection techniques

Occasionally, localized steroid injections to the posterior aspects of the apophyseal and costovertebral joints are required. This follows failure of response to manipulation or mobilization, and is only rarely indicated. If steroid injections help, but only temporarily, sclerosant injections to the supraspinous and capsular ligaments may give longer lasting relief. Occasionally, sclerotherapy is used to procure relative stability in a case of recurrent dysfunction.

Subcutaneous sodium salicylate or lignocaine injections may be used to treat patches of skin turgor which are part of a generalized fibromyalgia syndrome.

REHABILITATION/PREVENTION

Postural correction is as important for the thoracic spine as it is for the cervical and lumbar spines. This is considered further in Chapter 5. Two other aspects of prevention should be addressed.

(1) It is known that bone density may be increased by regular exercise. The prevention of postmenopausal osteoporosis, and therefore the reduction in the incidence of spinal fractures, should be commenced well in advance of the menopause. Promotion of the importance of prevention of osteoporosis, in addition to the cardiorespiratory benefits from exercise, should be an essential part of a therapist's counselling role.

(2) A number of sporting activities require a considerable degree of thoracic rotation. In some sports, such as golf, it is obvious that axial rotation is an essential component of the overall body movement involved in striking the ball. Regularly performed spinal rotational exercises help maintain a satisfactory level of shoulder turn; this reduces the likelihood of injury and helps to maintain or improve technique. In other sports, for instance racket sports and those involving throwing, the spinal component may not be so obvious, though it is just as important. Explosive power at the shoulder is dependent initially upon satisfactory torsion of the trunk. Lack of attention to flexibility exercises leads to application of maximum torque at inappropriate joint angles, resulting in overload and joint dysfunction. Dysfunction may then be apparent in the spine, or at the shoulders. *Flexibility exercises for the trunk and shoulder girdles prevent injury.*

REFERENCES

Bourdillon, J.F. (1992) *Spinal Manipulation*, 5th edn, Butterworth-Heinemann, Oxford.

Bruckner, F.E., Greco, A. and Leung, A.W.L. (1989) 'Benign thoracic pain' syndrome: role of magnetic resonance imaging in the detection and localisation of thoracic disc disease. *Journal of the Royal Society of Medicine*, **82**, 81–3

Burwell, R.G. and Dangerfield, P.H. (1992) Pathogenesis and assessment of scoliosis. In *Surgery of the Spine – a Combined Neurosurgical and Orthopaedic Approach* (eds G.F.G. Findlay and R. Owen), Blackwell Scientific Publications, Oxford

Fraser, D.M. (1990) T3 syndrome. In *Back Pain – an International Review* (eds J.K. Paterson and L. Burn), Kluwer Academic Publishers, Lancaster

Maigne, R. (1980) Low back pain of thoracolumbar origin. *Archives of Physical Medicine and Rehabilitation*, **61**, 389–95

Stoddard, A. (1977) *Manual of Osteopathic Practice*, Hutchinson, London

4
Lumbar spine and sacroiliac joints

Pleasure is oft a visitant, but pain clings cruelly to us . . .

Keats, *Endymion* (1818)

APPLIED ANATOMY

Vertebrae

Usually, there are five lumbar vertebrae, which are larger and stronger (reflecting their weight-bearing function) than the cervical or thoracic vertebrae (Fig. 4.1). Transitional vertebrae at L5 are not uncommon. A considerable degree of sacralization of L5 may effectively reduce (anatomically and functionally) the number of typical lumbar vertebrae to four; conversely, the sacrum may be lumbarized, yielding six lumbar vertebrae (and discs). Another developmental abnormality which is frequently found on X-rays is spina bifida, in which the laminae fail to unite dorsally behind the cauda equina; associated abnormalities of the dural sac or the nerve

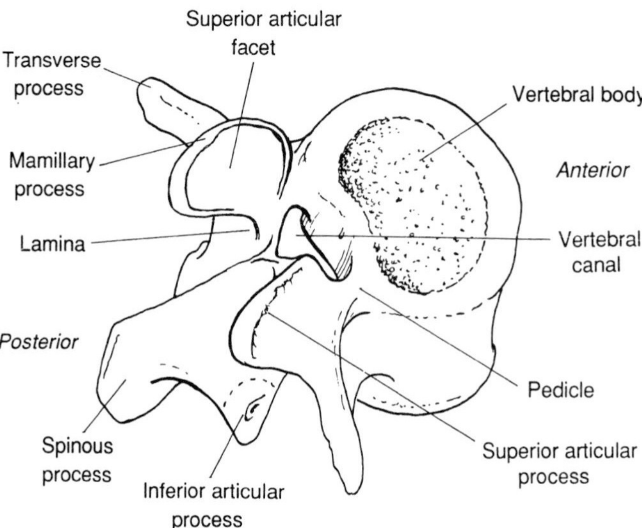

Fig. 4.1 A typical lumbar vertebra

roots are found in advanced cases. Spina bifida occulta, a relatively minor anatomical defect, is seen more frequently in patients with a spondylolysis, but is probably not associated with an increased risk of other 'mechanical' back problems.

The spinous processes project almost horizontally backwards; in the transverse plane their tips are aligned with the inferior margins of the vertebral bodies, and (approximately) with the facet joints. Identification of vertebral level by palpation of the spinous processes may be difficult because of the lumbar lordosis. To do so, the spine should be flexed (either in the sitting position, or with a pillow under the abdomen in the prone position), and the posterior superior iliac spines (PSISs) identified at the dimples of Venus. A line between the PSISs indicates the level of the lumbosacral joint. The L5 spinous process is palpable in the hollow 1–2 cm proximally. The L4 spinous process and the L4/5 facet joints lie approximately on a line drawn between the iliac crests (Fig 4.2).

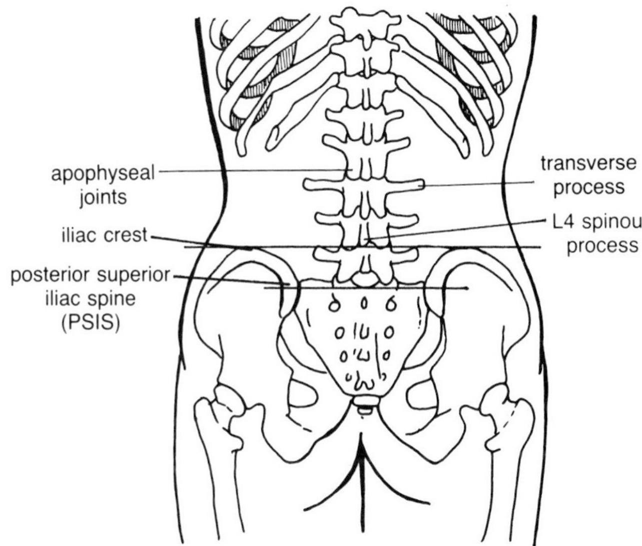

Fig. 4.2 The surface anatomy of the lumbar spine is demonstrated. A line between the PSISs indicates the level of the lumbosacral joint. The L4 spinous process and the L4/5 facet joints lie approximately on a line drawn between the iliac crests.

The transverse processes are short and relatively thin apart from at L5 where the iliolumbar ligaments are attached. The exceptional stresses at the lumbosacral joint have resulted developmentally in considerably increased strength of the L5 transverse processes.

The articular processes are somewhat curved or biplanar although relatively 'flat' joints are also described (Fig. 4.3). The superior processes are concave and face posteromedially; the inferior processes are closer to each other, are convex on their articular surfaces, and face anterolaterally (Fig. 4.4). In the proximal lumbar spine their orientation with respect to the sagittal plane is less than 45°. At the lumbosacral junction the inferior facets of L5 are set at a greater angle

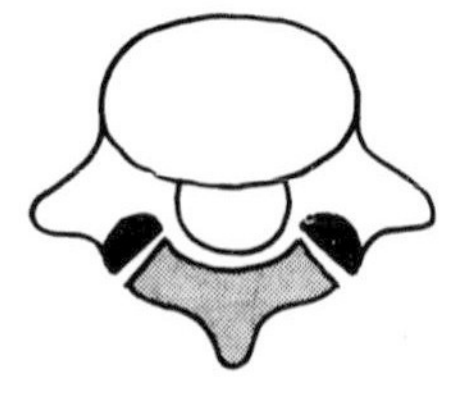

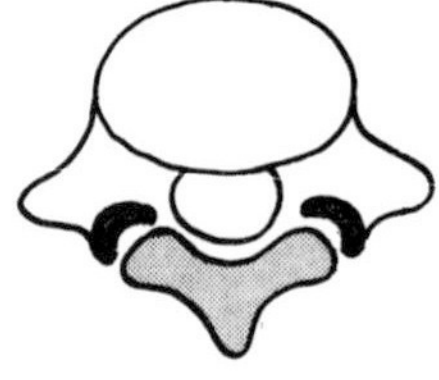

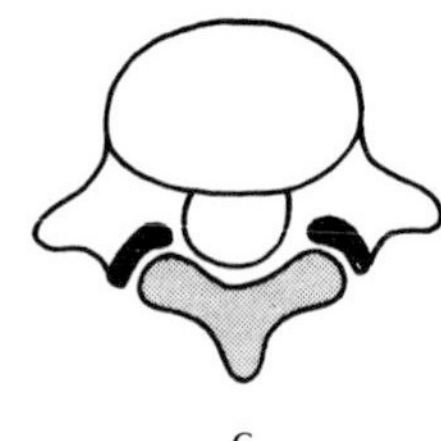

Fig. 4.3 Variations in curvature of the lumbar apophyseal joints. (a) flat joints; (b) 'C' shaped joints; (c) 'J' shaped joints. (After Bogduk, N. and Twomey, L.T., 1987, *Clinical Anatomy of the Lumbar Spine*, Churchill Livingstone, New York.)

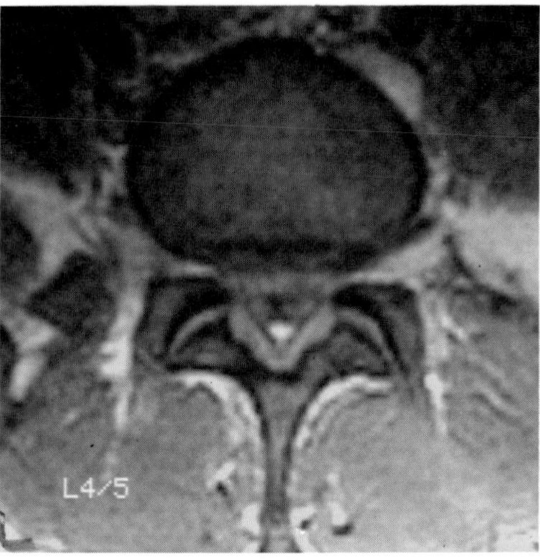

Fig. 4.4 MRI scan of the lumbar spine revealing the disposition of the articular surfaces of the apophyseal joints at L4/5.

to the sagittal plane (that is, they are more coronal in their orientation and they create a 'flatter' joint). They articulate with the superior facets of the sacrum which face considerably backwards (Fig. 4.5). Articular tropism (asymmetrical orientation of the facet joints) is not uncommon, particularly at L5 (Fig. 4.6). This may be responsible for

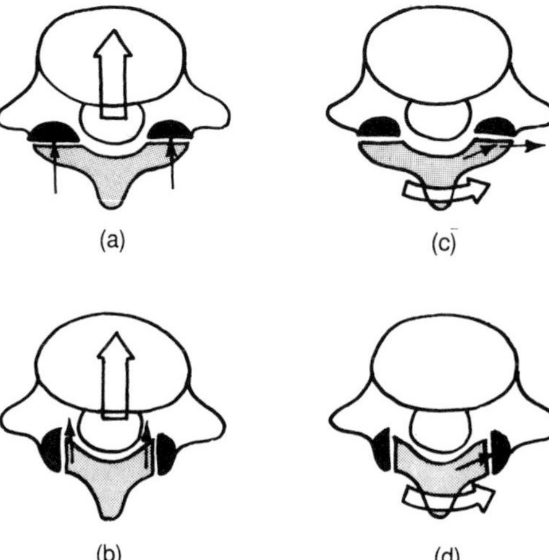

Fig. 4.5 Variations in orientation of lumbar apophyseal joints. (a) joints orientated in the coronal plane strongly resist forward displacement; (b) joints orientated in the sagittal plane are less able to resist forward displacement; (c) joints orientated in the coronal plane are less able to resist rotation; (d) joints orientated in the sagittal plane strongly resist rotation. (After Bogduk and Twomey, 1987.)

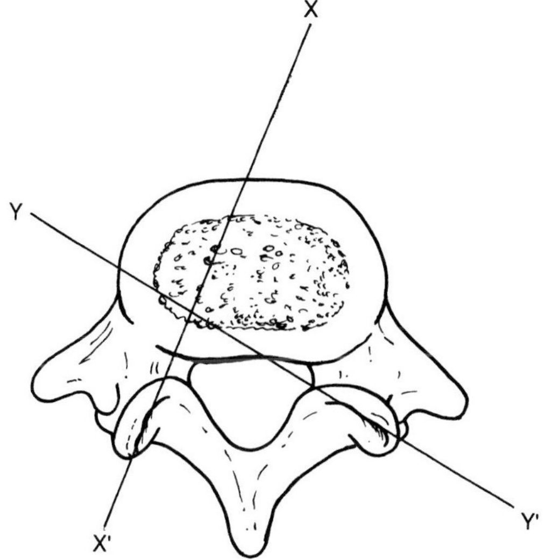

Fig. 4.6 Tropism of the fifth lumbar vertebra X–X′ = plane of sagittally orientated facet; Y–Y′ = plane of coronally orientated facet.

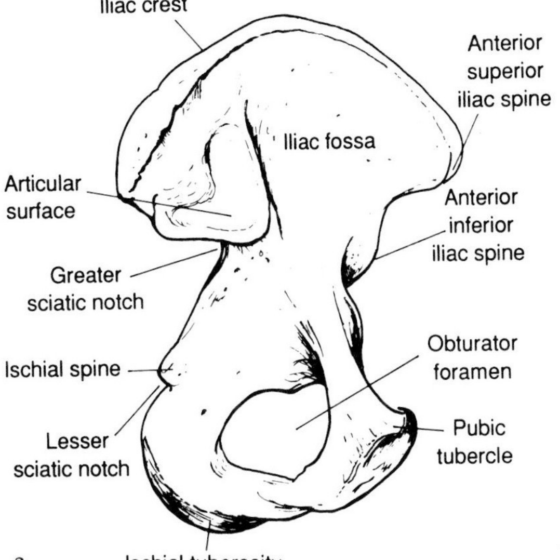

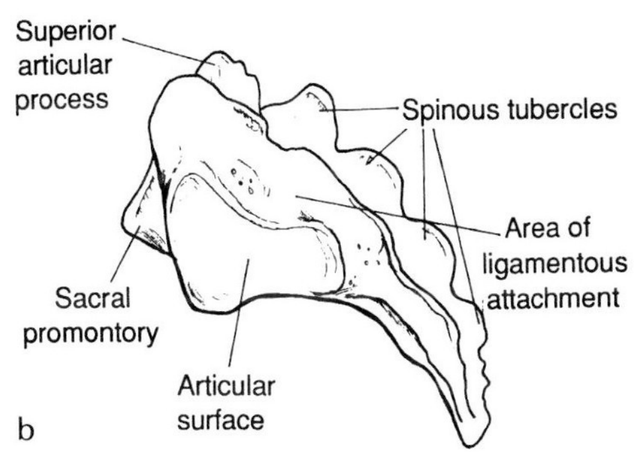

Fig. 4.7 The left innominate bone (a) and the left lateral view of the sacrum (b) demonstrating the articular surfaces.

the transmission of abnormal stresses to the lumbosacral joint. These zygo-apophyseal (facet) joints, formed from the articular processes of adjacent vertebrae, are synovial joints and, in the lumbar region, have been found to contain intra-articular structures known as meniscoids. These structures contain capsule, or synovium, or fat, and project, presumably dynamically, into the joint cavity. It has been postulated, without confirmation, that meniscoids may be responsible for intra-articular facet joint derangement by causing joint 'locking'. Under normal circumstances their function may be protective of the joint.

The sacrum consists of five fused vertebrae and is heart- or triangular-shaped. It articulates with the L5 vertebra superiorly, the coccyx inferiorly, and the innominate bones laterally. From within the spinal canal the nerve roots emerge through the anterior and posterior sacral foramina. The sacral canal is open inferiorly at the sacral hiatus, which is guarded by a ligament. The clinical importance of the sacral hiatus lies in its use as the site for caudal epidural injections. Its position may be palpated as the depression between the sacral cornua. Laterally, the auricular surface of the sacrum is pitted and covered with articular cartilage (Fig. 4.7). Inferiorly, the sacrum articulates with the coccyx which consists of four fused vertebrae, yet performs no useful function.

Lumbar lordosis

The lumbar lordosis develops during the first 1–2 years of childhood in response to extension of the legs and the need to maintain the upright posture (Fig. 1.1). It is achieved by the anatomical configuration – the wedge shape – of the lumbosacral disc and the 5th lumbar vertebra. The lumbosacral angle, the angle between the inferior border of the L5 vertebra and the upper border of the sacrum, approximates to 15°. The extent of the overall lumbar curve is such that, in the upright position, the L1 vertebra lies directly above the sacrum. The lordotic angle, made between the upper border of L1 and the upper border of the sacrum, averages 70°. The angle between the superior surface of the sacrum and the horizontal – sometimes referred to as the **pelvic angle** – also reflects the lumbar lordosis (Fig. 4.8). Prevention of forward slip of L4 on L5, and L5 on S1, is by the orientation of their facet joints, and the strength of the annuli fibrosi and the lumbar ligaments. The postural muscles include the erector spinae, the abdominals (which are subject to weakness), the hip flexors and the hip extensors.

Scoliosis and pelvic tilt

In the coronal plane, a pelvic tilt, from whatever cause, is associated with a lumbar scoliosis. Scoliosis may be **compensatory**, when it is usually due to leg length inequality. Alternatively, a pelvic tilt and

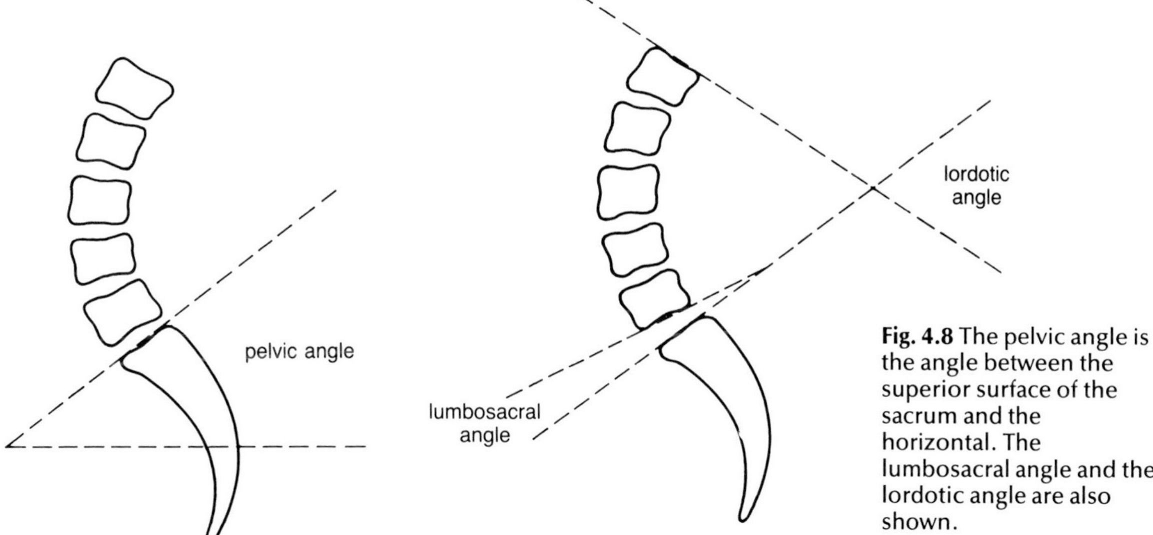

Fig. 4.8 The pelvic angle is the angle between the superior surface of the sacrum and the horizontal. The lumbosacral angle and the lordotic angle are also shown.

'sciatic' scoliosis may be associated with back pain which is caused by an intervertebral disc prolapse. When **structural**, on the other hand, a thoracolumbar scoliosis is usually idiopathic, and often presents in early adolescence (Fig. 3.10). Further discussion of scoliosis is found in Chapter 3.

Spinal and root canals

There is enormous variation in the size and shape of spinal canals. Porter (1986) has emphasized the importance of the mid-sagittal and interpedicular diameters in the pathogenesis of spinal disorders. Spinal canals range from dome-shaped to trefoil-shaped, the latter caused by posterolateral indentations of the neural arches (Fig. 1.25). Individuals with the trefoil-shaped canal are at greater risk of spinal stenotic syndromes: pathological changes in the soft tissues, for instance hypertrophy of the ligamentum flavum, combine with osteophytic encroachment from the facet joints to give rise to nerve root entrapment.

In an adult the spinal cord ends (as the filum terminale) at the level of L1. Distally, the neural content of the lumbar spinal canal consists of the lumbosacral nerve roots which, because of their resemblance to the tail of a horse, are known, collectively, as the cauda equina (Fig. 4.9). Within the lumbar spinal canal these spinal nerve roots are invested by the meninges. Extensions of the dura, in the form of root sleeves, surround the emerging nerve roots, which consist of paired motor and sensory roots, in the root (syn. 'radicular') canals. Caudal to the dorsal root ganglion, the sensory and motor roots unite to form the spinal nerve.

From the lateral aspect of the dural sac within the spinal canal, the distal nerve roots run obliquely downwards and laterally, winding

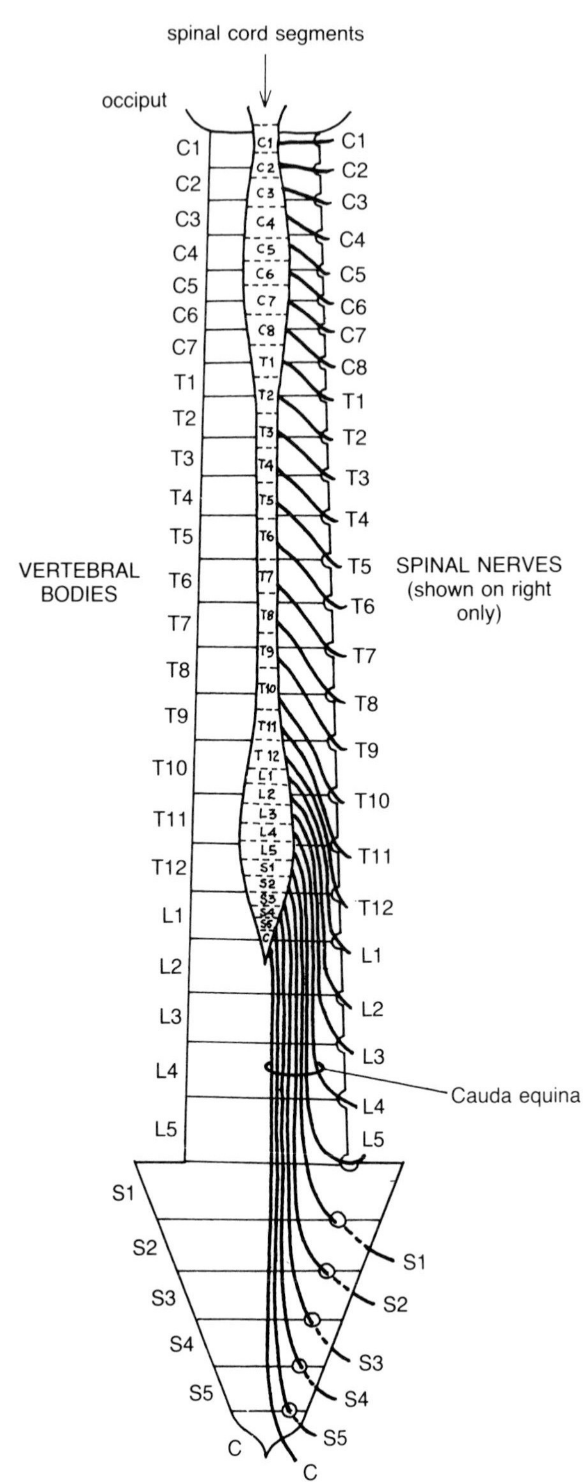

Fig. 4.9 Diagrammatic representation of the spinal nerves in relation to vertebral levels. The cauda equina is demonstrated. (From Grieve, G.P., 1988, *Common Vertebral Joint Problems*, 2nd edn, Churchill Livingstone, New York.)

around the medial aspect of the pedicle. In a trefoil spinal canal, this anatomical position is referred to as the lateral recess (of the spinal canal). The intervertebral foramen, through which the spinal nerves emerge, is bounded anteriorly by a disc and adjacent parts of the vertebral bodies, posteriorly by a lamina and apophyseal joint, and above and below by pedicles (Fig. 4.10). At the level of the foramen

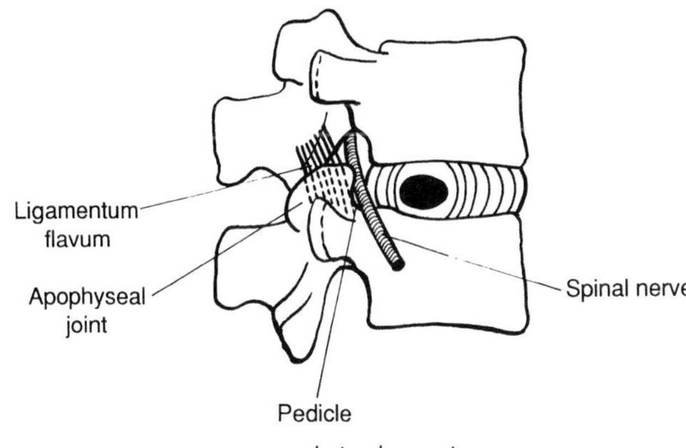

Fig. 4.10 The boundaries of the intervertebral foramen of the lumbar spine are demonstrated (lateral view).

the dural sleeve encloses the nerve tissue more tightly, though there is less tethering to the bony surrounds than there is in the cervical spine. The dural sleeve becomes contiguous with the epineurium of the spinal nerve beyond the foramen. Mechanical deformation of the nerve roots may occur in the root canals as a result of swelling, for instance from tumour or disc herniation; neural ischaemic changes too may arise as the radicular arteries and nerves are vulnerable within the dural sleeves in the canals.

The sinuvertebral nerves are given off by the common spinal nerves (Fig. 1.8). They are mixed nerves, having sensory components and also contributions from the grey rami communicantes of the autonomic nervous system. They re-enter the spinal canals to supply the contents of the spinal canal, providing ascending and descending branches which interlink over several segments. Histological studies have demonstrated that the outer halves of the annuli fibrosi are innervated by nerve fibres from the sinuvertebral nerves; although confirmation is lacking, it is presumed that the nerve endings have a nociceptive function. The apophyseal joints too are rich in free nerve endings, the connections of which are to the medial branches of the dorsal rami. Rami communicantes from the sympathetic chain (situated along the anterolateral border of the vertebral bodies) are distributed to the lumbar ventral rami.

Muscles acting on the lumbar spine

The lumbar erector spinae, consisting of iliocostalis and longissimus, form the superficial group of muscles attached posteriorly to the lumbar spine, and contribute substantially to the prominence of the paravertebral contour (Fig. 1.10).

Recent studies (Macintosh and Bogduk, 1987) have demonstrated that the lumbar components and thoracic components of the erector spinae function independently. The lumbar muscles pass between the lumbar vertebrae and the ilium; the thoracic iliocostalis and longissimus form the erector spinae aponeurosis which attaches to the ilium, sacrum and lumbar and sacral spinous processes. The erector spinae extend and side flex the lumbar spine, and contribute to posterior translation of one vertebra on another.

Medial to the erector spinae is the multifidus which consists of fascicles spanning several vertebrae (Fig. 1.11). The longer fascicles arise from the spinous processes and insert distally into mamillary processes, the iliac crest, and the sacrum. Some of the deeper fibres attach to the capsules of the apophyseal joints adjacent to the mamillary processes; they may have a *stabilizing* role in addition to contributing to trunk extension.

A third group of muscles, having a segmental stabilizing role, are the intertransversarii and interspinales (best developed in the cervical spine) and the rotatores (best developed in the thoracic spine).

The quadratus lumborum is deep to the erector spinae; it is a thick muscle of quadrilateral shape attached inferiorly to the iliolumbar ligament and adjacent area of the iliac crest, and superiorly to the 12th rib. Additionally, there are attachments to the anterolateral aspects of all the lumbar transverse processes. When contracting unilaterally, it laterally flexes the spine; when contracting with the opposite muscle, it extends the spine. It is covered by the deeper (anterior and middle) layers of the thoracolumbar fascia (Fig. 1.12).

Three layers of fascia cover the erector spinae, multifidus and the quadratus lumborum. Medially, they originate from the spinous processes and the transverse processes; laterally, they fuse. The posterior layer of this thoracolumbar fascia covers the back muscles, and is continuous with the transversus abdominis via a lateral raphe. A description of the abdominal muscles, and an outline of the function of the thoracolumbar fascia in the biomechanics of bending and lifting, are to be found in Chapter 1.

The sacroiliac joints

The sacroiliac joint (SIJ) is a synovial joint formed between the auricular ('earshaped') surface of the ilium (part of the innominate bone) and the corresponding portion of the lateral mass of the sacrum (Fig. 4.7). The ilial auricular surface is divided by a central crest; the sacral articular surface has a corresponding furrow. Posterior and superior to the auricular surfaces is the strong interosseous ligament which is attached, on the ilial side, to its tuberosity (Fig. 4.11). The posterior sacroiliac ligaments too have considerable strength, resisting forward movement of the sacral promontory, and inferior movement

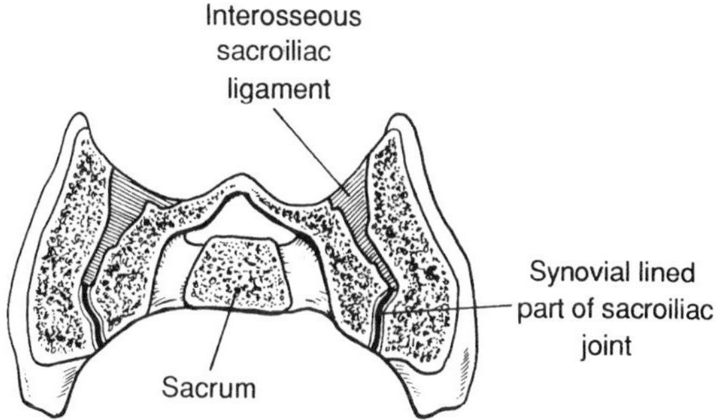

Fig. 4.11 Horizontal section through the sacrum and the sacroiliac joints.

of the sacrum on the ilium. By comparison, the anterior ligament, on the pelvic side of the joint, is broad and flat and relatively less strong.

Accessory ligaments impart added stability to the sacroiliac joint. The sacrospinous ligament extends from the lower segments of the sacrum and the coccyx to the ischial spine, thereby creating greater and lesser sciatic foramina. Superficial to the sacrospinous ligament is the extensive sacrotuberous ligament, extending from the sacrum below its auricular surface (and also from the ilium below the PSIS and the PIIS) to the ischial tuberosity; at its distal attachment it is closely associated with the long head of biceps femoris (Fig. 4.12).

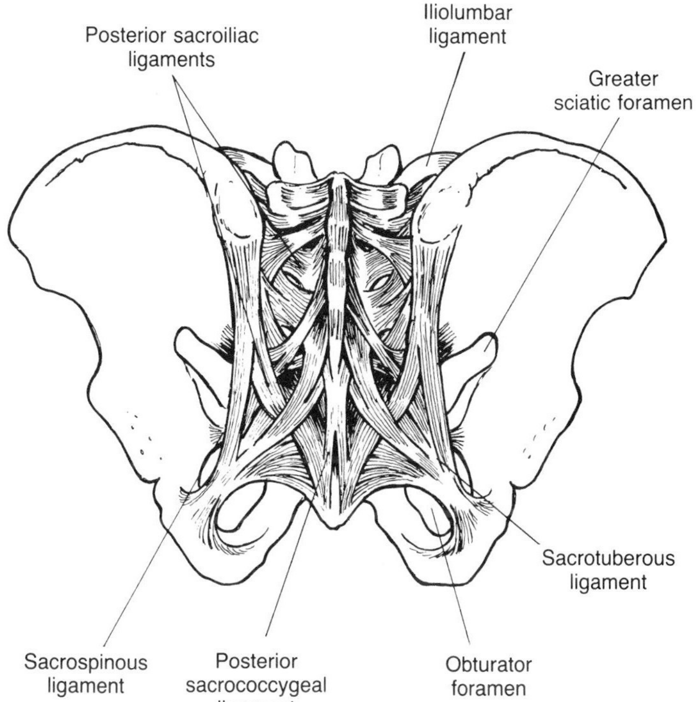

Fig. 4.12 The ligaments associated with the posterior aspect of the sacroiliac joints are demonstrated.

Although the iliolumbar ligaments, extending bilaterally from the transverse processes of L5 (and to a lesser extent from L4) to the ilium, are considered primarily to be important strengtheners of the lumbosacral joint, the proximity of the lumbosacral joint and the sacroiliac joints (and their functional interdependence) allows these ligaments to be considered here. Indeed, some of the fibres of the iliolumbar ligament cross the SIJ anteriorly, where they are in close apposition to the anterior sacroiliac ligament (Fig. 4.13). The iliolumbar ligament is very strong, preventing forward movement of L5 on the sacrum.

In the upright position, the body weight is slightly in front of the sacroiliac joints. Anterior rotation of the sacral promontory is resisted by the sacroiliac ligaments, aided by the sacrospinous and sacrotuberous ligaments (which prevent backward rotation of the apex of the sacrum).

The innervation of the ventral side of the SIJ is thought to be extensive, between L3 and S2; posteriorly, the innervation is from S1 and S2. Overall, S1 innervation is dominant, explaining the commonly experienced posterior thigh pain in sacroiliac lesions.

There are no muscles which attach to both the sacrum and the innominate. There are important muscles, however, which act over the joint. The iliopsoas flexes the hip, and exerts a major influence on lumbopelvic function. The piriformis also crosses the SIJ, arising from the anterior surface of the sacrum via several slips of muscle, traversing the sciatic notch, and inserting on the greater trochanter. It externally rotates and abducts the hip. It is in close apposition to the sciatic nerve, and may (in the 'piriformis syndrome') give rise to sciatic irritation. It thus enters into the differential diagnosis of posterior thigh pain. Confusingly, not only may sacroiliac pathology produce similar symptoms, it may also be associated with piriformis muscle spasm.

BIOMECHANICS

The anterior pillar of the lumbar spine consists of the vertebral bodies, which are specifically designed for weightbearing, and the intervertebral discs. Longitudinally applied (axial compression) loads are resisted by the flatness of the superior and inferior surfaces of the vertebral bodies, and by their internal stress-absorbing features. An outer rim of cortical bone surrounds a cancellous cavity in which vertical and horizontal bony trabeculae provide additional weight-bearing strength and dissipation of forces. Should the bony integrity be overcome by axial compression loading, an anterior wedge fracture, usually at T12, L1 or L2, is the usual result.

The intervertebral discs allow movements between vertebral bodies and, because of their inherent deformable and resilient (viscoelastic)

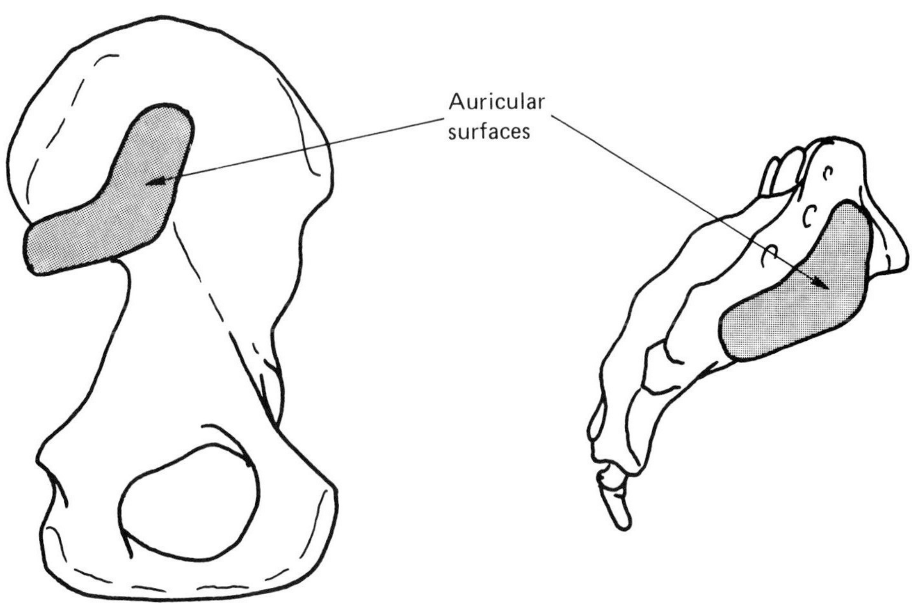

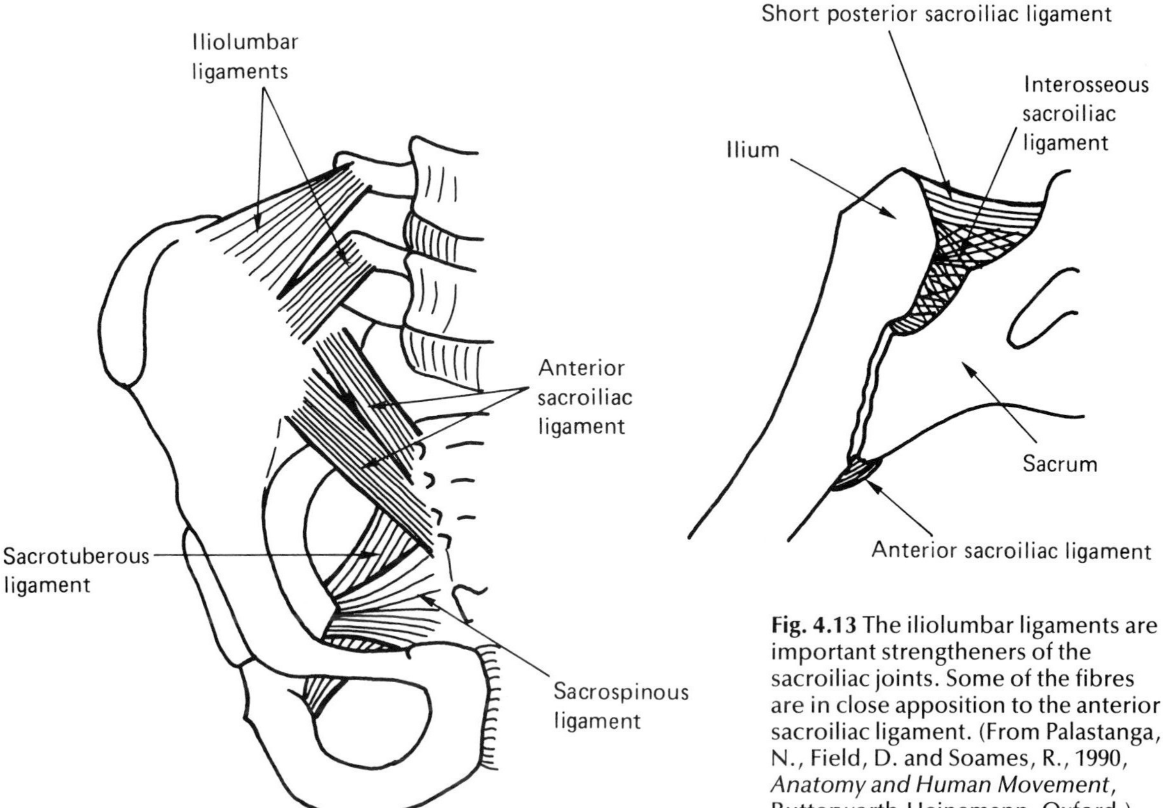

Fig. 4.13 The iliolumbar ligaments are important strengtheners of the sacroiliac joints. Some of the fibres are in close apposition to the anterior sacroiliac ligament. (From Palastanga, N., Field, D. and Soames, R., 1990, *Anatomy and Human Movement*, Butterworth-Heinemann, Oxford.)

nature, allow transmission of forces. Analysis of the microstructure of the disc reveals the typical constituents of all collagenized connective tissues: collagen fibres, a proteoglycan matrix and water. There are significant differences between the annulus and nucleus however.

(1) The **annulus fibrosus** is composed of concentric rings of collagen fibres which make up 50–60% of its dry weight, and elastic fibres which constitute up to 10%. Proteoglycans, constructed from glycosaminoglycans and core protein, make up about 20% of the dry weight in the form of aggregates. The collagen lamellae, made up predominantly of type 1 collagen in the outer fibres, are responsible for the tensile properties of the annulus, resisting the pressure imposed by the nucleus.

(2) The **nucleus pulposus** contains a high (70–90) percentage of water. Proteoglycans make up approximately 65% of the dry weight, and collagen (entirely type 2) approximately 15–20%. The fluid content is important; its presence is responsible for the biomechanical function of deformation, which is often likened to the bulging of a balloon filled with water. Deformation occurs on compression, when the balloon stretches in all directions, though the overall volume remains the same. The tension within the nucleus is produced by, and significantly affected by, the water-binding capacity of the glycosaminoglycan macromolecules.

In summary, the shock-absorbing function of the disc is due to the transmission of compression forces radially to the annulus, and superoinferiorly to the cartilaginous vertebral end-plate. Movements of the lumbar spine are resisted by the annulus. In forward flexion, for instance, the nucleus is compressed anteriorly and deformed posteriorly, thereby dissipating the forces maximally towards the posterior rim of the annulus.

The posterior pillars of the lumbar spine are the neural arches (laminae, articular processes and spinous processes), which are connected to the vertebral bodies by the pedicles and the transverse processes. As a consequence of the lumbar lordosis, the anterior longitudinal ligament contributes to the absorption of stress during weightbearing. The apophyseal joints probably do not contribute much to the absorption of such axial compression loads unless the spine is extended, or the discs are degenerate.

Although biomechanical studies of the lumbar spine tend to concentrate upon the part played by the discs and the apophyseal joints, both the laminae and the pedicles also play important roles in shock-absorption and stability. The laminae, in particular, are prone to injury if bending and rotational forces are not overcome. The pars interarticularis (otherwise referred to as the isthmus) is that part of the lamina which is interposed between the superior and inferior articular processes. At L5, body weight is transferred through the pars to the lumbosacral joint. If forces are excessive the pars may sustain a 'fatigue' or stress fracture (spondylolysis). Translatory moments may then be sufficient to produce a spondylolisthesis – a forward movement of the vertebral body (and the proximal spine) at the fracture site.

The sacroiliac joints too are shockabsorbers, particularly during jumping and other forms of vigorous exercise, they act as torque-converters during walking and running.

Movements – lumbosacral

The global movements of the lumbar spine are flexion and extension (sometimes referred to as sagittal rotations), (axial) rotations and side flexions. Some of these movements are invariably coupled (see below).

Flexion

Essentially, this is an unfolding of the lumbar lordosis – a summation of movements at each vertebral level. Flexion at L5/S1 is probably the least, but substantial variations occur throughout the population. A considerable loss of flexibility is usually seen in old age. It is probable that the degree of flexion within the lumbosacral spine is no greater than 50° (Fig. 1.16). During toe touching exercises, hip flexion contributes to the overall range of movements to a significant degree; it follows that reduction in the ability to touch one's toes may be due to tightness of the hamstrings. Clearly, estimation of flexibility of the trunk by measuring the extent to which the finger tips run down the shins is useful when comparison is made with the same measurement in the same subject on another occasion, but is not a true quantitative assessment of lumbar flexion.

Of considerable importance in the consideration of forward flexion is the concomitant anterior translation (shear) of the cephalic vertebra over the caudal vertebra and intervening disc (Fig. 1.15). Impaction of the articular surfaces of the facet joints arrests further translation. Tension in the capsules of the facet joints and the posterior ligamentous system restrains the upward and forward movements of the inferior articular processes during flexion from the upright position. Normal function of the facet joints, in association with normal disc biomechanics, is reflected in a smooth lumbopelvic rhythm on flexion; as will be described later, a disturbance of this rhythm is a manifestation of segmental instability.

It is probable that the effects of shear are maximal at L4/5, the site at which degenerative spondylolisthesis usually occurs. At this level the orientation of the facets, the relative weakness (compared with L5/S1) of the ligaments, and the larger disc space result in less effective resistance to shear forces.

The length of the lumbar spinal canal increases during flexion; of practical significance is the resulting increased tension on the dura mater.

Extension

During extension from the flexed to the upright position, posterior translation of the cephalic upon the caudal vertebrae occurs. From the (neutral) upright position, the range of extension is normally 10–20°. Hyperextension is restrained by impaction of the inferior articular processes against the laminae of the vertebrae below. Additional tension is provided by the anterior longitudinal ligament and the anterior margins of the annuli. The posterior longitudinal ligament, dura mater and ligamentum flavum are all lax in the extended position; the root canal and intervertebral foramina have reduced diameters.

Axial rotation

The combination of forces during rotation is more complex than appears at first sight, as some accompanying shear forces are applied to the discs. The range of rotation is limited to a few degrees only, and is minimal in extension as a result of the apposition of the articular surfaces of the facet joints. Movement is limited principally by impaction at the facet joints on the side to which rotation takes place, assisted by tension in the annuli fibrosi.

Side flexion

Enormous variations occur in the range of side flexion, as well as in sagittal flexion and extension, in different individuals. On average, there may be approximately 20–30° each side. At the lumbosacral joint the iliolumbar ligaments prevent much movement. Side flexion throughout the lumbar spine is greater in the upright than in the flexed position. It is accompanied by axial rotation to the contralateral side in the upper four lumbar joints; at the lumbosacral joint, however, axial rotation and side flexion are to the same side. (Some authorities consider that coupling is in the same direction during flexion throughout the lumbar spine, but in opposite directions on extension.) During side flexion the apophyseal joints on the ipsilateral side become impacted, and the intervertebral canals narrowed.

Accessory movements (joint play)

Translatory movements, otherwise referred to as shear in the transverse plane, have already been described as accompanying flexion and extension in the sagittal plane. Clinically, these movements may be demonstrated at individual segmental levels by the application of manual compression or springing to the spinous processes when the patient lies prone. This is the basis of the segmental compression test which provides information on segmental mobility (in the form of extension and translation). Application of pressure to the lateral aspect of a spinous process ('lateral' or 'transverse' springing) produces a localized rotational movement which is the basis for both segmental mobility assessment and also for Maitland-type mobilization.

Rotation in varying degrees of flexion is conveniently produced with the patient in a side lying position. To procure segmental rotation, overpressure at the (apparent) limit of range is necessary.

Joint play at the lumbosacral joint in a patient lying supine may be demonstrated by side tilting (side flexing) when the spine has been flattened, the knees flexed and hips flexed (see 'Examination: facet stress tests').

Movements – sacroiliac

Two aspects of this contentious subject are clear to the author:

1 Despite the relatively great stability afforded to the sacroiliac joint by its ligamentous system and articular surfaces, a few degrees of movement may be demonstrated.
2 Biomechanically, this movement is complicated; the situation is further confused by the plethora of terminology.

Sacroiliac biomechanics are based on the concept of multiple axes of motion; to some extent, the model shown in Fig 4.14 is an attempt to explain the clinical findings of dysfunction. **Nutation** indicates forward (ventral) movement of the sacral base (promontory) between the ilia, around an axis which is approximately transverse.

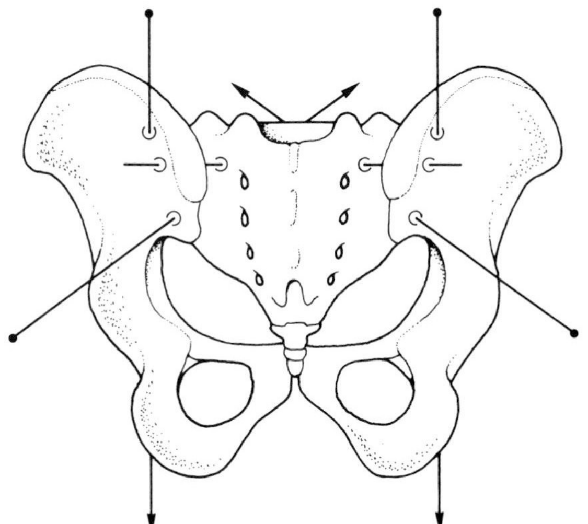

Fig. 4.14 Axes of motion in the sacroiliac joints. (From Dvorak *et al.*, 1984, *Manual Medicine*, Springer-Verlag, Berlin.)

Counternutation is the reverse movement. These movements occur during trunk bending and straightening in two-legged standing, and have been found to be of greater range in women compared with men (Brunner *et al.*, 1991). Unilateral nutation occurs in walking, and is then asynchronous with the contralateral SIJ. Movement around other axes occurs in walking, so that the sacrum may be considered to rotate and side bend (in opposite directions).

The innominate may rotate forwards around a vertical axis, producing 'gapping' between the PSIS and the sacrum; movements around this axis are otherwise referred to as in-flare and out-flare. Superoinferior translatory movements give rise to superior (cephalic) shear, and inferior (caudal) shear.

The commonly used anatomical reference point during clinical assessment of sacroiliac mobility is the PSIS (posterior superior iliac spine); movements of the PSIS may then be recorded in respect to the adjacent sacrum. **Sacroiliac dysfunction** often manifests as apparent unilateral 'locking' in nutation, such that the PSIS appears to be inferior and the ASIS superior, giving the appearance of 'pelvic torsion'; this is equivalent to the 'posterior innominate', resulting from anterior sacral torsion around an oblique axis, in osteopathic circles (though the true biomechanical situation is somewhat more complicated – sacroiliac afficionados should read Bourdillon (1992) for further information). SIJ hypomobility on the affected side is found on mobility assessment.

PATHOANATOMY AND PATHOPHYSIOLOGY

The distinction between age-related changes and pathoanatomical changes in the lumbar spine is often subtle and, unless gross macroscopic changes are evident, often somewhat arbitrary.

Age-related changes

Significant changes occur in the intervertebral discs throughout adult life. Within the nucleus, the concentration of proteoglycans decreases, the collagen content increases and the water content drops: the nucleus gradually desiccates. In the annulus too, the collagen content increases, and the elastin content decreases: the annulus stiffens, that is becomes less resilient. Cracking may occur as the annulus gradually takes an increasing share of axial loading. The vertebral bodies too become less capable of absorbing shock; the vertebral end-plates deform, and the superior and inferior surfaces of the vertebral bodies become concave. As a consequence of repeated stresses throughout adult life, **adaptive** changes occur; junctional osteophytes (either claw type or traction spurs) arise at the junction of the vertebral bodies and the discs, a condition referred to (when seen radiographically) as **spondylosis** (Fig. 1.26).

Additionally, the posterior pillars are not exempt from the ravages of time: thinning and fibrillation may occur in the articular cartilage of the apophyseal joints. Radiographically, narrowing and irregularities of the apophyseal joints, and surrounding subchondral sclerosis, are considered to constitute the typical degenerative changes of **osteoarthrosis**.

It is quite clear however that there is *no* statistical correlation between episodes of back pain and spondylosis, and it is relatively unusual for osteoarthrosis of the apophyseal joints to give rise to significant symptoms; consequently, the practice of considering these conditions to be specific disease entities should be abandoned.

Pathoanatomy

Disc prolapse

Repeated stresses, particularly torsional, upon the disc result in radial tears of the annulus. These are seen frequently at post mortem, and usually involve the posterolateral portions of the disc (the site at which nuclear herniation is common). If the injury to the annulus is severe enough the nucleus may herniate through the fissure. This often results from trunk flexion as the nucleus is displaced posteriorly in this position. Conversely, the disc is at less risk in lumbar lordosis as the posterior part of the annulus is compressed, and the nucleus displaced anteriorly.

Posterior (central) prolapse of the nucleus gives rise to the characteristic features of a 'locked back'; the fixed forward flexion and fixed side flexion cause a 'pelvic tilt'. The fixed flexion posture of the patient is explained by the fact that the tension within an established posterior prolapse of some size is increased during extension of the spine, when the posterior longitudinal ligament is lax.

Typically, continued compression of and extrusion of the nuclear material results in its propulsion from a central position, where it is restrained in flexion by the posterior longitudinal ligament, to a posterolateral, or frankly lateral position (Fig. 4.15a). Depending upon the size of the protrusion, and the capacity of the spinal canal (Porter, 1978), nerve root entrapment may then ensue (Fig. 4–15a, d). Irrespective of the proximity of the herniation to adjacent nerve roots, stretching of the dura over this space-occupying lesion within the spinal canal is a probable source of nociceptor stimulation (Fig. 4.15c); increased dural tension is then found in postures in which the lumbar lordosis is reduced. Occasionally, a massive posterior prolapse may compress the cauda equina and constitute a surgical emergency; should bladder dysfunction be ignored, and surgery delayed, a neurogenic bladder may result.

A fragment of disc may become **sequestrated** if it loses its connection with the herniated nucleus pulposus. Migration of the fragment in a cephalic or caudal direction in the spinal canal may occur. Although, at one time, it was felt that an established sequestrated fragment demanded surgical excision, it is probable that spontaneous resolution occurs in the majority of cases.

As a result of compression loading in adolescence, **disc failure** may result in vertical or peripheral (usually anterior) extrusion of the nucleus through the vertical end-plate, forming (radiographically) a

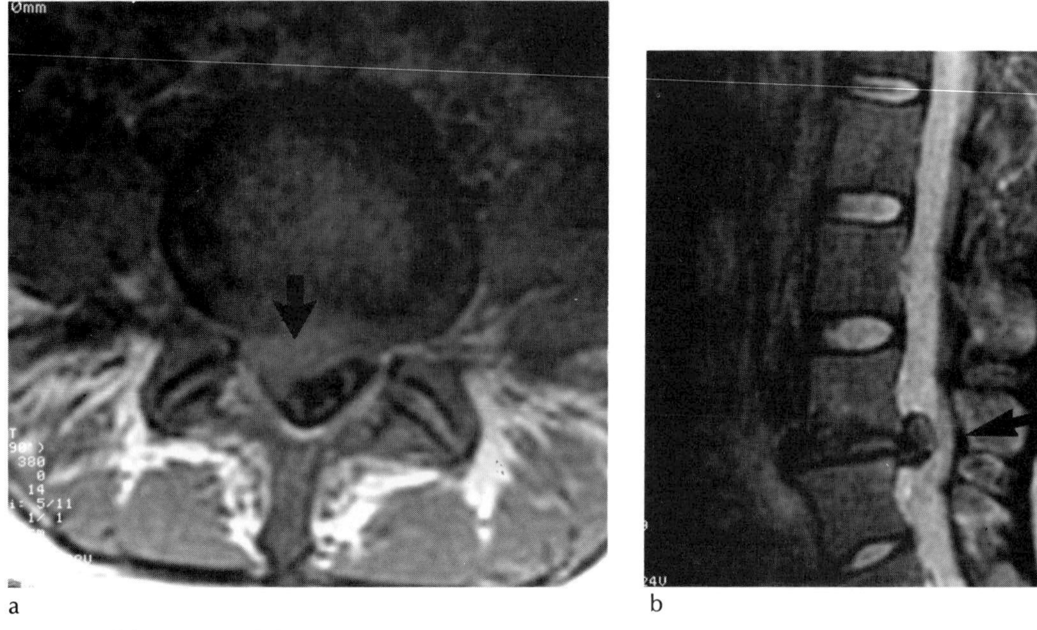

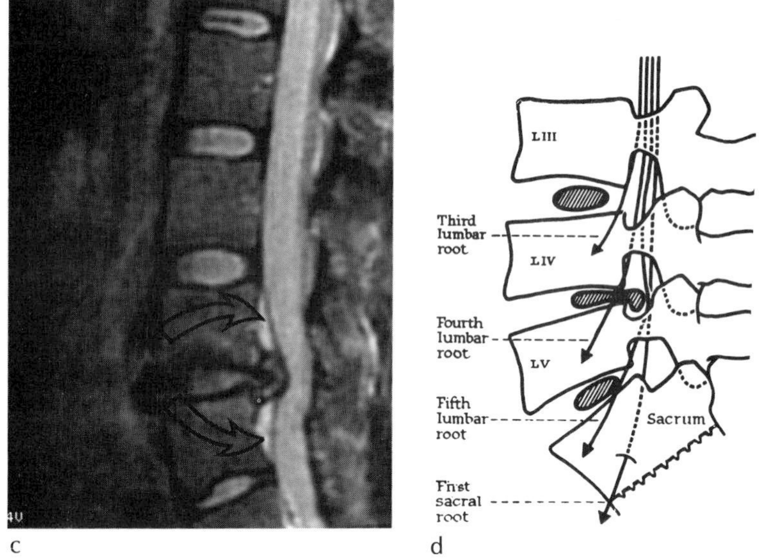

Fig. 4.15 (a–c) MRI of the lumbar spine. The axial image (a) reveals a right posterolateral disc protrusion at L4/5 with impingement upon the L5 and S1 roots and deformation of the thecal sac. The sagittal images (b, c) reveal disc degeneration, a large disc protrusion and overlying stretching of the dura. (d) Diagrammatic representation of a large L4/5 disc prolapse compressing the L5 and S1 roots (from Hutson, M.A., 1990, *Sports Injuries: Recognition and Management*, Oxford University Press, Oxford by permission of Oxford University Press).

Schmorl's node (Fig. 1.23). Posterior nuclear herniation too may arise in adolescence though it is more common from the third decade onwards.

Disc degeneration

Disc degeneration in relatively young adults has recently been identified by the use of MRI scanning. Disc narrowing is accompanied by loss of signal indicating reduced water content in the nucleus (Fig. 4.15). The increasing use of MRI is an interesting development, the more particularly as a number of patients with a clinical diagnosis of chronic ligamentous strain may be shown to have one or more degenerate lumbar discs. In these patients, it is logical to assume that nociceptive stimulation arises in those tissues which are subjected to repetitive overload – the peripheral fibres of the annuli fibrosi or the posterior ligamentous system, for instance. It has also been propounded that, although the nucleus is devoid of nerve endings, small amounts of nuclear material may be extruded through a radial fissure into the epidural space (without any significant or demonstrable herniation), thereby creating afferent stimulation. This is conjectural.

However, the prevalence of *asymptomatic* degenerate discs in the population, as determined by MRI scanning, is beginning to be appreciated. Powell *et al.* (1986) have demonstrated that asymptomatic disc degeneration was present in over one-third of women, aged 21–40, who were investigated by MRI for unassociated obstetric or gynaecological indications. Boden *et al.* (1990) also noted degeneration or bulging of a disc in 35% of asymptomatic subjects (male and female) aged 20–39 years.

Discography, CT-discography and the combination of MRI and discography all have their advocates in the demonstration of a correlation between abnormalities in a disc and *symptomatic* disease. As yet, none is satisfactory. A further consideration is the association between disc degeneration and disc bulging, and the possible subsequent development of nuclear herniation. Further longitudinal studies are required in order to evaluate the usefulness of these relatively expensive investigations in clinical situations other than in established disc prolapse and associated nerve root entrapment, in which scanning already has an established role prior to surgery.

The facet joint

A different pathological model is required to account for the frequency of clinical problems which are associated with the posterior pillars. The combination of flexion and torsion places substantial strains upon the facet joints, as a result of which acute dysfunction may occur. Although it is logical to invoke the concept of structural (pathoanatomical or pathophysiological) changes in those situations in which the onset of low back pain is acute, and disability is considerable, the nature of these changes is conjectural. Meniscoid locking (intra- or extra-articular) and intrusive articular cartilage fragments have been proposed, although proof is lacking. Clinically, dysfunction usually responds to manual therapy or anti-inflammatory injections to the joint, though this method of treatment could equally well stimulate a neurophysiological response (see below).

Sacroiliac dysfunction not uncommonly complicates lumbar spinal joint dysfunction, such that it is a *sine qua non* for a comprehensive examination of the lower back to include both the lumbar spine and the sacroiliac joints.

Segmental instability

Some situations arise in which there appear to be features of combined disc prolapse and facet joint dysfunction. The coexistence of such pathoanatomical and pathophysiological entities is not surprising in view of the interdependence of these structures in respect of stress dissipation. Over a period of time the three-joint complex may undergo excessive structural changes, resulting in multiple radial tears to the annulus, progressive inspissation of the nucleus, and increasing weakness of the restraining capsular ligaments of the facet joints. Loss of disc height is accompanied by offsetting (subluxation) of the facet joints, resulting in segmental instability. Clinically, the patient suffers from repeated bouts of back pain, and describes a 'weak back' which intrudes severely into his life style; the signs of instability are present on examination. Subsequently, increasing degenerative changes may occur in response to the excessive shear forces associated with abnormal spinal biomechanics.

Unless symptomatic stenotic changes in the spinal or lateral canals supervene, the prognosis for segmental instability is often an improving situation in late middle age and beyond, as the spine stiffens and the patient becomes less inclined to impart excessive strains upon it.

Spinal stenosis

It has been well established that both the incidence of myelopathy, when secondary to cervical spondylosis, and the incidence of common lumbar syndromes are higher when the mid-sagittal diameters of the spinal canals at the respective levels are narrow. Some patients have a congenitally narrow spinal canal. On the other hand, substantive hypertrophic changes, particularly to the inferior articular processes, may reduce the capacity of the spinal canal, giving rise to developmental **central** (or 'laminar') spinal stenosis. Cauda equina compression gives rise to sciatic symptoms ('neurogenic claudication') which are typically aggravated by increasing the lumbar lordosis (when the canal becomes narrower), for instance by walking downhill, and improved or relieved entirely by forward flexion of the spine (when the canal lengthens and widens). Various tests have been devised to differentiate between intermittent claudication (due to arterial insufficiency in the legs) and neurogenic claudication. For instance, cycling (performed on a 'static' cycle for investigative purposes) is well tolerated in spinal stenosis, whereas, in the presence of intermittent claudication, the claudicant pattern of leg pain soon emerges; the discriminant value is reinforced if the patient leans forward in the saddle when cycling.

Alternatively, gross diminution in the available space for the nerve roots in the root canals, and at the intervertebral foramina, causes **lateral** canal stenosis. This is usually associated with disc narrowing, superior migration of the superior articular facets, and hypertrophic osteophytosis of these facets (Fig. 4.16a). Occasionally, gross reactive ossification around the facet joints is seen in relatively young adults when it is due to repetitive rotational stress during sport (Fig. 4.16b).

A spondylolisthesis, whether isthmic (that is, secondary to a spondylolysis), or degenerative, may also exert traction on the nerve roots by contributing to significant narrowing of the central or lateral canals.

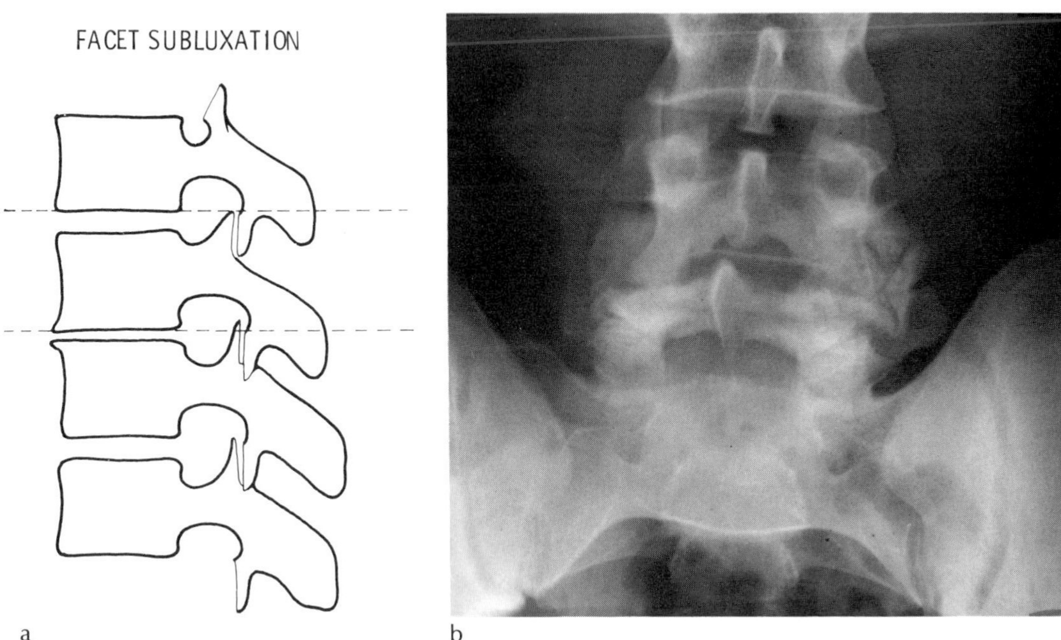

Fig. 4.16 (a) Disc narrowing is associated with superior migration of the superior articular facets. (b) Periarticular ossification (around the L4/5 apophyseal joints) in this professional soccer player is a reaction to repetitive rotational stress.

Spondylolysis

Overload of the pars interarticularis (isthmus) of a distal lumbar vertebra may give rise to a stress (fatigue) fracture. In the established case the fracture is seen radiographically as a lytic defect, when it is referred to as a spondylolysis. It is visible on a lateral X-ray of the lumbar spine if bilateral (Fig. 4.17), and on the relevant oblique view if unilateral, when its appearance is often referred to as a Scottie dog with a collar (see Fig. 4.18a, b). A pre-radiological stress injury may be revealed by bone scanning (scintigraphy).

Although spondylolysis was considered at one time to be congenital, it is now known to occur during childhood and adolescence. It has a peak incidence between the ages of 5 and 7, when there appears to be a definite (hereditary) diathesis. A further peak occurs in puberty and early adolescence when it is often symptomatic, and probably caused by sports overload – most often in sports such as gymnastics and high jumping which necessitate repeated hyperextension, though it is also seen in other sports as a

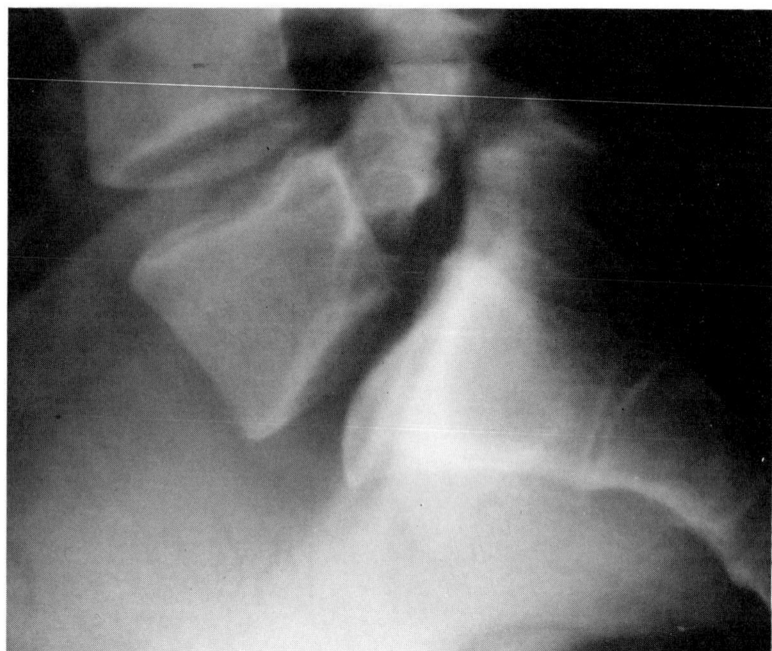

Fig. 4.17 On this lateral X-ray of the lumbar spine a spondylolysis at L5 is associated with a grade 1 spondylolisthesis.

result of repeated flexion and torsional stresses (Fig. 4.19). Its incidence varies between 2 and 6% in the general population, rising to 11% in selected groups (such as young female gymnasts – Jackson *et al.*, 1976). Overall, it is more common in males and, interestingly, there are extremely wide ethnic variations (for instance, a high incidence amongst Eskimos). It is most common at L5 but also occurs at L4 and L3. There is an increased incidence in patients with neural arch defects, such as spina bifida occulta, and in the presence of long transverse processes at L5. A variant of a spondylolysis is an elongated and narrowed isthmus which is probably also a response to overload.

Spondylolisthesis

A significant minority of patients with a spondylolysis progress to listhesis – a forward slip of the body of the vertebra at the site of the fracture (Fig. 4.17). This slip probably occurs within a few years of the fracture, and is unlikely to arise after the age of 18. It is graded according to the percentage, or degree, of forward displacement of the upper vertebra upon the lower. For instance, a grade I (up to 25%) slip is common, and often asymptomatic. A grade II (50%) slip is more worrisome, and is likely to be associated with tight hamstrings and a typical listhetic posture.

Over the age of 50, a spondylolisthesis may be secondary to degenerative changes in the lumbar spine, often at L4/5.

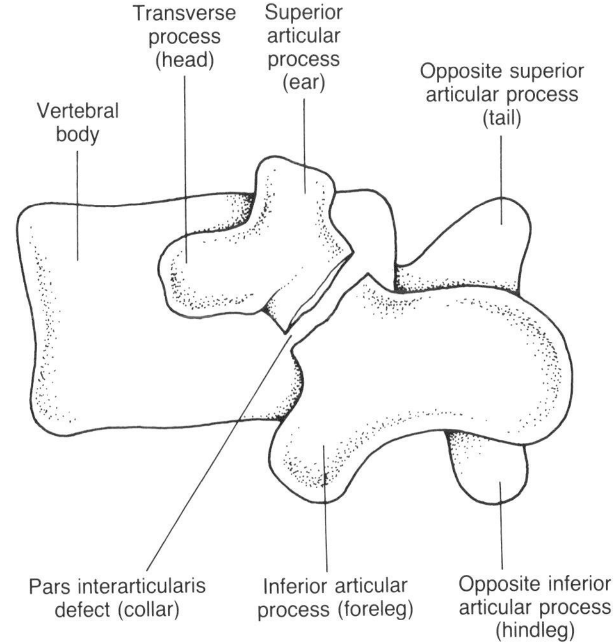

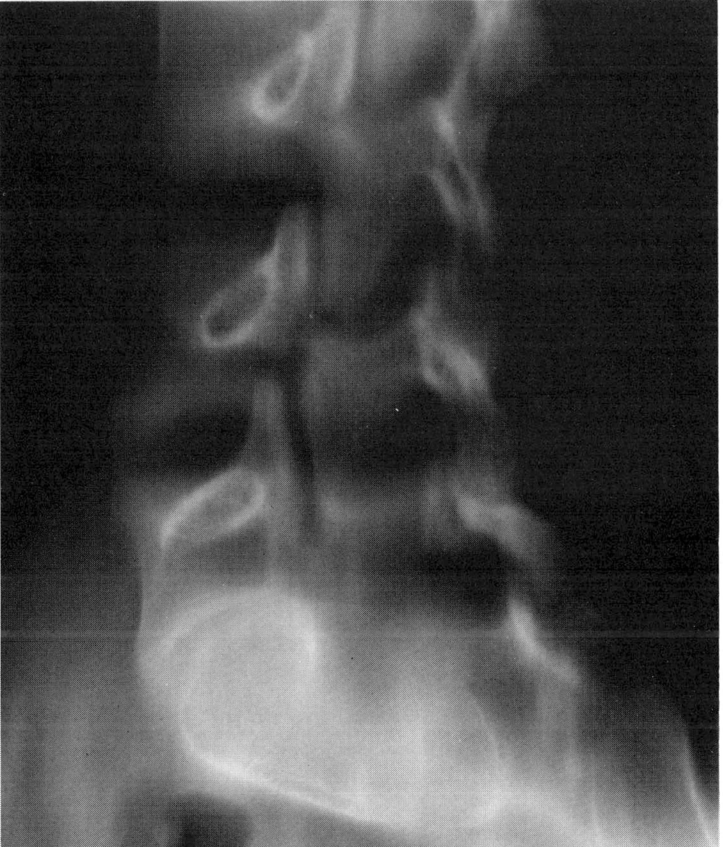

Fig. 4.18 (a) A stress fracture in the lumbar spine (spondylolysis) affects the isthmus (pars interarticularis) of the neural arch. A Scottie dog with a collar is seen on the oblique X-ray (Hutson, 1990 by permission of Oxford University Press). (b) A tomogram reveals a spondylolysis at L4.

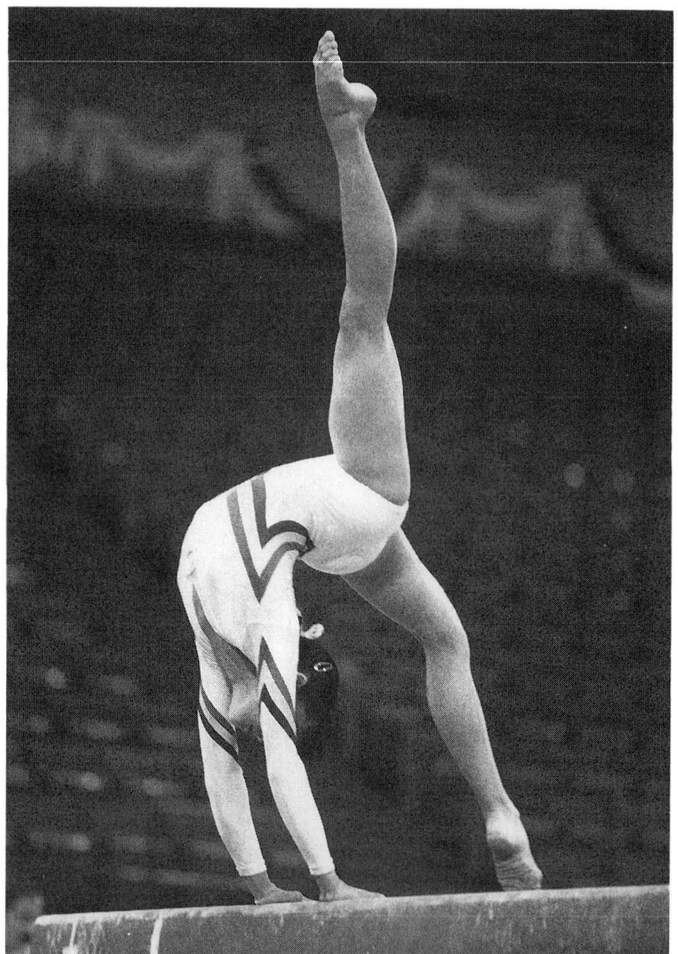

Fig. 4.19 There is a relatively high incidence of spondylolysis in sports such as gymnastics which demand repetitive hyperextension of the lumbar spine. (By permission of Supersoft Photography.)

Pathophysiology

Historically, it has been common practice to ascribe the cause of **radicular** symptoms to **compression** of the nerve roots. Undoubtedly, this occurs when the root canals or foramina are narrowed by hypertrophic osteophytosis or by space-occupying lesions such as tumours or disc protrusions. Under these circumstances, root compression is intensified, and symptoms are provoked, by spinal extension and ipsilateral side flexion, and by the development of oedema which is a secondary phenomenon.

Abnormal increases in **root tension** may also provoke symptoms in susceptible individuals. Experimental traction on nerve roots which have previously been affected by disc herniation has been shown to provoke sciatica (Macnab). Mechanical stimulation of nerves elsewhere in the body, however, usually gives rise to dysaesthesiae only. Thus, other factors which might be involved in the causation of sciatica at nerve root level have been sought – dural pressure, chemical stimulation, autoimmune reactions and ischaemia, for instance. Increased tension on the nerve root by neck flexion and by straight leg raising is accompanied by **dural tension**. The dura is innervated by the sinuvertebral nerve and is sensitive to both mechanical and chemical stimulation. Transient relief from sciatica due to disc prolapse may be gained by caudal epidural injections of local anaesthetic, and permanent improvement is often found with the addition of steroids. It is probable, therefore, that dural irritation plays a significant part in the pathogenesis of radicular pain. **Chemical stimulation** and a subsequent inflammatory reaction may be caused by the release of chemicals from a nuclear extrusion (McCarron *et al.*, 1987).

Disturbances with nutrition of a nerve root may well result from vascular impairment. Intraneural oedema and fibrosis, associated with reduction in axonal transmission, are most likely to arise in situations in which the root is subjected to repeated mechanical pressure. Chronic inflammatory changes and venous obstruction are probably self-perpetuating in some patients, but may respond (as in acute lesions) to epidural procaine and steroid injections.

PAIN SOURCE AND PAIN PERCEPTION

Source

Free nerve endings have been identified in all tissues other than bone and the nucleus pulposus (Bogduk *et al.*, 1991; Wyke, 1987). Various structures in the lumbar spine have been demonstrated to be the potential source of lumbar pain by noxious or mechanical stimulation. Kellgren (1939) invoked low back and **referred** pain by injecting the interspinous ligaments with hypertonic saline. Feinstein mapped out areas of referred pain, which he noted to be of an overlapping segmental type yet differing from conventional dermatomes, following paravertebral injections of hypertonic saline; areas of hypoaesthesia and deep tenderness were detected within the areas of referred pain (Feinstein *et al.*, 1954). Hackett (1956) also produced pain in the lower limbs by injecting the sacroiliac and lumbosacral ligaments. McCall *et al.* (1979) and Mooney and Robertson (1976) have produced pain in the lower back, buttock and thigh by injecting the apophyseal joints. Fairbank *et al.* (1981) also identified the apophyseal joints as the source of pain in a proportion of patients suffering from their first attack of low back pain who were subjected to, and responded to, local anaesthetic injection into the maximally tender lumbar apophyseal joints under X-ray control.

Smyth and Wright (1958) induced buttock and thigh pain by traction on the dura. Epidural injections of local anaesthetic have been known to reduce or abolish pain, in the presence of disc prolapse, for many decades (Cyriax, 1982).

Wiberg (1947) demonstrated the development of low back pain by pressure on the annulus fibrosus. The relatively modern technique of discography depends, in part, on pain induction following intradiscal injection (even occurring in an apparently normal disc as a 'false positive' result). Rydevik *et al.* (1984) have shown that the nerve roots, particularly the dorsal roots, are sensitive to ischaemia. Troup (1986) has emphasized that both compression of and tension upon nerve roots cause pain.

Porter (1986) has emphasized the importance of the arterial supply to the cord, and the complexity of the venous channels in the epidural space, in the pathogenesis of spinal stenosis.

Pain perception

The nociceptive system converts the stimulation of nerve endings, via various neurotransmitters, to the perception of pain. It is clear that the strength of pain perception in different individuals is not proportional to the stimulus. Modification of the impulses on their way through the sensory afferents to the posterior horn, and onwards to higher centres, takes place at various levels. Some control is exerted by the neurotransmitters – opiate-like substances of the endorphin class. Self-regulation is possible; a well-recognized elevation of endorphins is produced by regular exercise, for instance. The gate theory of Melzack and Wall (1965) is based on the modulation of the activity of this nociceptive system by stimuli from other sources, peripheral or central. This theory explains the modification of pain perception by the stimulation of mechanoreceptors, for instance by the application of pressure, heat, massage and vibration. Regrettably, perhaps, in other subjects, pain enhancement may occur as a result of a summation or 'facilitation' mechanism.

CONCEPTS – DYSFUNCTION AND ILLNESS

Osteopathic diagnosis

In spite of the well-recognized pathoanatomical and pathophysiological changes which may contribute substantially to the perception of pain via the nociceptive system, their presence in many patients with spinal complaints may be largely irrelevant. For instance, spinal joint dysfunction is one of the commonest causes of spinal pain but its incidence does not correlate well with radiographic degenerative changes or known structural pathoanatomical disease processes. In respect of pre-existing changes, however, loss of shock-absorption in the motion segment should be considered to be one of the numerous factors involved in the aetiology of joint dysfunction.

This concept of reversible spinal (joint) dysfunction – a neuromuscular or neurophysiological disorder – and its causal relationship to the interaction between the stresses imposed upon the individual and the individual's vulnerability is not new but is certainly gaining in respectability. It combines a *functional* approach to the diagnosis of musculoskeletal lesions with a *holistic* approach to management (based, nevertheless, upon segmental spinal mobilization allied to restoration of normal muscle function). There is little difference between the condition described here as spinal (facet) joint dysfunction and the 'osteopathic lesion'.

Illness behaviour

Low back disability has increased alarmingly over the past three decades, yet there is no sound evidence that low back and radicular pain, or pathological changes, have increased in incidence. The conclusion to be drawn is that *the pattern of illness or pain behaviour has changed.* Various factors may be identified to explain this concept.

(1) Iatrogenic disease

Medical practitioners find it convenient to explain back pain by reference to a slipped, ruptured, or prolapsed disc – based on a radiologist's report of 'disc narrowing' or 'degeneration'. This often delays accurate diagnosis and appropriate management. In a proportion of cases the emotive label of 'disc injury' or 'rupture' suggests culpability, and leads to a determined effort by the patient towards retribution. In this respect, the scenario is similar to some cases of 'repetitive strain injury', in which an employer may be held liable for the condition.

(2) Inappropriate management

This is a further iatrogenic source. Bed rest is often advocated as the primary therapeutic strategy for moderately severe back pain. Not only is there scant evidence for the usefulness of this modality (admittedly disc pressures are lower, though a significant proportion of patients have more pain on lying), but the debilitating effects may be profound. Many patients remain disenchanted with the quality of medical advice they receive.

(3) Socioeconomic factors

Both medical assessment and treatment are influenced more by the patient's distress and illness behaviour than by the actual physical disorder (Waddell 1987). The basis for this view, which is difficult to fault, is that socioeconomic factors have appeared to play an increasing role (at least in post-war Britain). Abnormal (inappropriate or exaggerated) behavioural reactions to examination are often a response to interacting social and physical factors, rather than a true 'malingering' or 'litigation-minded' attitude. In some cases the 'sick role' adopted by patients (a concept beloved of sociologists) is obvious to relatively untrained observers. 'Acceptable' reactions are observed, however, in the majority of patients, for whom management of the physical aspect of their illness becomes relatively more straightforward.

Waddell advocates a holistic approach to the management of low back pain, using a 'biopsychosocial' model which includes physical, physiologic, and social elements rather than a disease, or pathological model which (he considers) often depends on a nominal rather than a substantive diagnosis. These views on an active approach using ergonomics, exercises and behavioural therapy should, however, be allied to greater expertise amongst physicians and therapists in the art of making diagnoses based on detailed examination procedures (the thrust of this text), thereby avoiding the pitfall of constructing non-specific strategies based on the concept of 'low back syndromes'.

HISTORY

Much may be learnt from the first contact with the patient, and from his account of the history of the condition. Of particular value is the style of presentation of the history, and the patient's responses to further questioning and to the subsequent examination. These behavioural characteristics have already been referred to, and are elaborated upon in the section on Examination below. In addition to the general comments made in Chapter 1 in respect of the history, the following points are worthy of note.

Attitudes

The attitude of the clinician or therapist is the most important factor in the establishment of a rapport with the patient. Once the initial feeling of awe or uncertainty has been overcome the patient seeks, consciously or unconsciously, signs of interest and empathy from the examiner. Although the back problem may be seen as a challenge, the comment of Porter (1986) is appropriate: 'The clinician's heart should be gladdened, not saddened, by the patient with backache'. Successful management demands positivity on the part of the clinician and, particularly, the therapist.

Back pain characteristics

Onset

Patients may recall a sudden onset of pain on forward flexion of the trunk, possibly with a twisting element. Alternatively, there may be an insidious onset when they often *associate* pain with, and ascribe causation (rightly or wrongly) to circumstances such as a change of car or to a specific event such as an epidural injection during the second stage of labour. In respect to child-rearing, the female lumbar spine and pelvis are subjected to considerable strains. MacArthur *et al.* (1990) have confirmed an association between obstetric epidural anaesthesia and long-term backache, after normal and abnormal vaginal deliveries, and emergency caesarian sections. Irrespective of the type of delivery, the puerperium necessitates repetitive trunk flexion over a cot. Following caesarian section an additional stress upon the spine is the postoperative period which is spent in a strange (hospital) bed with weakened abdominal muscles.

The relationship with trauma, for instance an industrial accident or an RTA, may have an obvious bearing on culpability and litigation. In its own right, a rear-end vehicle collision, or a heavy fall (on a slippery floor) on to the coccyx, may give rise to joint dysfunction, ligament strain or disc disturbance.

Past history

It is particularly important to establish a pattern, should one exist, to the past history of backache or back pain. This is of specific relevance to the second phase of management – re-establishment of stability.

Site

In acute 'lumbago', and particularly if there is an associated pelvic tilt, pain may be felt across the lower back and around the iliac crests. Radiation to both thighs is not uncommon. A massive disc prolapse causing cauda equina compression commonly gives rise to low back pain and bilateral sciatica, and symptoms of bladder dysfunction, such as dribbling.

Once the acute phase is over, pain tends to become predominantly unilateral. Pain felt in the sacroiliac region is particularly common, but should not be assumed necessarily to be of sacroiliac origin – one of the commonest errors in a casual approach to low back problems. Patients are often seen in the subacute phase when their complaints are of pain felt in the sacroiliac region radiating to the buttock and posterior thigh. Without a careful examination routine this may prove to be one of the most difficult scenarios in musculoskeletal medicine to interpret – the differential diagnosis is extensive. It is this type of situation in which a historical perspective is paramount. Direct questions need to be asked, such as was there preceding lumbosacral pain, pelvic tilt, or marked restriction in flexibility?

If pain radiates to the thigh or beyond, its location and character should be recorded as accurately as possible. Referred pain is usually aching in type and diffuse in nature – that is, difficult to localize. Radicular pain is sharper or more intense, and more specific to a dermatome. It is nearly always felt below the knee (apart from L3 root compression when pain is felt in the anterior thigh). Even so, it is unwise to rely on a constant distribution of radicular pain.

Usually, L4 radicular pain is felt predominantly in the anterolateral thigh and knee (mimicking hip joint pain), and also in the anteromedial shin. L5 radicular pain radiates along the posterolateral aspect of the upper and lower leg to the dorsum of the foot and hallux. S1 radicular pain is felt posteriorly in the limb, radiating to the heel and lateral border of the foot. Dysaesthesiae – burning, tingling, and 'pins and needles' – and numbness are common accompaniments, whatever the dermatome.

Associations

The association between back pain and everyday activities is noted. With respect to lumbar flexion, patients may be uncertain as to whether their symptoms are worse on bending when they have learnt to maintain their lumbar lordosis; if asked about the inconvenience of putting on socks, stockings, or tights, however, this often prompts an admission of pain when due to disc prolapse or facet joint lesions.

Although recumbency is often expected to relieve 'mechanical' back and leg pain, nocturnal pain is troublesome in a significant percentage of patients; for instance, sciatica due to lateral canal stenosis (often with a superimposed disc bulge) may be very painful at night. However, in comparison with spinal malignancy which enters into the differential diagnosis when pain interrupts sleep, a relationship with posture during daily activities may be established. Diffuse backache which has been present for months, possibly with a history of sciatic aching alternating from one leg to another, and with marked morning stiffness and a tendency to be easier with exercise, is typical of ankylosing spondylitis.

Many patients with chronic ligamentous insufficiency are happiest when 'pottering about' rather than when immobile. The relationship to activity and inactivity, for instance in the 'cocktail party' syndrome and the 'theatre-goers' syndrome, should be deduced at this stage.

The apparent claudicant nature of spinal stenosis should be established, if necessary by direct questioning on the relationship of back or leg pain to walking. A useful ancillary question is: 'What makes it easier?'. If sitting is the most comfortable and restful position, the diagnoses of spinal stenosis and L3/4 disc herniation (giving rise to L4 root entrapment) spring to mind.

A positive impulse pain (that is, pain on sneezing, coughing or straining) suggests a diagnosis of disc herniation, though it may be positive in relatively severe facet dysfunction too. The relationship to sport, recreational exercise and occupation may be revealing. Exercise-dependent backache in the adolescent suggests a possible spondylolysis. Exercise-related backache in the middle-aged suggests degenerative changes in the apophyseal joints. An association between low backache and prolonged sitting, either in the workplace or in a car, is very common. However, as sitting is biomechanically disadvantageous to most of the soft tissue components of the lumbar spine, discomfort on sitting does not have a very high discriminant value. An ergonomic analysis demands further detailed questioning, of particular relevance to secretaries or VDU operatives, for instance, who spend their working days sitting at desks.

Any symptoms which suggest visceral or systemic disturbances are noted.

EXAMINATION

Standing

(1) Posture

The obvious discomfort of a patient with a list or pelvic tilt (Fig. 4.20) indicates a probable disc prolapse. Some patients prefer to stand, rather than sit, to be interviewed, and usually adopt an attitude of least discomfort by leaning on a proffered chair. When undressed, a

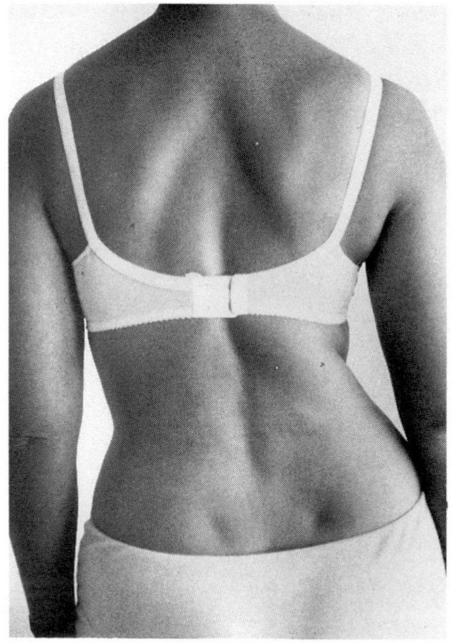

Fig. 4.20 A list or pelvic tilt of this magnitude indicates a probable disc prolapse.

scoliosis is usually obvious, but may be confirmed by the observation of asymmetry of the skin creases at the waist. A fixed flexion posture may be present, when a virtually simean attitude may give the patient the most ease.

Asymmetry of the two innominates, in the form of a pelvic torsion, is a common finding; for instance, the anterior superior iliac spine may appear to be higher and the PSIS lower on the same side. Pelvic torsion may be congenital or due to a (treatable) sacroiliac dysfunction. Often the lower of the two PSISs has a less obvious dimple overlying it, possibly due to a little surrounding oedema, thereby emphasizing the asymmetry.

Dural tension is tested by flexion of the neck; reproduction of low back or leg pain is pathognomonic of a disc prolapse.

(2) Spinal mobility

The patient is asked, in turn, to forward flex his trunk and return to the upright position, to extend and return, then side flex to the right and finally side flex to the left (Fig. 4.21). Forward flexion of the trunk is a most valuable test. The 'normal' range of flexion may be unknown to the examiner though the patient is usually able to tell whether it is restricted or not. For the purpose of comparison with future examination findings (that is, to monitor progress), the most practical method of assessment is to record the topographical level down the legs (for instance, 'toes' or 'mid-shins', Fig. 4.21a)) to which the fingers reach. More accurate measurements of distances or angles are unnecessary as the ability to bend forwards is also dependent upon pelvic rotation and hamstrings flexibility.

Of greater value, perhaps, is the rhythm (or loss of it) with which flexion is accomplished. Does the lumbar lordosis unfold, or is it maintained, for example? Deviation to left or right, accompanied by paraspinal muscle spasm, indicates a probable disc herniation.

a

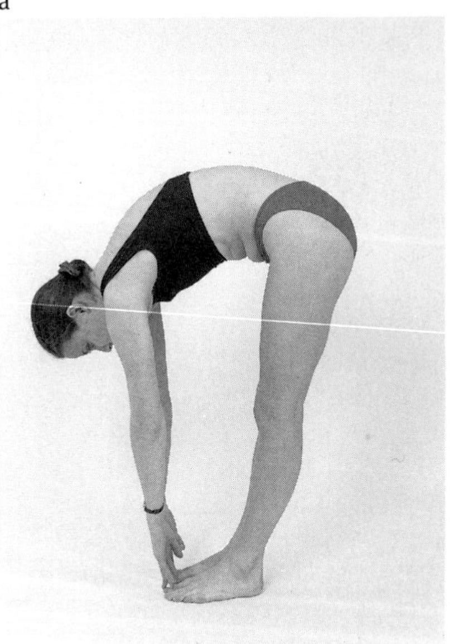

b

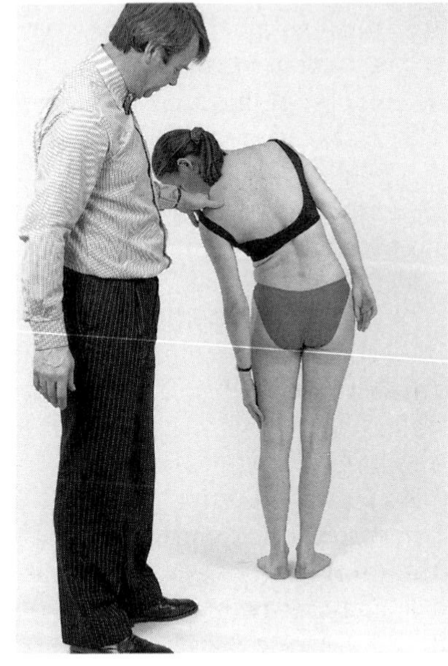

Fig. 4.21 (a) Trunk flexion – 'fingers to toes'. (b) Trunk side flexion.

Although a 'jerk' or 'catch' may be present on forward flexion, it is usually more obvious during recovery from the flexed position. This hesitancy may be accompanied by temporary deviation to one side or the other, and is indicative of segmental instability. In the more severe case, a patient (often in his fifties or sixties) may use his hands, placed on the knees and thighs, to 'climb up his legs'. The patient is asked whether flexion is painful, and also where the pain is felt. Lumbar flexion increases nerve root tension.

Extension from the upright position may be restricted, or lost altogether. The examiner wishes to know whether extension reproduces the back or leg pain. When sciatica is due to lateral canal stenosis, the affected nerve is 'pinched' by extension and by ipsilateral flexion.

Side flexions are tested (Fig. 4.21b). Not uncommonly, some degree of fixed side flexion (indicating loss of side flexion to the other side) accompanies the loss of lordosis in a patient with a pelvic tilt. Ipsilateral side flexion is often painful and restricted in the presence of a posterolateral disc prolapse, particularly if the nerve root is compressed.

(3) Palpation

The ledge, which is caused by the prominent spinous process at the level of a spondylolisthesis, is best felt in the standing position. In sacroiliac disorders of a 'mechanical' nature, the PSIS may be exquisitely tender to palpation.

(4) Sacroiliac mobility

The movement of each innominate bone, in turn, is assessed by noting its relationship to the sacrum during ipsilateral hip (and knee) flexion to 90° (the **standing hip-flexion test**). The examiner uses his thumbs, placing one on the sacrum at the S1 level and the other on the PSIS. Movement of the PSIS in a caudal direction is the normal finding when the hip is flexed (Fig. 4.22a); if this movement is restricted, or if the PSIS moves in a cephalic direction, when compared subsequently with the other side, 'blockage' or dysfunction of the SIJ is present (Fig. 4.22b).

The patient is then asked to flex her spine while the examiner's thumbs are placed on each of the two PSISs. If dysfunction exists, the thumb on the PSIS of the affected side will rise relative to the normal side. This test is the equivalent, in the standing position, of the Pièdallu test (see below) performed in the sitting position. A positive test for dysfunction on the affected side denotes 'adherence' of the ilium to the sacrum, whereas normal posterior rotation of the ilium on the sacrum is reflected in a caudal movement of the PSIS. These tests are sometimes referred to as the standing (or sitting) forward flexion tests (FFTs).

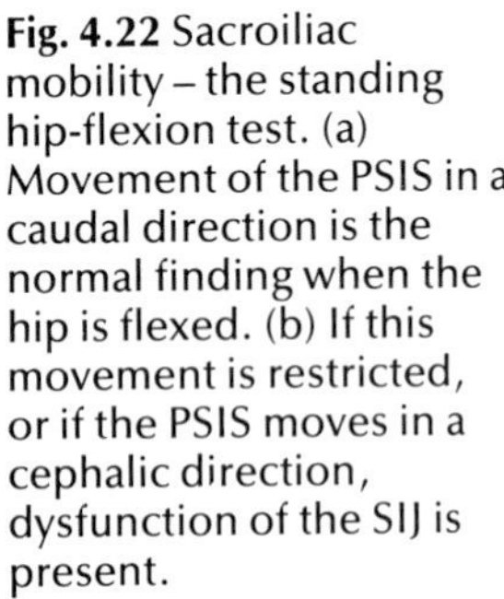

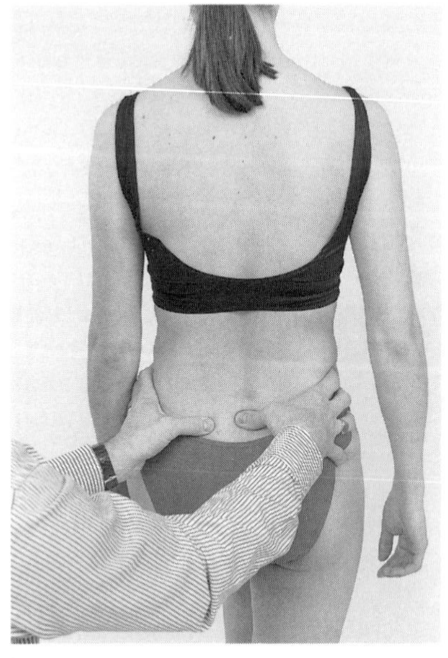

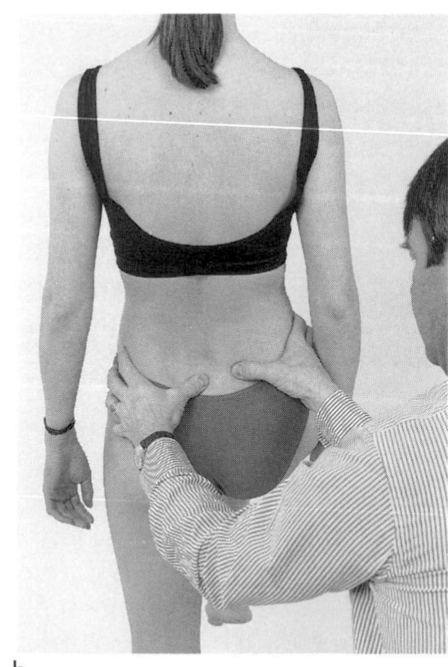

Fig. 4.22 Sacroiliac mobility – the standing hip-flexion test. (a) Movement of the PSIS in a caudal direction is the normal finding when the hip is flexed. (b) If this movement is restricted, or if the PSIS moves in a cephalic direction, dysfunction of the SIJ is present.

A further test may be performed by noting the lateral movement of the ischial tuberosity on ipsilateral hip flexion, and then comparing with the same test performed on the other side. Restricted lateral movement of the ischial tuberosity is a sign of sacroiliac dysfunction.

(5) Unilateral hyperextension test

This is a useful test when there is a suspicion of a recent spondylolysis. The spine is extended, first when standing on one leg, then on the other (Fig. 4.23). The test is positive, indicating a probable stress

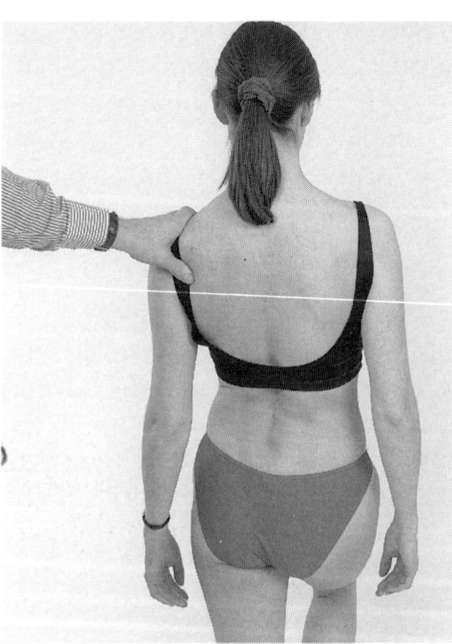

Fig. 4.23 Lumbar spine – the unilateral hyperextension test.

injury to the pars interarticularis of one of the lower lumbar vertebrae, if unilateral low back pain is accentuated when weightbearing on the affected side.

(6) Calf muscle power

The most sensitive gauge of calf power is to ask the patient to stand on one leg, thence on to tiptoe. Raising and lowering of the leg may be repeated in quick succession up to six times, and compared with the other leg. In this context, weakness denotes an S1 root palsy.

Supine

(1) Comfort

If a disc herniation, particularly at the L3–4 level, has caused a loss of lordosis, the patient may be unable to lie flat without flexing one or both hips.

(2) Leg length

Although criticized as being a crude method of assessment, 'eyeballing' the difference in leg lengths at the medial malleoli, after satisfying oneself of level ASISs, is probably as good a clinical method as any other. 'Apparent' leg length inequality may disappear if the patient is asked to sit up – a sign of sacroiliac dysfunction.

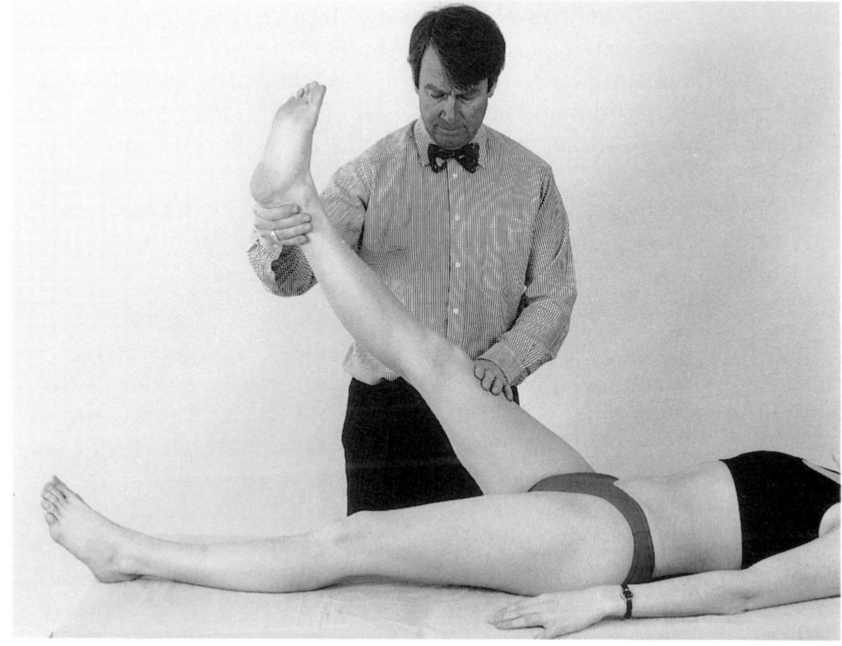

Fig. 4.24 Lumbar spine – straight leg raise.

(3) Straight leg raise (SLR)

When used as a test for neural tension (tension on the L5 and sacral nerve roots, and their dural investments) this test has considerable discriminant value (Fig. 4.24). Its sensitivity in a patient with a disc herniation is dependent upon a careful examination technique, and a relaxed patient; when degenerative changes cause root entrapment in the elderly, it is less sensitive.

Its specificity may be improved by modifications such as the bowstring test, and by passive dorsiflexion of the ankle, if the test is equivocal initially. The bowstring test is useful if hamstring tightness (for instance, when secondary to recent injury) is considered to be a possibility. The knee should be flexed a little once painful limitation of SLR has been reached, and the popliteal nerve is then stretched by direct pressure upon it. Further pain represents a positive bowstring test (indicating positive neural tension). Alternatively, passive dorsiflexion of the ankle may be used instead of popliteal nerve pressure.

To prevent movement at the lumbosacral and sacroiliac joints during straight leg raise, the buttock should not be allowed to rise from the couch. Even so, pain in the buttock and thigh may be felt at the end-range of SLR with some sacroiliac lesions, particularly chronic ligamentous strain. With experience and care, the SLR test, when taken in conjunction with the bilateral SLR test (lumbosacral stress test – see below), has considerable predictive value.

Often there is little doubt in respect of genuine restriction of SLR, which may be measured as the angle imparted by the leg against the horizontal; for instance, painful restriction to 45° or less is an unequivocal sign and strongly suggests a herniated nucleus pulposus. Sequential measurements during treatment for an HNP (herniation of the nucleus pulposus) are a sensitive guide to progress. Crossover (syn. 'crossed leg', 'crossed sciatica') pain is pathognomonic of a disc prolapse – pain reproduction by SLR of the non-affected contralateral leg.

If there is doubt in respect of the conclusions to be drawn from the SLR test, a diagnostic epidural injection may then be of some help.

(4) Lumbosacral stress test (bilateral SLR)

Using Mennell's nomenclature and ideology, this test, which is performed when the examiner holds both legs by the ankles or heels and raises them into the air, stresses the lumbosacral joint initially (Fig. 4.25). By increasing the height of the outstretched legs, the lumbar spine becomes increasingly flexed, and stress is imparted to the proximal lumbar joints. It is not a test for neural tension. Although stress is also imparted to the sacroiliac joints, its principal use is to detect strain at the lumbosacral segment (when it is usually due to degenerative changes, or joint dysfunction), and thus to have a discriminant value in those patients who experience painful

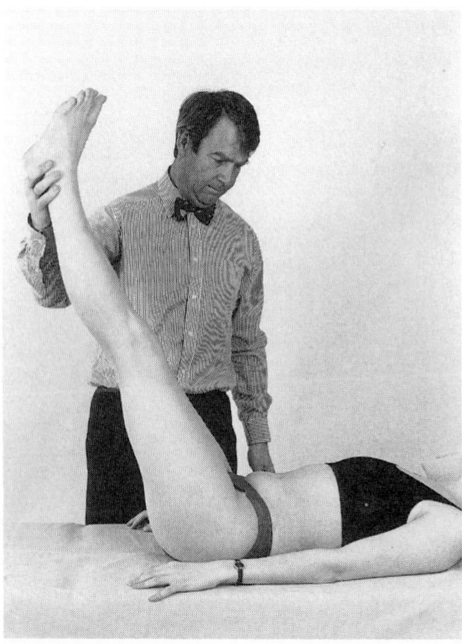

Fig. 4.25 Lumbar spine – the lumbosacral stress test.

restriction of trunk flexion from the standing position. It is perhaps remarkable that, under certain circumstances, (unilateral) SLR may be unrestricted at 80–90° each side yet the lumbosacral stress test is painful at 60°.

Under other circumstances, these findings may be reversed: a patient with a unilaterally restricted SLR due to neural tension may exhibit a greater range of bilateral SLR .

(5) Hip mobility and sacroiliac stress

Passive hip flexion should be assessed; its importance is twofold. First, in conjunction with passive internal rotation, it is a sensitive test for early hip joint disease. Secondly, the combination of painful restriction of hip flexion and restricted SLR – the 'sign of the buttock' according to Cyriax (1982) – implies pathology in the buttock, for instance gluteal bursitis, rather than root irritation.

Passive external rotation, internal rotation, abduction and adduction of the hip are tested with the hip flexed to approximately 45° and the knee flexed to 90°. The capsular pattern of restriction of hip joint mobility, found in osteoarthritis of the hip, for instance, is early loss of flexion, internal rotation and abduction; pain at end-range is usually felt in the groin. Painful restriction of internal rotation, in isolation, may be an early sign of hip disease (particularly if the discomfort is felt in the groin), or of SIJ dysfunction (when the discomfort is usually felt over the SIJ, but sometimes in the groin), or of piriformis muscle spasm (in which case the discomfort is felt in the buttock).

Patrick's test is occasionally useful. The hip is flexed, abducted and externally rotated, so that the lateral malleolus rests on the contralateral knee. It is usually used as a screening test for hip disease, but pressure on the medial aspect of the ipsilateral knee may aggravate SIJ pain.

The most useful stress test for sacroiliac ligamentous strain, however, is one that is eponymously associated with M. J. Ongley and may be referred to as the MJO test; it is otherwise referred to as the **hip flexion-adduction test**. Initially, the hip is flexed to 90° and adducted; axial compression along the length of the femur stresses the sacroiliac ligaments, and particularly the iliolumbar ligaments (Fig. 4.26). The test may be repeated in greater degrees of hip flexion; when

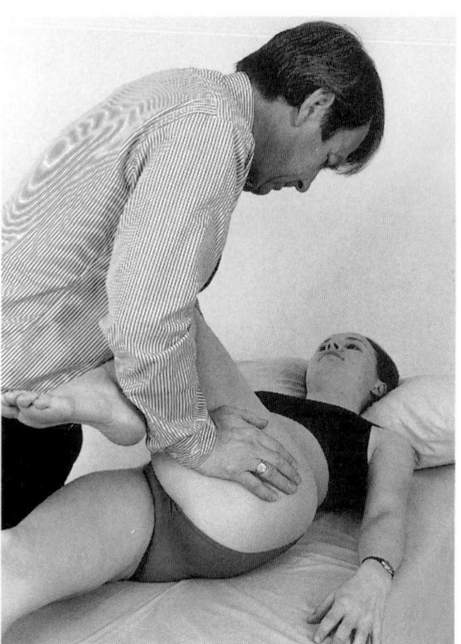

Fig. 4.26 Sacroiliac joint – the hip flexion-adduction stress test.

the thigh points towards the contralateral shoulder, stress is applied to the posterior sacroiliac ligament, and in further hip flexion to the sacrotuberous ligament. Reproduction of the patient's pain, felt in the SIJ region or buttock, incriminates SIJ ligamentous strain. Pain in the groin indicates either SIJ or hip pathology.

The SIJ stress test is also positive in sacroiliitis. Historically, the pelvic compression test, performed by applying backwards pressure on the two ASISs, has been advocated as a test for sacroiliitis. Interestingly, although painful in sacroiliitis, it tends not to be painful in chronic ligamentous strain of the SIJ.

Downing's test for sacroiliac mobility is occasionally used but is less reliable. It depends upon the identification of a change in apparent leg length on forcefully internally rotating, then externally rotating the hip, when the hip and knee are flexed to 35–45°. If SIJ mobility is normal, shortening is seen on internal rotation, and lengthening (or more appropriately, reversion to apparent leg length equality) on external rotation.

(6) Facet stress tests

The lumbar apophyseal joints may be stressed in flexion and side flexion using the patient's thighs to create leverage. The examiner holds the thighs close to his body and produces increasing lumbar flexion, first with side flexion to the left, then to the right (Fig. 4.27). Effectively, these tests add side flexion and torsional stress to passive lumbar flexion (which, independently, is procured by the lumbosacral stress test).

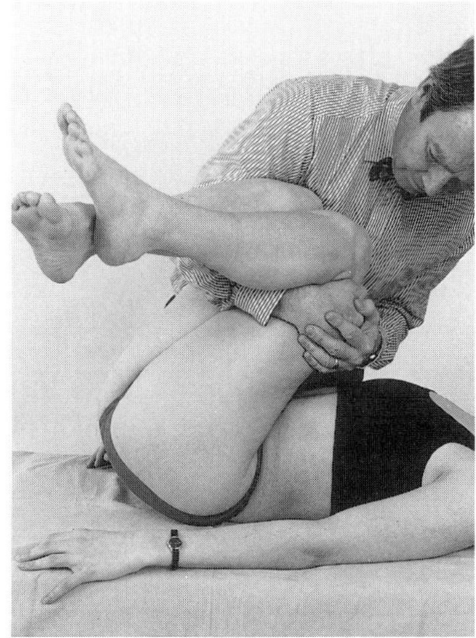

a

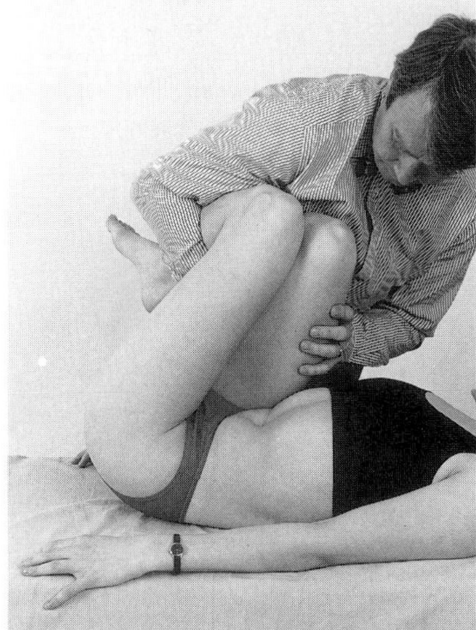

b

Fig.4.27 Lumbar spine – facet stress tests. (a) Flexion and side flexion to the left. (b) Flexion and side flexion to the right.

(7) Neurological signs

In the supine position the signs of muscle denervation are sought by assessment of power in the following groups:

Hip flexors (psoas, rectus femoris) L2,3,4.
Foot dorsiflexor (tibialis anterior) L4,5.
Hallux dorsiflexor (EHL) L5.
Foot evertors (peronei) L5, S1.
Knee jerk L4.

The plantar (Babinski) reflexes are routinely assessed. Occasionally, a neurological condition which gives rise to an upper motor neurone lesion, such as multiple sclerosis, causes aching in the legs, and enters into the differential diagnosis of leg pain(s). Cloniform ankle jerks and extensor Babinski reflexes are found.

Cutaneous anaesthesia may be sought if additional evidence is required in respect of nerve root compression, but a careful assessment of muscle power has greater sensitivity and predictive capacity.

Prone

(1) Comfort

A patient with fixed flexion of the lumbar spine, often associated with an L3/4 disc prolapse and femoral nerve root entrapment, will not be able to lie without rolling over to one side to flex the hip of the affected leg.

(2) Femoral (nerve) stress test (FST)

The FST is performed by passively flexing the knee (Fig. 4.28); it places the L3 and L4 nerve roots under tension and is therefore painful (positive) in the presence of a posterolateral disc protrusion at the L3/4 level. Occasionally, a positive crossover sign may be present (when pain in the anterior thigh is caused by a contralateral FST).

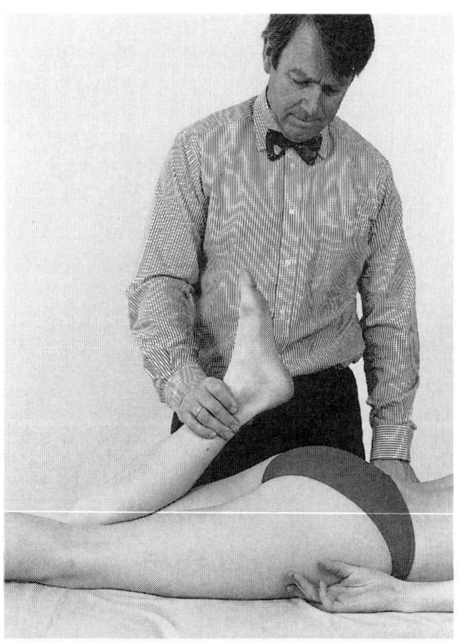

Fig. 4.28 Lumbar spine – the femoral (nerve) stress test.

(3) Bilateral FST

This is performed by simultaneous flexion of both knees and pressure on the anterior aspects of the ankles to push the heels to the buttocks, and is really an extension stress (provocation) test for the lumbar

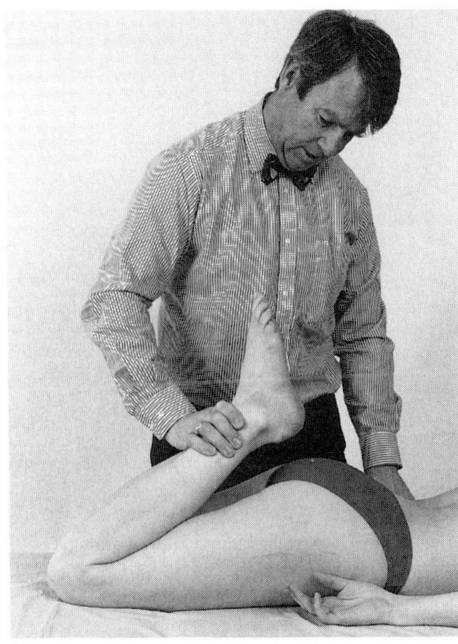

Fig. 4.29 Lumbar spine – the bilateral femoral stretch test.

spine (Fig. 4.29). In common with the lumbosacral stress test, it is somewhat non-specific, creating sacroiliac torsion as well as facet joint stress.

(4) Hip joint rotation

Hip joint rotation, medial and lateral, may be assessed with the hip in the neutral (also described as the 'extended') position. Occasionally, discomfort on passive medial rotation of the hip is found with sacroiliac dysfunction, presumably due to associated piriformis muscle spasm, but is an unreliable sign.

(5) Joint play assessment

- **Segmental compression test** – vertebral springing. Segmental mobility and discomfort are assessed by springing each lumbar vertebra with the ulnar border of the hand, or using the thumb and index finger (Fig. 4.30).
- **Lateral springing.** Thumb pressure on each spinous process, first from one side then the other, provides the basis for further assessment of discomfort and segmental joint play (Fig. 4.31).

(6) Tenderness

Tenderness overlying the PSISs and posterior aspects of the sacroiliac joints is sought. Overall, skin rolling is less likely to evoke positive signs in the lumbar region in comparison with the thoracic region

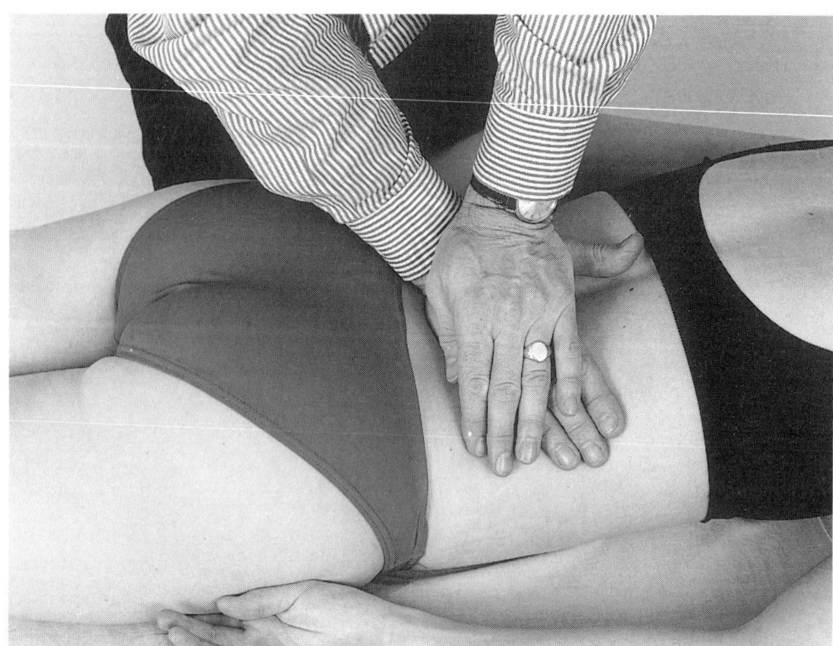

Fig. 4.30 Lumbar spine – joint play assessment: segmental compression test.

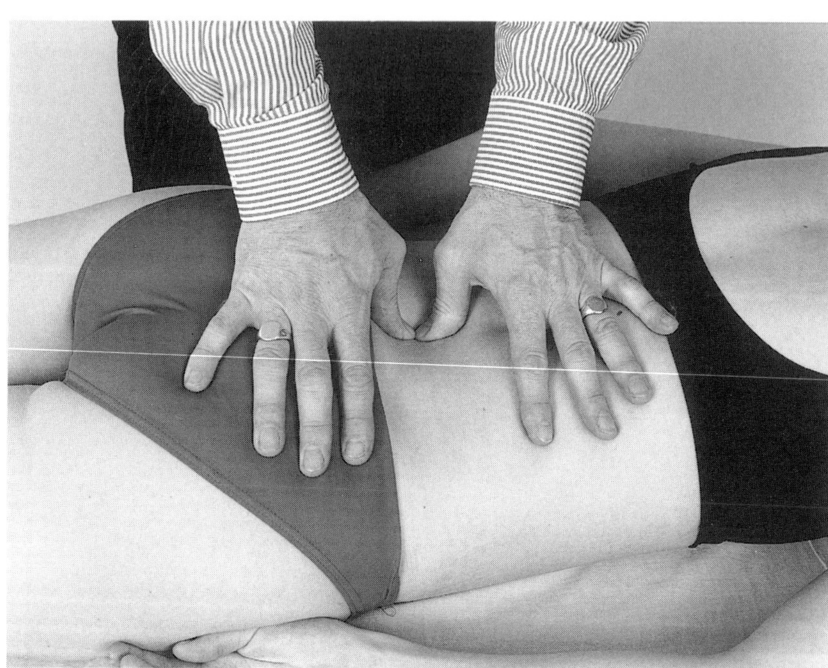

Fig. 4.31 Lumbar spine – joint play assessment: lateral springing.

though, occasionally, both skin drag and paravertebral hyperaesthesiae are marked features. Trigger points, if present, are usually found in the muscles of the buttock, either lateral to the mid- or upper sacrum (possibly in the piriformis) or below the iliac crest (in the glutei). Deep pressure over the lumbar facet joints may elicit a painful response in facet joint lesions.

(7) Neurological assessment

Muscle power of the following groups is assessed:

Knee flexion (hamstrings) S1,2.
Knee extension (quadriceps) L4.
Glutei (buttocks squeezed together) S1.
Ankle jerk S1.

(8) Sacrococcygeal joint

The sacrococcygeal joint should be assessed if there is a complaint of coccydynia. The joint may be sprung by the application of anteriorly directed pressure over the distal coccyx, whereupon pain may be elicited. However, the lumbosacral region must always be assessed

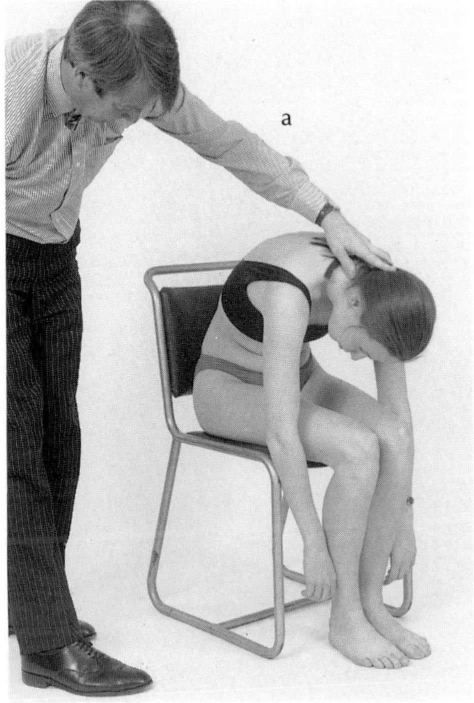

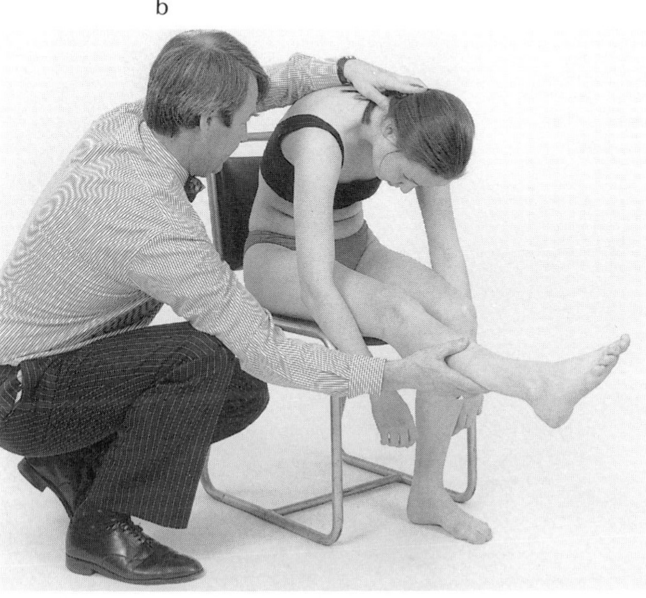

Fig. 4.32 Lumbar spine. (a) Slump test. (b) Reinforced slump test.

additionally as combined lesions are common, particularly after a fall on to the base of the spine.

Sitting

(1) Slump test

The patient slumps into a sitting position in a chair, flexing the neck (Fig. 4.32*a*). This is a test for dural tension; exacerbation of lumbar pain indicates pressure from a disc protrusion on the dura. An extension of this test involves a simultaneous SLR (flexion of a hip with an extended knee), thereby placing further tension unilaterally on the L5 and sacral nerve roots (Fig. 4.32*b*). These tests are useful if the neural tension tests in the standing and lying positions are equivocal, and offer a greater degree of sensitivity.

(2) Mennell sacroiliac test

The patient sits on a couch and slumps back against the examiner. The examiner uses one arm to rotate the thoracolumbar spine and place a torsional strain on the sacroiliac joint of the side towards which the spine is rotated (Fig. 4.33); then he uses his free hand to spring backwards on the ASIS of the side of the pelvis which has lifted from the couch, thereby creating a torsion on that SIJ. This test is used to detect discomfort; that is, it is a provocation or stress test. It may also be used subsequently to mobilize the SIJ.

a

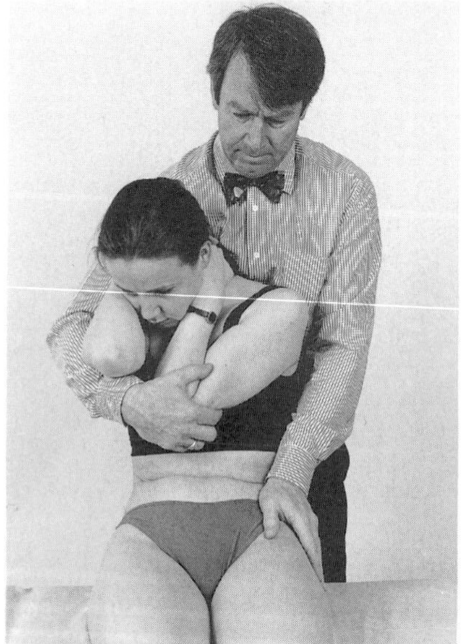

b

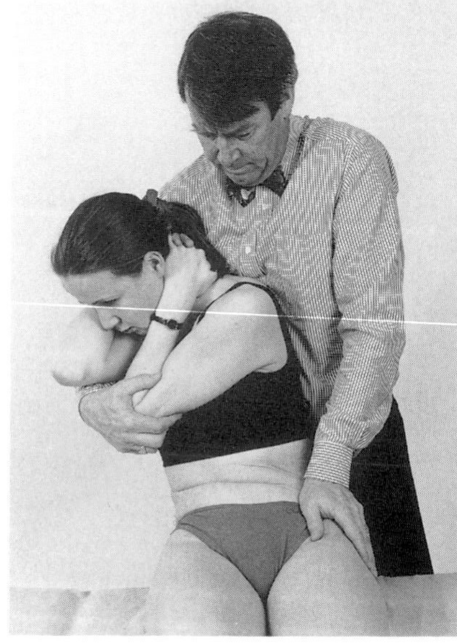

Fig. 4.33 Sacroiliac joint – the sitting sacroiliac stress test. (a) Prior to application of SIJ torsion. (b) Application of torsion.

(3) Piėdallu SIJ test

The patient sits with legs over the edge of a couch, and bends forwards. The relationships of the PSISs are noted by the examiner, using his thumbs (Fig. 4.34). This is an equivalent test to that performed by forward flexion of the trunk from the standing position.

a

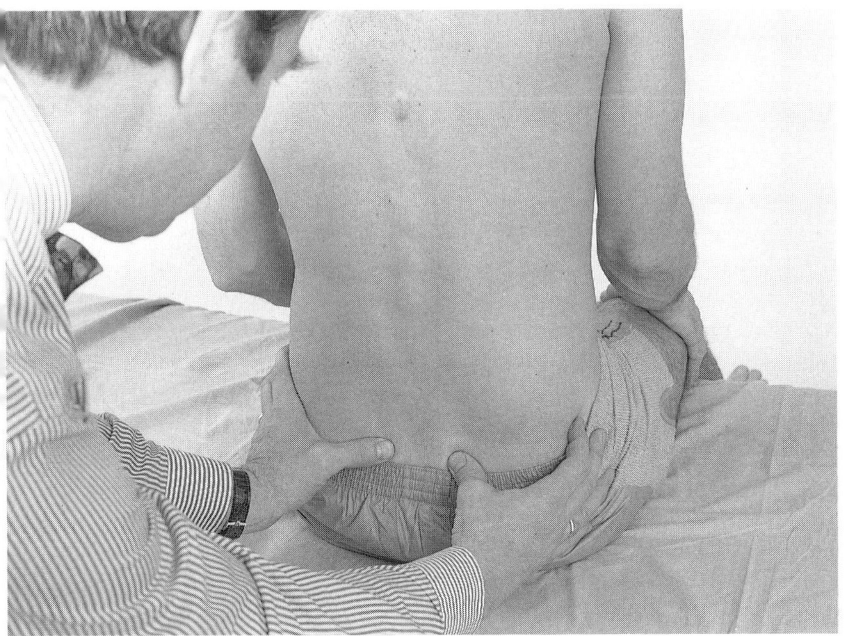

b

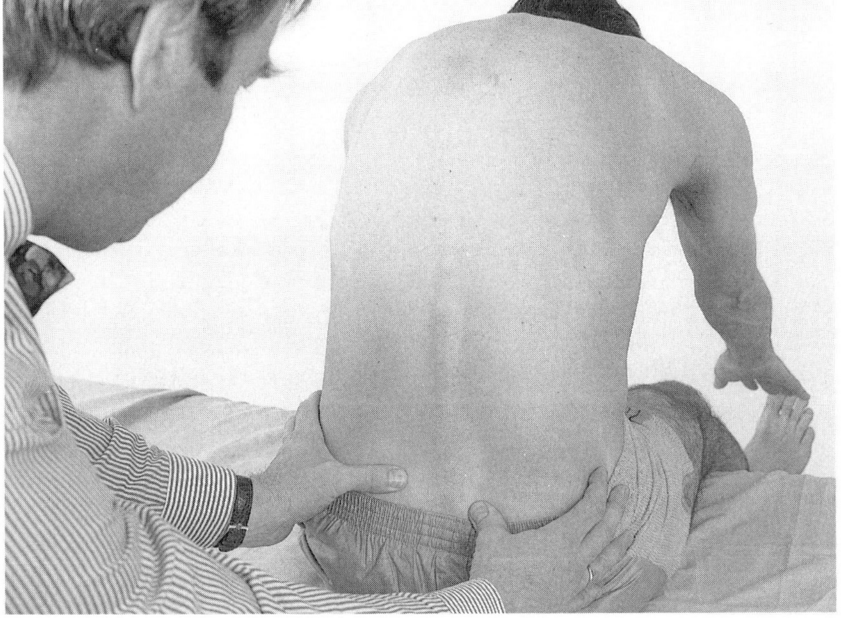

Fig. 4.34 Sacroiliac mobility – the Piėdallu SIJ test. (a) The sitting position. (b) Demonstration of left SIJ dysfunction on trunk flexion.

(4) 'Deception test'

A patient with significant restriction of SLR due to nerve root tension will not be able to sit upright with legs outstretched on the couch. Occasionally, attempted deception by the patient is found when the SLR is apparently reduced when supine, yet unrestricted in the sitting position.

INTERPRETATION

Acute conditions

Disc protrusion

A central disc protrusion usually gives rise to fixed flexion of the lumbar spine, often with pelvic tilt and 'sciatic' scoliosis. Characteristically, when a protrusion at the lower two lumbar levels moves posterolaterally, resulting in sciatica, the prominent features on examination are positive dural tension signs (restricted SLR, for instance) and restricted flexion of the spine in the standing position. Neurological examination may be normal, a situation that is not incompatible with disc protrusion and root irritation. The presence of dysaesthesiae in the history suggests root entrapment, which may be confirmed by the signs of motor denervation in the affected limb. In this situation, in which the signs confirm a root palsy, a sound clinical examination alone has a high sensitivity and specificity in respect to HNP. Should there be doubt regarding the diagnosis, or in the absence of clinical improvement over a month or so of treatment, CT scanning or MR imaging are required for confirmation (see below, 'Investigations').

- **L3 root compression**. Occasionally, a laterally positioned disc protrusion at L3/4 compresses the L3 nerve root. Pain is felt in the anterior thigh as far as the knee, and is often accompanied by hypoaesthesia. The hip flexors are weak and the knee jerk depressed. The FST is painful.
- **L4 root compression**. The L4 nerve root is compressed by a posterolateral protrusion of the L3/4 disc. Pain radiates from the anterolateral thigh to the anteromedial aspect of the lower leg. The articular signs in the standing position are usually reversed – restriction of extension rather than flexion – and the FST is markedly restricted and painful. Weakness of the quadriceps and an absent knee jerk are the usual neurological findings.
- **L5 root compression**. L5 root compression is usually due to a posterolateral herniation at L4/5 (Fig. 4.15), but occasionally may be affected by a laterally placed L5/S1 herniation or by degenerative changes in the L5 root canal. Pain radiates down the lateral aspect of the leg, and over the dorsum of the foot to the big toe. Weakness of the extensor hallucis longus (EHL) is the most sensitive finding, and may be the only indicator of a

root palsy at this level. In severe cases a typical foot drop may result, a situation that warrants an urgent orthopaedic opinion as surgical decompression may encourage restoration of normal neurological function. Tendon reflexes are usually not affected, but the SLR is painfully restricted.

- **S1 root compression**. This results from a posterolateral L5/S1 disc prolapse and is the most common root affected by disc herniation in the lumbar spine. Occasionally, a large posterolateral protrusion at L4/5 is responsible (Fig. 4.15*a*, *d*). Pain radiates posteriorly down the leg to the heel and the sole, and the lateral border of the foot as far as the lateral toes. Hypoaesthesia may be felt in the heel or the little toe. The ankle jerk is diminished or absent and may be the only neurological finding. A careful examination often reveals weakness of the hamstrings and/or glutei, even in the relatively 'minor' case; in the full root syndrome the patient is unable to rise on to tiptoe when standing on one leg, and gait is clearly abnormal.

Disc bulge

Lesser degrees of disc prolapse, possibly involving the annulus rather than the nucleus, may give rise to back and leg pain. The inflammatory response at the interface between the disc and the dura may play an important role in the pathogenesis of root irritation. The more subtle signs of dural tension, such as the slump test, may be decisive in establishing the diagnosis.

Disc degeneration

Degenerative changes within the nucleus, as demonstrated by MRI or discography, do not give rise to nociceptive stimulation (because of the absence of afferent nerve endings in the nucleus). Low backache may, sometimes, be due to degenerative changes affecting the outer lamellae of the annulus, though there are no specific tests available to confirm this. It is possible that annular degenerative changes are responsible for backache in those patients who are labelled as having chronic ligamentous strain (see below). Clinical examination is negative unless frank disc prolapse or sacroiliac ligamentous strain supervene.

Acute segmental dysfunction

It is probable that when patients experience recurrent bouts of pain, during which marked pelvic tilt and loss of extension (and often reduced flexion) are features, there are combined lesions of disc prolapse and facet joint dysfunction (or 'locking'). The pelvic tilt, and corresponding scoliosis, may be changed in orientation by manipulation, suggesting the presence of a central 'pulpy' (that is, nuclear) disc prolapse. Dural tension signs are often negative, however, from which one may conclude that locking of the facet joints is also an essential feature in this three-joint segmental dysfunction.

Facet (syn. 'spinal joint') dysfunction

Lesser degrees of restriction in mobility in the standing position, and the absence of dural tension signs, are features of facet dysfunction. The diagnosis is clinched by the detection of positive segmental signs (for instance, on vertebral springing) and by stress (provocation) tests. Dysfunction may occur at any level of the lumbar spine. The thoracolumbar junction should be included in the examination; lesions at this level may give rise to buttock and groin pain, and may coexist with lower lumbar or sacroiliac dysfunction.

Spondylolysis

A (recent) stress fracture of the pars interarticularis rarely gives rise to significant restriction in mobility. Extension of the trunk and the unilateral hyperextension test are painful. Deep tenderness may be found. Exercise-dependent pain is a characteristic feature of the history, and further investigations (X-rays, bone scan and possibly CT scan) are necessary to establish the diagnosis and provide a historical perspective.

Sacroiliac dysfunction

Hypomobility of the SIJ is often recurrent and secondary to ligamentous insufficiency. Mobility tests, which compare the two sacroiliac joints, confirm the dysfunction. Since sacroiliac dysfunction may exist independently, or coexist with lumbar lesions, routine tests for SIJ mobility should be employed in all cases of backache. Usually, there is little restriction in overall trunk mobility. The sacroiliac stress tests are not necessarily positive (see below).

Chronic conditions

Lumbar instability

This is characterized by frequent, at least recurrent, bouts of low back pain, often with a discogenic element. Between painful bouts there may be no apparent abnormalities on examination. A critical assessment of lifestyle factors must be made, including the overall level of physical conditioning.

The more specific condition of lumbar **segmental instability** is characterized by persistent, and possibly permanent, weakness of a motion segment which manifests as pain experienced *during* spinal movement. The examination findings which are virtually pathognomonic of segmental instability are a hitch, or arc, of pain on trunk flexion, or during recovery from flexion in the standing position. Different interpretations have been put forward to explain this sign. Excessive translatory movements probably occur, in which case muscle imbalance may be a contributory factor; alternatively, a small disc bulge and/or capsular weakness of the apophyseal joints may be present. Involvement of these joints is suggested by positive (painful) facet stress tests.

Facet joint lesions

- *Chronic joint dysfunction.* In this condition, which is equivalent to a chronic strain of the apophyseal joints, there is often a history of relatively minor injury, for instance whiplash due to an RTA (in which a neck strain may have appeared to be more troublesome initially to the patient). A nagging ache persists, and examination confirms the typical signs of joint dysfunction, usually at the lumbosacral level: positive facet stress tests, and pain and tenderness on segmental springing are characteristic features.
- *Facet joint arthrosis.* The 'grumbling' or 'weak' back is characterized by aching and morning stiffness *after* excessive physical activities in the older population. The findings are an overall reduction in global movements, a markedly painful lumbosacral stress test, positive segmental compression tests, and deep tenderness over the apophyseal joints.

Spinal stenosis

In central spinal stenosis there are often no significant signs on routine (static) examination. Dynamic assessment should be made by means of a walking or cycling test. Reduced arterial pulsation in the legs suggests arterial insufficiency, from which spinal stenosis should be differentiated.

In lateral canal stenosis the principal signs on examination are those resulting from compression of a nerve root at the intervertebral foramen: extension and ipsilateral flexion of the spine reproduce root pain. Dural tension tests are often not markedly positive, and may be negative. Neurological signs may be positive, and very occasionally may reveal multi-root pathology. In this latter situation, in which the pattern of motor weakness and abnormalities of the reflexes suggests involvement of more than one root, the differential diagnosis may be metastases, and the overall appearance of the patient should be taken into account.

Chronic sacroiliac (ligamentous) strain

Almost exclusively, this condition is confined to females in their child-rearing years. Exceptionally, it is found in athletes undergoing rigorous and lengthy training programmes. Upon a background of nagging ache in the sacroiliac region, buttock, posterior thigh and groin, there are recurrent bouts of sacroiliac dysfunction. The signs of chronic ligamentous strain are a positive sacroiliac stress test and tenderness overlying the PSIS and the posterior sacroiliac ligaments. The condition may be uni- or bilateral. Lumbar articular signs are negative unless there is additional lumbar facet strain. Sacroiliac mobility tests are only abnormal if the SIJ is hypomobile at the time of examination. Correction of the hypomobility does not cure the underlying ligamentous insufficiency, the most reliable treatment for which is sclerotherapy combined with a fitness programme (see Chapter 5).

Chronic (lumbosacral) ligamentous strain

A minority of patients with backache, predominantly males in their thirties and forties, suffer from chronic ligamentous strain. There are no detectable structural abnormalities (for instance, no spondylolisthesis) and the history is typical of ligamentous strain – increasing discomfort on immobility, manifesting as the 'cocktail party' syndrome or 'theatre-goer' syndrome. Unlike chronic sacroiliac ligamentous strain, the SIJ tests are negative and, indeed, *all* signs of lumbosacral dysfunction are negative. This is perhaps the only 'dustbin' diagnosis to be made in patients with low back pain in respect of the lack of confirmation of the condition on physical examination. It is uncommon, and may respond to sclerotherapy.

Spondylolisthesis

Disc degeneration and prolapse, nerve root compression, chronic ligamentous strain and spinal stenosis are all more common in the presence of a spondylolisthesis. In the absence of these secondary features, the only physical finding in a patient with an asymptomatic listhesis may be a palpable step in the lumbar spine. If the slip is 50% or more, the sacrum tends to assume a vertical position and the patient exhibits a typical posture with tight hamstrings and apparent loss of extension of the hips.

Ankylosing spondylitis

Spondyloarthropathies affect the sacroiliac joints initially (giving rise to sacroiliitis) and, subsequently, the rest of the spine to a variable degree. The signs of sacroiliitis are essentially the same as those for chronic sacroiliac strain – yet with one subtle difference. On performing the conventional sacroiliac stress test (the hip flexion-adduction test in the supine position) in a patient with sacroiliitis, there tends to be a 'springy' reaction which is associated with pyriformis muscle spasm. The history, of course, is quite characteristic and should lead the examiner towards the correct diagnosis.

In the early stages of the condition radiological confirmation of sacroiliitis may be lacking, yet a clinical diagnosis may often be made with reasonable confidence.

Associated conditions

- **Trigger points** are usually secondary to a primary disorder of the lumbar spine, or sacroiliac joint, and resolve when the primary condition is treated adequately (for instance, by lumbar traction or by mobilization). Occasionally, TPs persist on resolution of joint dysfunction, in which case they require treatment in their own right.
- **Myofascial syndromes** (myotendinoses) typically give rise to deep tenderness in the buttock or around the greater trochanter of the femur. Usually, they are associated with adverse postural characteristics, of which by far the most common is prolonged sitting, either at a desk (for instance, in typists or VDU operators) or in a motor car. There is an absence of articular signs on examination. Within the affected muscle it may be possible to demonstrate a 'knotted' feeling, irritability (for instance to repeated palpation), a jump sign, and abnormal function (for instance, shortening). Besides postural stresses, other predisposing factors include fatigue, psychological stress and coexistent debilitating conditions.
- **Pyriformis syndrome** may occur as a primary condition, or in association with sacroiliac disorders (either sacroiliac dysfunction or sacroiliitis). Passive internal rotation of the hip is painful, and usually restricted in range. Resisted external rotation is painful, and possibly weak. Tenderness and muscle tension are felt lateral to the sacrum and adjacent to the trochanteric attachment.

Pathophysiologically, piriformis muscle spasm may be considered to be a variety of trigger point; thus, piriformis syndrome may be treated as such. The popularization of the diagnosis suggests that it is the most likely explanation for localized buttock tenderness, whereas a careful examination more often reveals TPs in the glutei.

INVESTIGATIONS

A *sine qua non* in respect of the establishment of a definitive diagnosis in a patient with back pain is the fact that a sound history and an expert clinical examination are essential prerequisites, and that radiologocal or imaging investigations are usually not helpful. Two facts are worth repeating:

- Radiologically detected degenerative changes or minor congenital abnormalities in the lumbar spine do not correlate well with clinical problems.
- Discal abnormalities, for instance degeneration (as demonstated on MRI or discography) or bulging or minor degrees of prolapse (as demonstrated by radiculography, CT, MRI, or discography), are present in a significant percentage of the non-symptomatic population.

In other words, these investigations are poor predictors of spinal or limb pain in the vast majority of cases.

Undoubtedly, however, there are circumstances in which it is prudent to exclude more sinister pathology, such as infection or neoplasm; thus, screening tests – ESR, blood chemistry, radiology, radionuclide scanning and imaging techniques – may be required on occasions. Additionally, confirmation of the nature and location of a space-occupying lesion giving rise to nerve root entrapment – usually an HNP, but not invariably so – is required if there is substantial doubt regarding the diagnosis, or if conservative management has failed and surgical intervention is likely.

Each of the techniques already referred to has its advocates; however, the trend has been towards non-invasive methods, amongst which **magnetic resonance imaging** (MRI) has not only been shown to give superior definition but also a lack of known side-effects. MRI is based on the responses of hydrogen protons to a strong magnetic field; for the spine, computerized imaging in multiple planes reveals early biochemical changes as well as physical changes. In many surgeons' practices, the use of MRI has largely superseded the invasive technique of radiculography. Good definition of the contents of the spinal canal is usually obtained, and a high sensitivity is to be expected in the presence of a sizeable posterolateral disc protrusion or sequestrated fragment (Fig. 4.15). Its drawbacks should also be appreciated – it is a 'static' examination (when compared with the more dynamic procedure of provocation discography), and the absence of a significant space-occupying lesion does not exclude a diagnosis of sciatic root irritation.

TREATMENT

Bedrest

A youngish patient with a very painful sciatica or lumbago due to a nuclear disc protrusion may find that any position other than lying flat is too painful to tolerate. Quite commonly, the spinal attitude in recumbency is critical: side lying on one side may be painful, for instance, while side lying on the other side with the hips flexed – the fetal position – may be the only comfortable position. Although intradiscal pressures are low, bed rest for longer than three days is best avoided unless absolutely necessary. It has a debilitating effect on the body generally, and there is little evidence that it has a significant effect on the rate of resolution of disc herniation. A more flexible strategy would be to titrate increased physical activity against overall improvement in the patient's conditon.

Lumbar traction

Daily sustained lumbar traction is the treatment of choice for a disc protrusion that has not extruded sufficiently to have given rise to positive neurological signs. Cyriax (1982) popularized the use of outpatient traction using a standard wooden couch and fittings. Currently, there is a variety of couches dedicated to horizontal traction, and a variety of appliances that rely on gravity traction or inversion traction. For maximal effect, traction should be given daily for 30 minutes; it may be necessary to continue treatment for up to three weeks. Distraction forces of between 35 kg (for light females, for instance) and 75 kg (for heavy males) are required. These forces should be achieved gradually over a few sessions; in 'hyperacute' lumbago great care should be exercised, otherwise reducing the traction gives rise to very painful twinges. If horizontal traction (which is the most effective type) is used, the supine position may need to be modified for comfort, for instance by flexion of the hips and knees (Fig. 4.35).

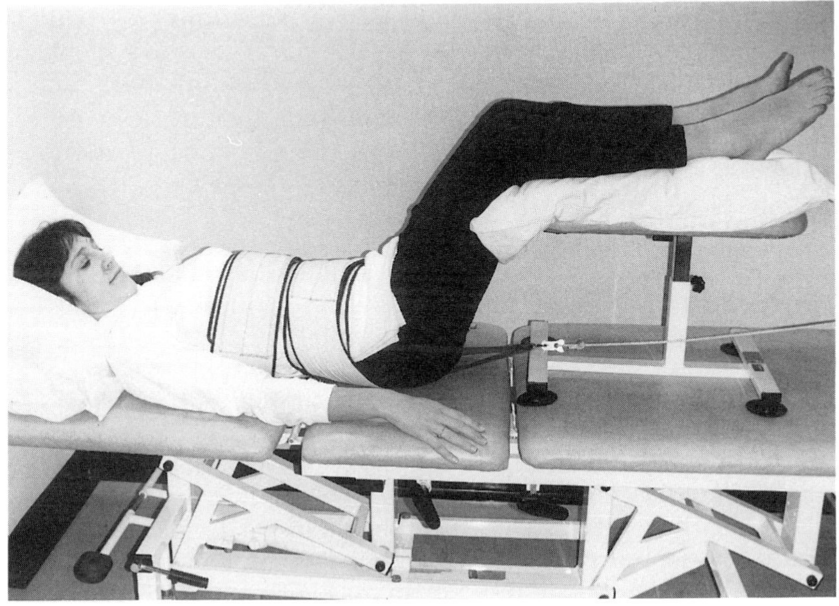

Fig. 4.35 Daily outpatient lumbar traction is given for prolapse of the nucleus pulposus.

There are no absolute contraindications, though chest discomfort from the harness may disturb some patients. Traction is ineffective when sequestration of a disc fragment has occurred; and it is usually unsuccessful, unless combined with epidural injections, in the presence of signs of a root palsy, whether due to a sequestrated or herniated disc. It has no significant effect on other conditions, although intermittent traction has its advocates for mobilization of stubborn facet joint dysfunction.

Epidural injections

The practice of caudal epidural anaesthesia was established by James Cyriax as a potent strategy in the management of sciatica and hyperacute lumbago. He advocated its use particularly when a posterolateral disc prolapse was associated with a nerve root palsy. Recently, its efficacy has been established in a prospective analysis using confirmation of disc herniation by CT scanning (Bush and Hillier, 1991).

Most orthopaedic physicians now use procaine 0.5% or lignocaine 0.5%, combined with a deposteroid such as methylprednisolone acetate 40 mg, in a total volume of 20–25 ml. Injections are given via the sacral hiatus (Fig. 4.39) at one- to two-weekly intervals, and repeated as many times as is necessary – usually between two and five in total. In the order of 85% of patients with neurological signs due to disc protrusion are helped by caudal epidural injections; the evaluation of improvement is based both on subjective parameters (for instance, a pain scale) and on objective parameters (in particular, improvement in dural tension signs).

During more than 20 years' experience of this practice, the author has found very few side effects, usually consisting of transient lightheadedness, in more than 5000 treatments. The patient should be informed that the treatment is anti-inflammatory in nature, and is used to accelerate the healing process; it is not used solely to provide immediate (anaesthetic) relief of symptoms.

Manipulation/mobilization

The indication for manipulation is joint dysfunction though it is possible that relatively small disc protrusions (for instance, giving rise to buttock and posterior thigh pain only) may respond to serial manipulations. An absolute contraindication is the possibility of impending (or established) cauda equina compression, suggested by altered sensation in the saddle area or bladder dysfunction, as the consequences may be awesome in respect of irreversible neurological sequelae (and subsequent litigation).

On the grounds that it is probable that dysfunction has a neurophysiological rather than a pathoanatomical basis, the distinction between manipulative and mobilization techniques is somewhat artificial. Joint dysfunction in the lumbar spine and sacroiliac joints may be reversed by a wide variety of techniques which are described in detail in other texts (Bourdillon, 1992; Lewit, 1985; Mennell, 1960; Stoddard, 1977, for instance). The author uses the following techniques, which are accorded brief descriptions, as standard.

For **lumbar joint dysfunction**, the therapist applies and controls (segmental) rotational manipulation by the use of his forearms and hands (Fig. 4.36). The thrust is applied largely through the shoulders and arms, and localized by the fingers and thumb to the relevant spinous process. The amount of lumbar flexion or extension may be adjusted to suit the therapist's inclination and the patient's comfort. Relief is usually instantaneous, and is detected by the patient in the improvement in the comfortable range of spinal movements. This technique is also useful for the thoracolumbar junction, and the distal thoracic spine as far up as T9.

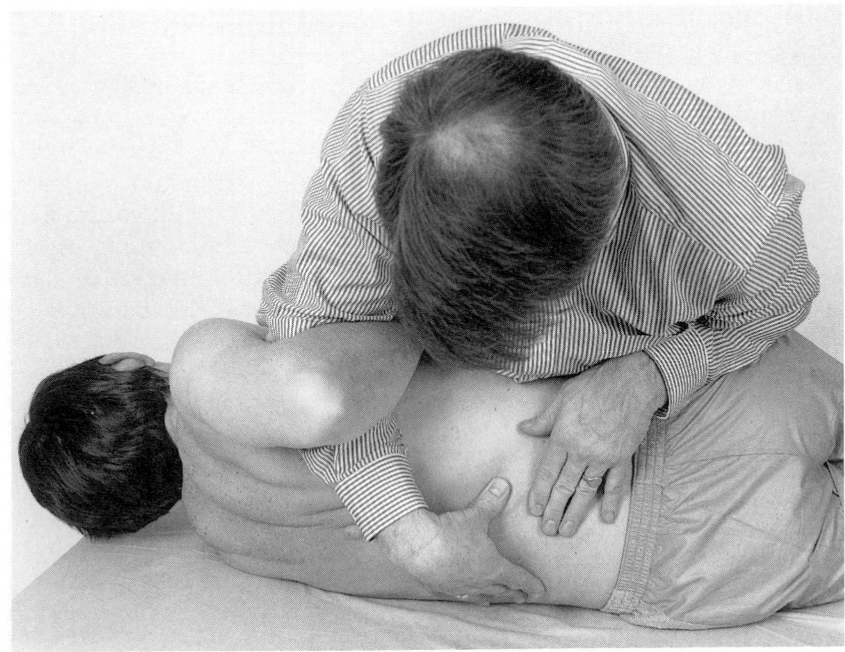

Fig. 4.36 Lumbar spine – a suitable rotational manipulation is demonstrated.

For sacroiliac dysfunction, a well-tried and trusted procedure involves a relatively non-specific rotational manoeuvre. Although rotational strain is also applied to the lumbar spine during the procedure, a significant counternutational force is applied to the sacroiliac joint. The thrust is made by applying the volar aspect of the forearm to the posterior ilium (Fig. 4.37). Although diverse types of hypomobility may be detected with increasing experience, the demonstrated technique is usually successful in reversing the signs of hypomobility described in this text. Immediate improvement in the patient's symptoms is usually found.

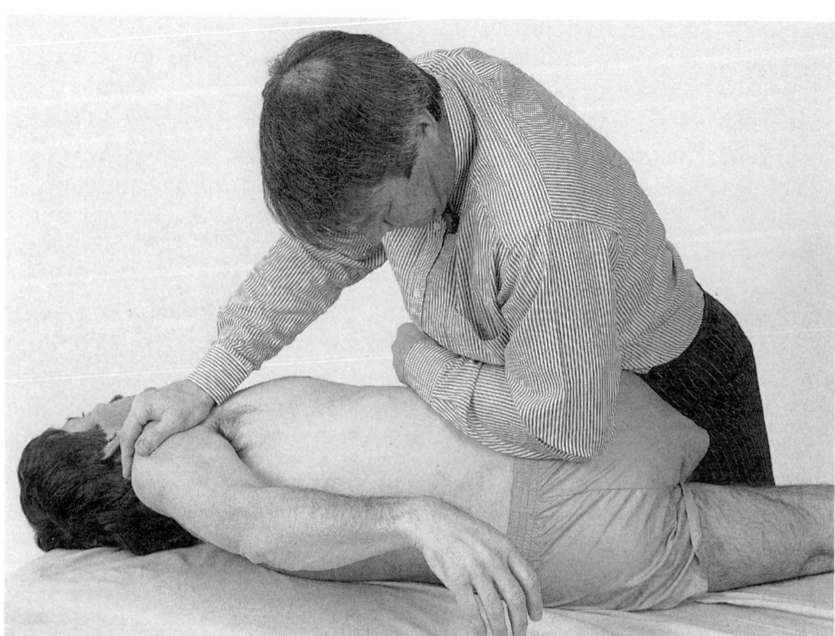

Fig. 4.37 Sacroiliac joint – a suitable rotational manipulation into nutation is demonstrated.

An alternative, somewhat more gentle, manipulation is an extension of the Mennell examining technique for the sacroiliac joint which is described under 'Examination; sitting'.

Self-mobilizing exercises

Pelvic tilting

Pelvic tilting, as described in Chapter 5 and demonstrated in Figure 5.3, is usually considered to be a specific exercise for flattening a prominent lordosis. However, when performed in a gentle, rhythmic fashion, either in the standing or supine positions, it is often useful in lumbar spinal joint dysfunction for 'loosening up' the back.

McKenzie concept

The McKenzie concept of centralization of pain is sometimes useful for disc bulges, either as a primary modality, or in conjunction with traction, for instance. The patient performs repeated active exercises, often (but not necessarily) into extension, in an attempt to reduce the size of a disc bulge (Fig. 4.38). Progress is monitored by the localization of pain which is expected to move from a lateral site (for instance, in the buttock) to a midline (for instance, lumbosacral) position as the condition improves.

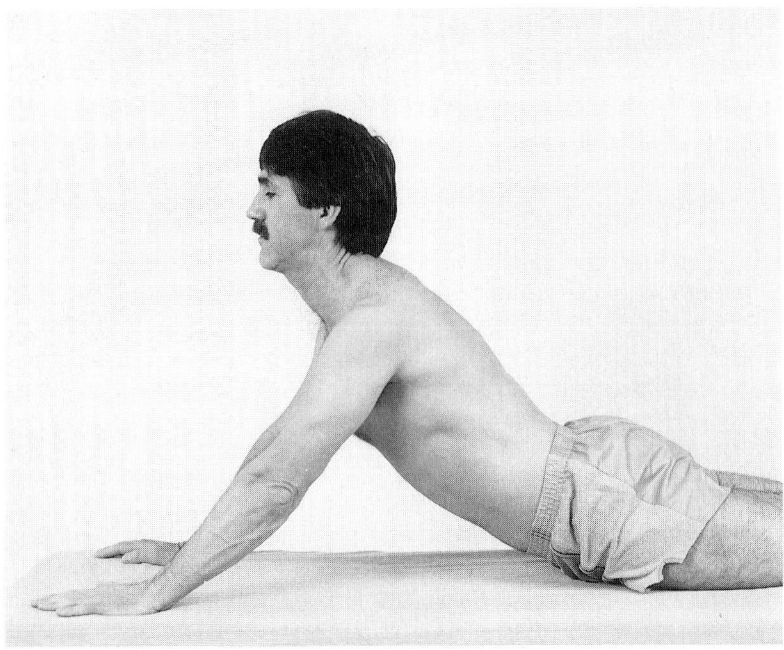

Fig. 4.38 Lumbar spine – self-mobilization: into extension.

Psoas stretch/sacroiliac relaxation

Relaxation of a tight psoas may assist the resolution of sacroiliac dysfunction. The use of postcontraction relaxation is particularly useful in this context. The patient lies supine with his contralateral hip maintained in full flexion by both his hands, and the leg of the affected side hanging over the edge of the bed or couch; gravity-aided extension of the hip occurs, once the thigh relaxes (Fig. 5.7). Passive hip extension is increased during the post-isometric relaxation phase which follows active (anti-gravity) flexion of the thigh, or resisted contraction of the hip flexors if assistance is available. Patients should be taught to follow this schedule at home. Otherwise, the hip may be forcibly stretched into extension (producing counternutation at the SIJ) by the patient, using his body weight in the upright position.

Flexibility exercises

In order to emphasize the importance of the rehabilitation and prophylaxis phases of management of spinal problems, flexibility exercises are included in some detail in the Rehabilitation section in Chapter 5. Range of motion exercises for maintenance of flexibility in ankylosing spondylitis are a crucial part of its *treatment*, however, and these are emphasized here: lumbar, thoracic, rib cage, and cervical exercises which are prescribed by the therapist are usually effective in preventing devastating and disabling spinal contractures.

Massage

Massage has little useful effect on paravertebral muscle spasm when this is secondary to an underlying disc disorder. For piriformis muscle spasm, psoas muscle spasm and other TPs the use of vigorous massage or acupressure may assist in the resolution of the underlying disorder – usually sacroiliac or lumbar spinal joint dysfunction. In general, massage has a (usually temporary) alleviatory effect on trigger points, and (often) exerts a somewhat more prolonged effect in myotendinosis. It should be followed by passive stretching of the affected muscle. Injections of local anaesthetic, intermittent cold-and-stretch techniques (Travell and Simons, 1992), or acupuncture are sometimes necessary for refractory TPs and areas of myotendinosis.

Additional injection techniques

Facet joint steroid injections

Intra-articular injections of steroid and local anaesthetic to the lumbar apophyseal joints, under X-ray control, may be used by orthopaedists for the purpose of diagnosis and management of chronic conditions, for instance symptomatic osteoarthrosis of the apophyseal joints, or segmental instability.

Facet dysfunction may also be treated by injections which are performed 'blind' (that is, without X-ray screening) – in effect, periarticular or facet block injections which are probably as effective as intra-articular injections. Their principal use is in those situations in which dysfunction has proved to be refractory to manipulative treatment.

If intra-articular or facet block injections of steroid and local anaesthetic give temporary relief only, treatment by sclerosant injections (see below) or radiofrequency denervation should be considered.

Root blocks

Paravertebral nerve root ('dorsal root ganglion') blocks of steroid and local anaesthetic are an alternative strategy to epidural injections in nerve root compression. They are given under X-ray screening for *exact* localization of the intervertebral foramen.

Sinuvertebral nerve blocks are given 'blind' (that is, without X-ray screening), the purpose being to introduce steroid and local anaesthetic *close to* the intervertebral foramen (Fig. 4.39). In the author's experience, they are extremely useful in the management of sciatica due to lateral canal stenosis – at least in those situations in which the soft tissue component of the stenosis is reversible.

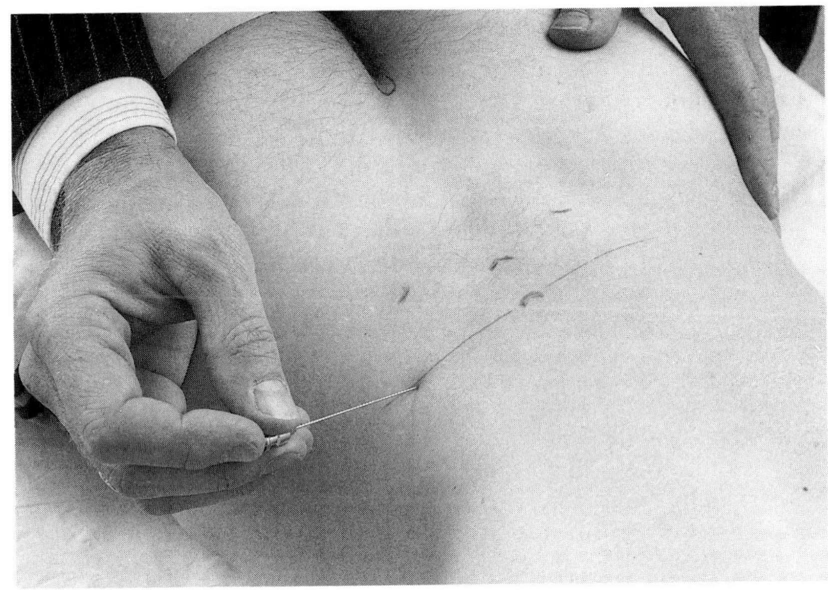

Fig. 4.39 With the patient in the prone position, the lateral approach for a sinuvertebral injection at the L4/5 level is demonstrated. The sacral hiatus (the site for a caudal epidural injection) is skin-marked.

Sclerotherapy (sclerosant injections)

Injections of P2G – 25% dextrose and 2% phenol – introduce irritant chemicals to the ligamento-osseous junctions in the lumbosacral and sacroiliac regions. Usually, the capsular ligaments of the apophyseal joints at L4/5 and L5/S1 (bilaterally) and those sacroiliac ligaments which are within reach of a spinal needle introduced over the lumbosacral interspace – iliolumbar, posterior sacroiliac and, possibly, the intra-articular interosseous ligament and proximal attachment of the sacrotuberous ligament – are treated following intravenous premedication with a sedative such as midazolam. A fibroblastic proliferative reaction is produced which is thought to increase collagen synthesis, and thus improve ligamentous competence. Ongley and co-workers (1987) have advocated the addition of a spinal manipulation, and an injection of steroid to surrounding trigger spots, to a series of sclerosant injection treatments (on six visits). The patient is then instructed in spinal flexion exercises. Other practitioners find that weekly injections of sclerosant solution on three or four occasions, followed by a walking or swimming schedule, is the strategy of choice.

An 85% positive response rate in chronic sacroiliac ligamentous insufficiency is to be expected. Lumbar instability, chronic lumbar ligamentous strain and spondylolisthesis may also be treated successfully, though the response rate is less predictable. 'Top-up' treatments at intervals may be required over succeeding years. Side-effects are few and infrequent; when given from a central puncture site overlying the lumbosacral joint, directing the needle laterally, the likelihood of intrathecal penetration is infinitesimally small.

Trigger point injections

Injections of local anaesthetic may be useful on occasions, particularly when directed to gluteal or trochanteric trigger points. Underlying lumbar or sacroiliac lesions must, of course, be identified and managed appropriately.

Sacrococcygeal/coccygeal injections

Localized intra-articular injections to the sacrococcygeal joint, or infiltrations around the coccyx, may be helpful in coccydynia. More often, management of an underlying lumbosacral lesion or sacroiliac lesion which is giving rise to referred pain at the coccyx is necessary.

Surgical management

The benefit of surgery for low back pain and sciatica at the present time has been proved in a scientific manner only for disc herniations giving root pain (Nachemson, 1989) and for cauda equina pressure with bladder dysfunction (a surgical emergency). Discectomy continues to be preferred to chemonucleolysis or percutaneous nucleotomy in many centres, and may be expected to offer a good result for confirmed disc herniation or sequestration following lack of response to conservative management.

However, the usefulness of fusion for segmental instability is contentious, due in no small measure to lack of agreement on the most satisfactory method of establishing the source of low back pain. The recent technique of utilizing external spinal skeletal fixation as a predictor for a good response to posterior fusion in chronic low back pain shows considerable promise (Esses *et al.*, 1989).

REHABILITATION AND PREVENTION OF INJURY

Not surprisingly, patients who are recovering from a recent back problem, in which there has been a significant disturbance of the three-joint motion segment complex, continue to feel vulnerable for some time after they have regained a normal range of spinal mobility. This situation is comparable to a destabilizing injury to a peripheral joint. It is particularly relevant to the distal two lumbar segments which effectively act as a lynch-pin in the dynamics of everyday movement and activity.

A detailed appraisal of the principles of rehabilitation – overall fitness, strengthening exercises, flexibility exercises and postural correction – is made in Chapter 5. Of special relevance to the lumbosacral spine is recognition of the need for abdominal muscle strengthening exercises. These should be commenced as soon as the patient's condition (and confidence) allows. Additionally, the maintenance of an appropriate degree of lumbar lordosis – that is, neither exaggerated nor flattened – is essential. Seemingly, a paradox may be encountered. On the one hand, pelvic tilting exercises are often a useful addition to muscle strengthening exercises to encourage pelvic rotation and reduction of an exaggerated lordosis (which is often a result of sagging of the abdomen). On the other hand, specific guidance is necessary to maintain the lordosis in situations, such as prolonged sitting, in which the spine slumps to a position in which the lordosis is threatened. Attention to sound ergonomic principles, therefore, is necessary, particularly in respect to the choice of office chair and its relationship to working surfaces, and the use of an appropriate back support when driving a car.

Notwithstanding the importance of self-help schedules to the majority of patients, the combination of adverse pathoanatomical and pathophysiological changes and the inevitability of adverse external biomechanical stresses may lead to persistent or increased vulnerability to further bouts of back pain. Consideration should then be given to treatment by sclerotherapy in an attempt to improve ligamentous stability. Occasionally, patients feel the benefit of a lumbar support, or more substantial corsetry. Maximum benefit may be gained when the use of the support is restricted to those situations in which excessive stresses are imposed upon the spine, for instance when gardening. Reliance upon a support should not become a substitute for the basic principles of physical conditioning which have already been described, and which are discussed further in Chapter 5.

REFERENCES

Boden, S.D., Davis, D.O., Dina, T.S. *et al* (1990) Abnormal magnetic-resonance scans of the lumbar spine in asymptomatic subjects. *Journal of Bone and Joint Surgery*, **72A**, 403–8

Bogduk, N., Tynan, W. and Wilson, A.S. (1991) The nerve supply to the human lumbar intervertebral discs. *Journal of Anatomy*, **132**, 39

Bourdillon, J.F. (1992) *Spinal Manipulation*, 5th edn, Butterworth-Heinemann, Oxford

Brunner, C., Kissling, R. and Jacob H.A.C. (1991) The effects of morphology and histopathologic findings on the mobility of the sacroiliac joint. *Spine*, **16**, 1111–17

Bush, K. and Hillier, S. (1991) A controlled study of caudal epidural injections of triamcinolone plus procaine for the management of intractable sciatica. *Spine*, **16**, 572–5

Cyriax, J. (1982) *Textbook of Orthopaedic Medicine*, vol. 1, 8th edn, Baillière Tindall, London

Esses, S.I., Botsford, D.J. and Kostuik, J.P. (1989) The role of external spinal skeletal fixation in the assessment of low-back disorders. *Spine*, **14**, 594–601

Fairbank, J.C.T., Park, W.M., McCall, I.W. *et al.* (1981) Apophyseal injection of local anaesthetic as a diagnostic aid in primary low-back pain syndromes. *Spine*, **6**, 598–605

Feinstein, B., Langton, J.N.K., Jameson, R.M. *et al.* (1954) Experiments on pain referred from deep somatic tissues. *Journal of Bone and Joint Surgery,* **36A**, 981–97

Hackett, G.S. (1956) *Ligament and Tendon Relaxation*, Charles C. Thomas, Springfield, Ill.

Jackson, D.W., Wiltse, L.L. and Cirincione, R.J. (1976) Spondylolysis in the female gymnast. *Clinical Orthopaedics and Related Research,* **117**, 68–73

Kellgren, J.H. (1939) On the distribution of pain arising from deep somatic structures with charts of segmental pain areas. *Clinical Science,* **4**, 35–46

Knuttson, B. (1961) Comparative value of electromyography, myelography, and clinico-neurological examination in diagnosis of lumbar root compression syndrome. *Acta Orthopaedica Scandinavia, Suppl.,* **49**.

Lewit, K. (1985) *Manipulative Therapy in Rehabilitation of the Motor System,* Butterworths, London

McCarron, R.F., Wimpee, M.W., Hudkins, P.G. *et al.* (1987) The inflammatory effect of nucleus pulposus. *Spine,* **12**, 760–4

MacArthur, C., Lewis, M., Knox, E.G. *et al.* (1990) Epidural anaesthesia and long term backache after childbirth. *British Medical Journal,* **301**, 9–12

McCall, I.W., Park, W.M. and O'Brien, J.P. (1979) Induced pain referred from posterior lumbar elements in normal subjects. *Spine,* **4**, 441–6

Macintosh, J.E. and Bogduk, N. (1987) The anatomy and biomechanics of the lumbar spinal erector spinae. *Spine,* **12**, 658–68

McKenzie, R.A. (1981) *The Lumbar Spine – Mechanical Diagnosis and Therapy,* Spinal Publications, Upper Hatt

Macnab, I. (1977) *Backache,* Williams and Wilkins, Baltimore

Maitland, G.D. (1986) *Vertebral Manipulation,* 5th edn, Butterworths, London

Melzack, R. and Wall, P.D. (1965) Pain mechanics: a new theory. *Science,* **150**, 331

Mennell, J.McM. (1960) *Back Pain: Diagnosis and Treatment using Manipulative Techniques,* Little, Brown and Company, Boston, Mass.

Mooney, V. and Robertson, J. (1976) The facet syndrome. *Clinical Orthopaedics and Related Research,* **115**, 149–56

Nachemson, A. (1989) Lumbar discography – where are we today? *Spine,* **14**, 555–7

Ongley, M.J., Klein, R.G., Dorman, T.A. *et al.* (1987) A new approach to the treatment of chronic low back pain. *Lancet,* **8551**, 143–6

Pièdallu, P. (1952) *Problèmes sacro-iliaques,* Homme sain No.2, biére edn, Bordeaux.

Porter, R.W. (1986) *Management of Back Pain,* Churchill Livingstone, Edinburgh

Porter, R.W., Hibbert, C.S. and Wicks, M. (1978) The spinal canal in symptomatic lumbar disc lesions. *Journal of Bone and Joint Surgery,* **50B**, 485–7

Powell, M.C., Wilson, M., Szypryt, P. *et al.* (1986) Prevalence of lumbar disc degeneration observed by magnetic resonance in symptomless women. *Lancet,* 1366–7

Rydevik, B., Brown, M.D. and Lundborg, G. (1984) Pathoanatomy and pathophysiology of nerve root compression. *Spine,* **9**, 7–15

Smyth, M.J. and Wright, V. (1958) Sciatica and the intervertebral disc. *Journal of Bone and Joint Surgery,* **40A**, 1401

Stoddard, A. (1977) *Manual of Osteopathic Practice,* Hutchinson, London

Travell, J.D. and Simons, D.G. (1992) *Myofascial Pain and Dysfunction: the Trigger Point Manual,* vol. 2, Williams and Wilkins, Baltimore, Md

Troup, J.D. (1986) Biomechanics of the lumbar spinal canal. *Clinical Biomechanics,* **1**, 31–43

Waddell, G. (1987) A new clinical model for the treatment of low-back pain. *Spine,* **12**, 632–44

Wiberg, G. (1947) Back pain in relation to the nerve supply of the intervertebral disc. *Acta Orthopaedica Scandinavia,* **19**, 211–21

Wyke, B.D. (1987) The neurology of low back pain. In *The Lumbar Spine and Back Pain,* 2nd edn (ed. by M.I.V. Jayson), Pitman Medical, London, pp. 265–339

5
Rehabilitation and prophylaxis

Our nature consists in movement; absolute rest is death.

Blaise Pascal (1623–1662). *Pensées*

The principles of management of soft tissue injuries to the spine are no different from those appertaining to injuries to the shoulder and pelvic girdles, and to the peripheral joints. Whatever the site of injury, the initial priorities are to reduce intra-articular derangements, control joint instability and reverse joint dysfunction; if appropriate, anti-inflammatory modalities of treatment may be introduced. As this phase proceeds, improvement in function tends to be proportional to loss of pain inhibition. For peripheral injuries, the therapist plays an important role in instituting mobilizing exercises for the relevant joints. For spinal conditions, this role is often more subtle as dysfunction is inclined to occur without any evidence of significant trauma and to persist without overt signs of gross loss of mobility; furthermore, spinal joint dysfunction often tends to be self-perpetuating as self-protective attitudes may provoke further segmental hypomobility and muscle tension. Subsequently, during the repair phase, **restoration of normal segmental function** is mandatory; additionally, an analysis of aetiological factors must be carried out at this stage, and adverse physiological characteristics corrected.

An analogy may be made with the management of a condition such as subacromial bursitis, which is often secondary to supraspinatus tendinitis. The first phase of treatment is anti-inflammatory, during which active shoulder abduction improves and a painful arc recedes. Strengthening exercises for the rotator cuff are instituted once subacromial dysfunction has resolved. Similarly, nerve root entrapment in the lumbar spine is treated by mechanical means (for instance, traction) and by anti-inflammatory means (for instance, epidural injections), prior to the commencement of strengthening exercises for the affected motion segment. Management is incomplete without this rehabilitation phase which is, of course, dependent upon sufficient healing during the repair phase following injury to suppress nociceptive afferent stimulation, and to allow adaptive processes to take place.

Prophylaxis is simply the projection of the principles of rehabilitation, including ergonomics, into the development of an appropriate lifestyle strategy for a particular individual. Effectively, 'rehabilitation' and 'prophylaxis' may be used interchangeably in this context. The following factors should be considered and will be enlarged upon:

1 Overall fitness (physical conditioning).
2 Flexibility exercises.
3 Strengthening exercises.
4 Postural characteristics and movement patterns.
5 Ergonomics.

PHYSICAL CONDITIONING

Endurance ('aerobic') exercise improves cardiorespiratory fitness which, to a large extent, is due to improved capacity of the peripheral muscles (not just the cardiac muscle) to utilize oxygen. Fitness training also has a non-specific 'toning' effect upon the physiological function of all the collagenized soft tissues, as well as improving bone strength. Therefore, patients should be encouraged to take regular exercise of a type that is appropriate to their age, inclination and their stage of recovery from injury or dysfunction. Indeed, this strategy should be commenced, if possible, *during* treatment for a painful condition; a positive outlook and an improved circulating endorphin level are helpful. Encouragement by the physiotherapist is important as some patients find it difficult to accept that, during treatment, 'rest' should mean restriction of provocative exercise or stress, but not absolute rest.

To some degree, the type of endurance exercise is not critical. For instance, cycling, brisk walking, jogging and low impact aerobics may all be appropriate in certain circumstances. Overall, swimming is the best form of regular exercise for the majority. It has the advantages of overcoming the effects of gravity on the spine, and of combining rhythmic spinal motion with aerobic muscle activity. The butterfly stroke is too stressful on the lower back for those (few) who can accomplish it. The breast-stroke also demands some hyperextension of the lumbar spine if performed vigorously, and of the cervical spine if performed by keeping the head consistently out of the water. The most appropriate strokes, as far as the spine is concerned, are the front and back crawls. Initially, during rehabilitation, diving should be excluded and, subsequently, should be performed with circumspection by those with sufficient inclination.

A 'tramline' situation may be described to patients. A moderate degree of regular aerobic exercise is desirable. If too infrequent or insufficient, the effect will be undetected; yet, in the pursuit of the target of fitness, sport such as squash rackets, which is very demanding of the spine, should be prohibited. Rowing machines should be used with caution because of the stresses imposed on the thoracic spine and the lumbosacral junction. The golf swing, involving more axial rotation than movement in the sagittal plane, may often be performed without discomfort, yet other activities associated with a round of golf may be provocative – for instance removal of golf clubs from the boot of a car, carriage of the clubs, placing the ball on the tee, retrieving it from the golf hole, and the occasional 'heavy' shot from the rough. Many jobs around the garden place excessive stresses upon a weak back, and are not usually contributory to aerobic fitness. Lawn mowing may involve a considerable amount of walking – a desirable activity – if the expanses of lawn are large, though the repetitive removal and emptying of a sizeable grass box impose considerable strains on the back, and should be eschewed during recovery from injury to the thoracic and lumbar spines.

When discussing fitness with an obese patient, the value of weight reduction should be promulgated.

FLEXIBILITY EXERCISES

Both soft tissues with a high collagen content, such as ligaments and joint capsules, and tissues with a low collagen content, such as muscles, depend on their inherent viscoelastic properties for normal function. Tensile strength is dependent upon elasticity, which is influenced primarily by regular levels of physical activity combined with regular stretching. Regrettably, a high percentage of the population of the Western hemisphere abuse their spines by subjecting them to periods of prolonged sitting and slouching, which contribute to shortening and weakening of important muscle groups. As a result, both the gradual loss of elasticity and muscle imbalance may be factors involved in the causation of spinal injury, or dysfunction, or chronic myotendinosis syndromes. Segmental joint dysfunction is associated with further loss of mobility, the persistence of which may be 'protected' by the unsuspecting patient by further voluntary reduction in exercise. Perpetuation of muscle tightness also occurs, unsuspectingly and involuntarily, as a result of the development of TPs and areas of myotendinosis. Clearly, ligaments and muscles need to be stretched after injury or surgery to regain their elongation potential, which is necessary not only for restoration of normal function but for prophylaxis against further injury by *improved capacity to dissipate forces* applied to the spine.

Jull and Janda (1987) have identified patterns of reaction by muscle groups to pain and pathology – either overactivation and tightness, or inhibition and weakness – which appear constant in the population. For instance, in the lumbopelvic region, the iliopsoas, the hamstrings, piriformis and erector spinae are prone to tightness, while the glutei and rectus abdominis are prone to weakness. In the shoulder–neck region, pectoralis major, levator scapulae, the sternomastoids and scalenes are prone to tightness while rhomboids, serratus anterior and the lower portion of trapezius are prone to weakness.

It is probable that muscle balance plays an important part in the dynamics of spinal movement, and in the maintenance of good posture. Imbalance – for instance, the combination of short, tight hip flexors, and weak glutei and abdominal muscles – allows the development of forward rotation of the pelvis, increased lumbar lordosis and fixed flexion of the hips. Frequently, the hamstrings are found to be tight, as a result of which excessive strain is imposed on the lumbar spine. Degenerative changes in the hip joints produce the same effect.

Confirmation of muscle tightness requires careful assessment and some experience on the part of the therapist; the hip flexors and extensors are particularly important groups in relation to low back pain, and pectoralis major and the fixators of the scapula in relation to neck and shoulder pain.

Low back stretching

For the low back, flexion exercises which stretch the erector spinae should be performed when lying horizontally; the supine position is usually adopted though the fetal position may be used. The spine is curled and held in this flexed position by grasping the thighs (Fig. 5.1a) or lower legs below the knees (Fig. 5.1b, 5.2a) with both hands and using them as levers . All stretches should be held for at least 5 seconds, but for not more than 10 seconds; this allows the stretch reflexes to be 'unloaded' and all viscoelastic (connective and muscle) tissues to undergo the **creep** phenomenon in which increased length is observed on constant loading. Alternatively, and safely, each thigh may be flexed individually (Fig. 5.2b). All repetitions should be performed five times with a 3–5 second gap in between. If both thighs

a

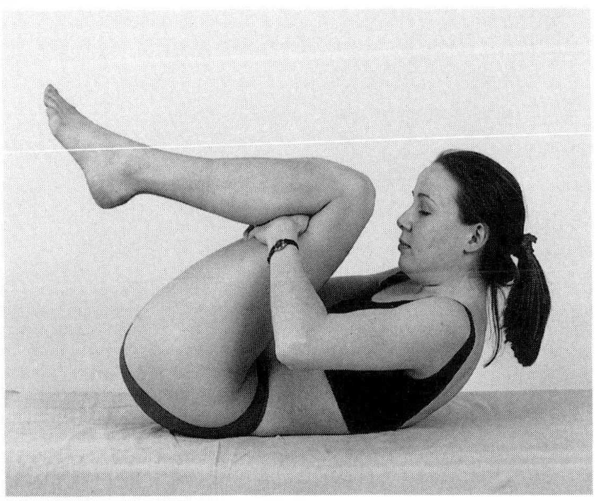

b

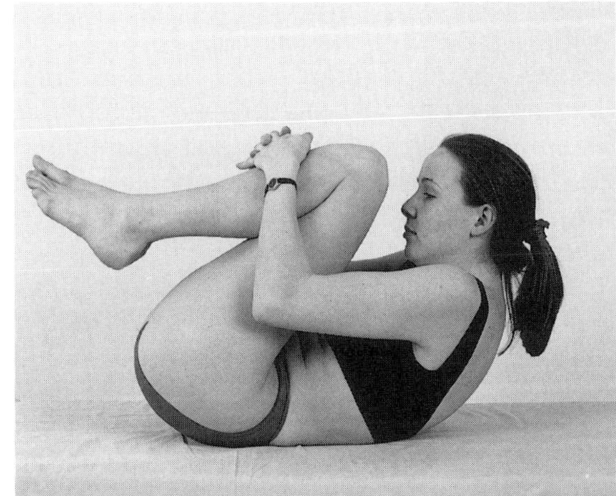

Fig. 5.1 Flexibility exercise – spinal flexion using (a) both thighs, (b) lower legs, as levers.

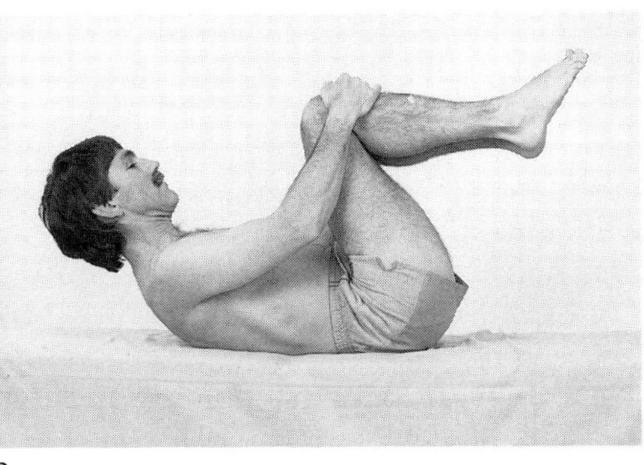
a

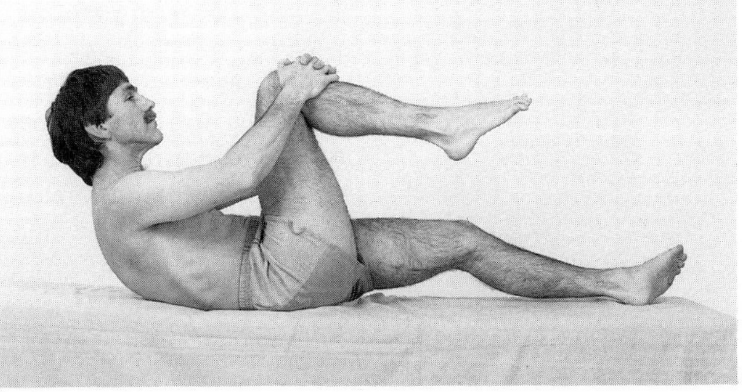
b

Fig. 5.2 Flexibility exercise in a less flexible subject – spinal flexion using (a) both thighs, (b) flexion of one thigh only.

are flexed, too rapid a return to the lordotic position should be avoided by completing the exercise one leg at a time.

Pelvic tilting

This exercise demands contraction of the abdominal muscles and glutei to produce backward tilting of the pelvis and flattening of the lumbar lordosis (Fig. 5.3); thus, it combines strengthening of muscles

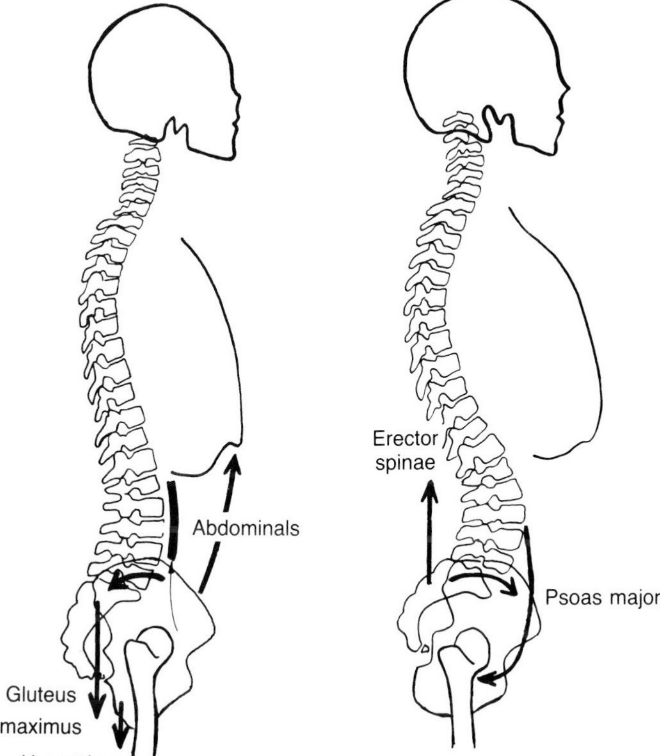

Fig. 5.3 Pelvic tilting – the glutei, hamstrings and abdominal muscles produce a backward tilt of the pelvis and flatten the lumbar lordosis.

which are prone to weakness with promotion of good lumbopelvi posture in those patients with a marked lordosis. For convenience, it i described here.

Initially, the exercise should be performed in the supine positio though, from a postural sense, it is important that, subsequently progression is made to the standing position (for example, whe leaning against a wall). When supine, the patient flexes her hips an knees slightly, and attempts to flatten her back on the floor (Fig. 5.4) For those patients who find the exercise difficult, the tactile sensatio during the intended movement may be improved by placing th examiner's hand, or the patient's hand, behind the small of their back Having flattened the lumbar spine, using the abdominal muscle predominantly, the patient is then encouraged to rotate the pelvi rhythmically by squeezing the buttocks and raising them from th floor, this part of the exercise requiring contraction of the glutei (and to a lesser extent, the hamstrings).

a

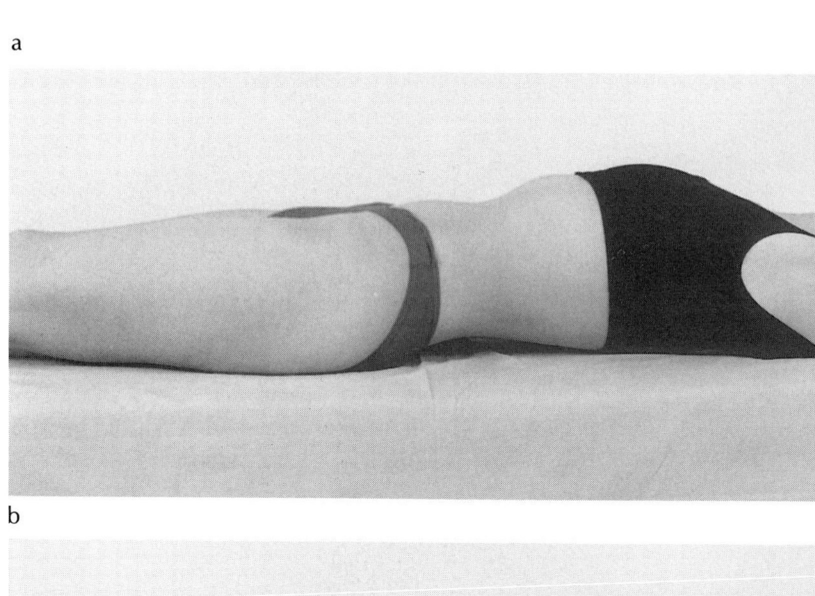

b

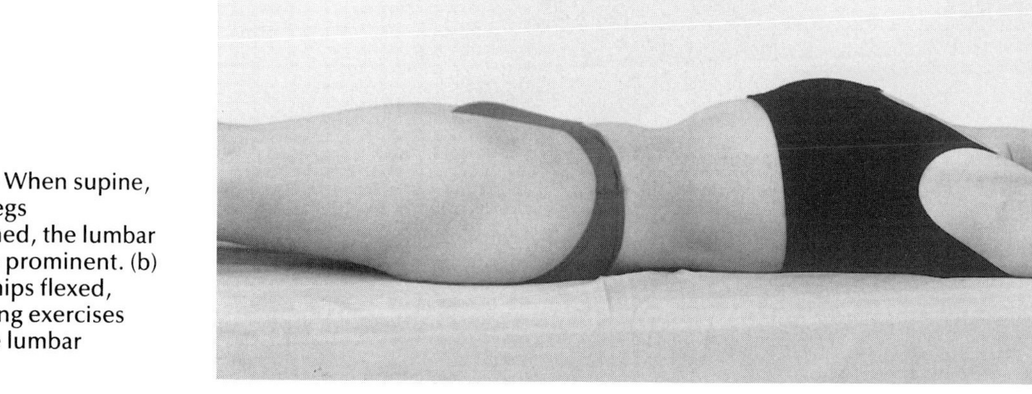

Fig. 5.4 (a) When supine, with the legs outstretched, the lumbar lordosis is prominent. (b) With the hips flexed, pelvic tilting exercises flatten the lumbar lordosis.

Hamstring exercises

Although the technique of hamstring stretching by bending forward from the upright position with a flat back may be learnt, it is safer for most patients that selective stretching is performed by raising the straight leg on to a plinth (Fig. 5.5a) and leaning forward (Fig. 5.5b). By this method the hamstrings are stretched by increasing flexion of the hip with the knee fully extended. Alternatively, for the younger patient, the position demonstrated in Fig. 5.6 may be adopted, in which the stretched leg is extended forwards along the floor, while the contralateral leg is internally rotated and abducted at the hip. Selective stretching may then be undertaken without concomitant flexion strain being imparted to the lumbar spine.

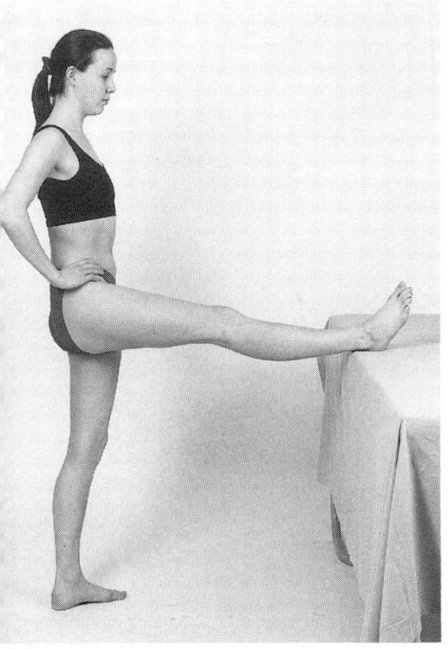

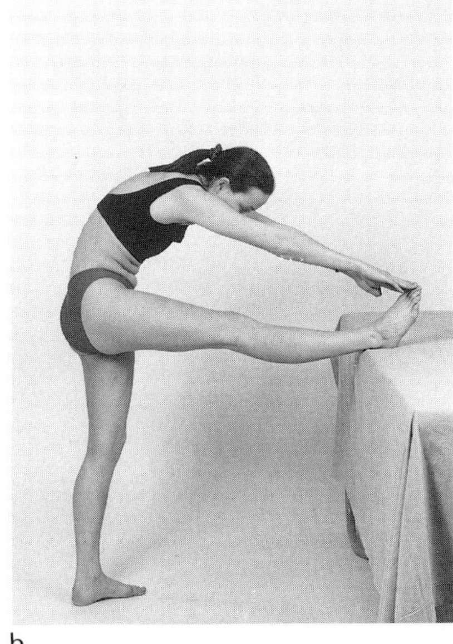

Fig. 5.5 Flexibility exercise – hamstring stretching. (a) Standing upright. (b) Leaning forwards.

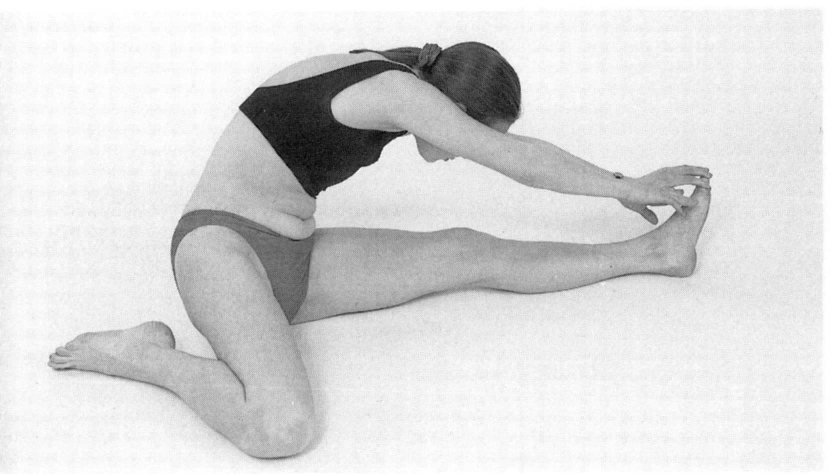

Fig. 5.6 Flexibility exercise – hamstring stretching and abduction/internal rotation of the contralateral hip.

Hip flexor stretching

Excessive tension in, and shortening of, the iliopsoas leads tc increased lumbar lordosis and flexion of the hips. Additionally excessive strain is placed on the sacroiliac joints. The easiest methoc of stretching is for the patient to lie supine with the thigh (of the leg tc be stretched) extended by hanging it over the side of a couch or bec (Fig. 5.7a). The contralateral hip should be flexed by the hands sc

a

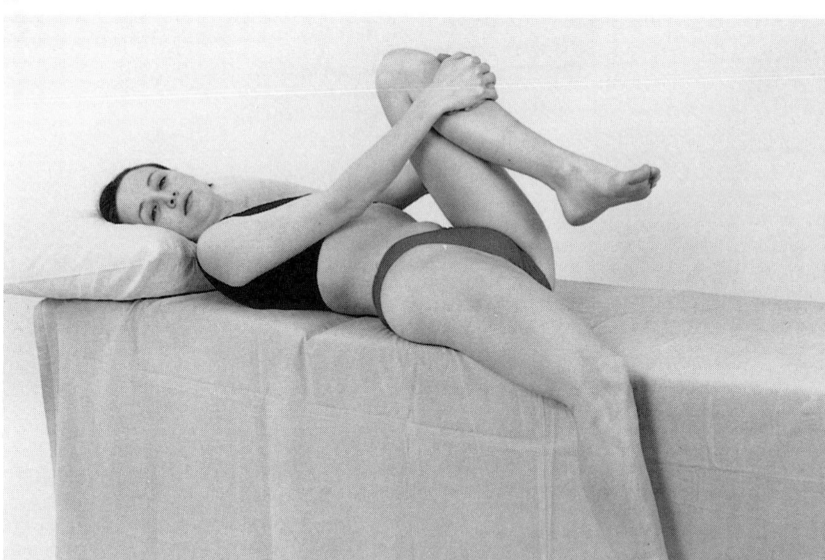

b

Fig. 5.7 Flexibility exercise – hip flexor stretching. (a) Gravity-aided. (b) Post-isometric relaxation.

that the lumbar spine is flattened. Gravity-aided relaxation of the hip flexors occurs. From this supine position postcontraction relaxation is particularly useful and easy to learn. The sequence of raising the knee by contraction of the hip flexors for 5 seconds, followed by 5–10 seconds of relaxation, is repeated five times. This should be performed regularly by patients within their homes. When a patient attends the clinic the therapist will be of further assistance by providing manual resistance to hip flexion, and subsequent gentle passive stretching of the thigh into extension (Fig. 5.7b).

The thigh may also be stretched into extension in the standing position by allowing the body weight to move forwards against the hip; in this position, however, it is difficult for most patients to avoid concomitant hyperextension of the lumbar spine.

Piriformis stretching

In the supine position, the knee is grasped and the lower leg used as a lever to procure flexion, adduction and internal rotation of the hip (Fig. 5.8). The latter movement is essential, otherwise the glutei are stretched preferentially (Fig. 5.9).

Trunk side bending

If trunk side bending is performed from the standing position, and combined with adduction of the elevated arm, the latissimus dorsi is stretched in addition to the quadratus lumborum (Fig. 5.10).

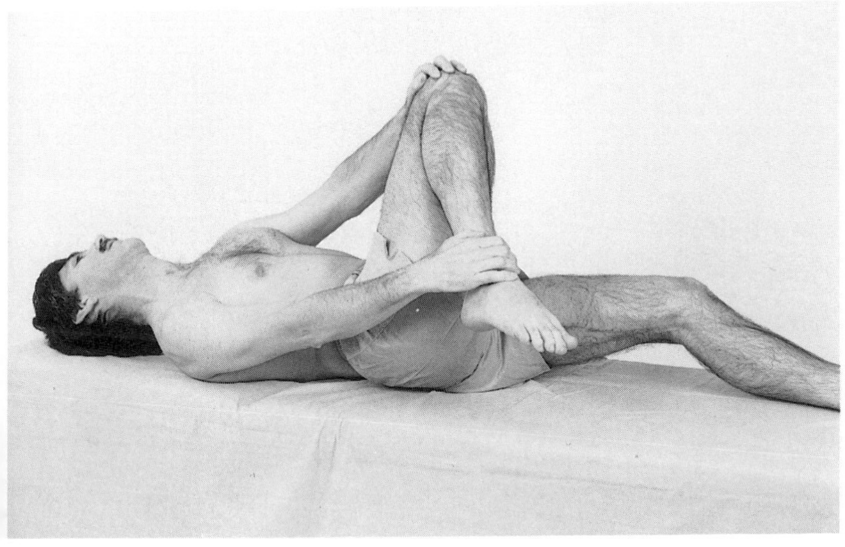

Fig. 5.8 Flexibility exercise – piriformis stretching.

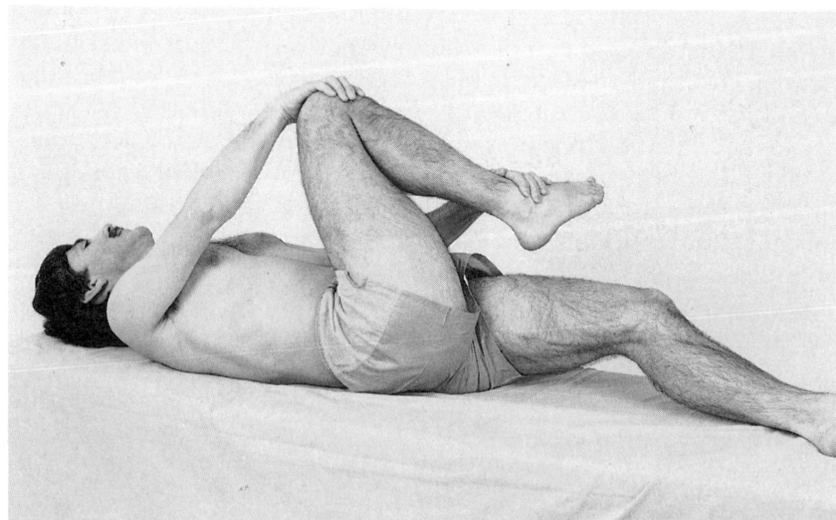

Fig. 5.9 Flexibility exercise – glutei stretching.

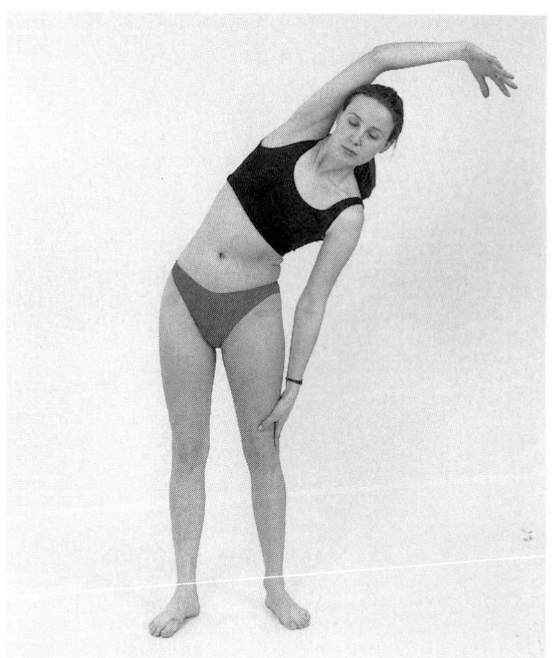

Fig. 5.10 Flexibility exercise – latissimus dorsi and quadratus lumborum stretching.

Thoracolumbar rotation/pectoralis major stretch

A useful exercise combines stretch of the pectoralis major with rotation of both the thoracic spine and lumbar spine in the supine position (Fig. 5.11). The right hip and knee are flexed, and the thigh allowed to drop over the left side of the body, by rotation of the thoracolumbar spine to the left. The right shoulder is abducted and externally rotated, and the elbow flexed to 90°; the critical part of the

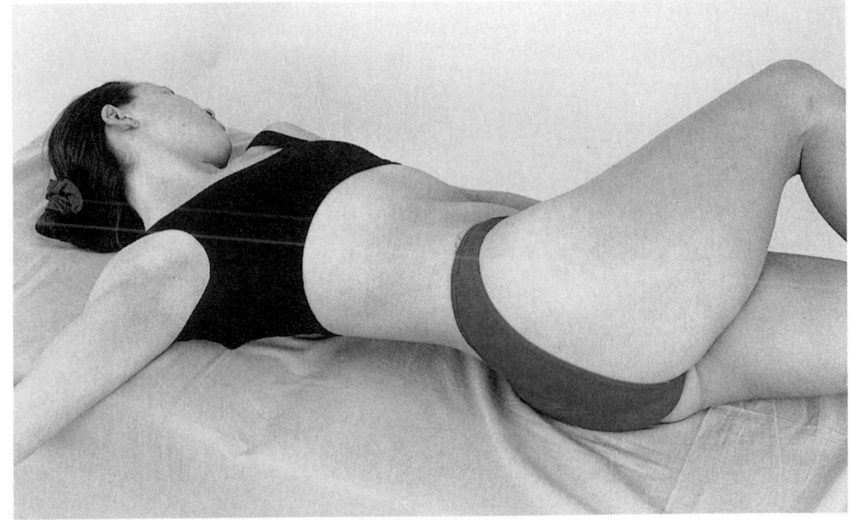

a

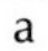

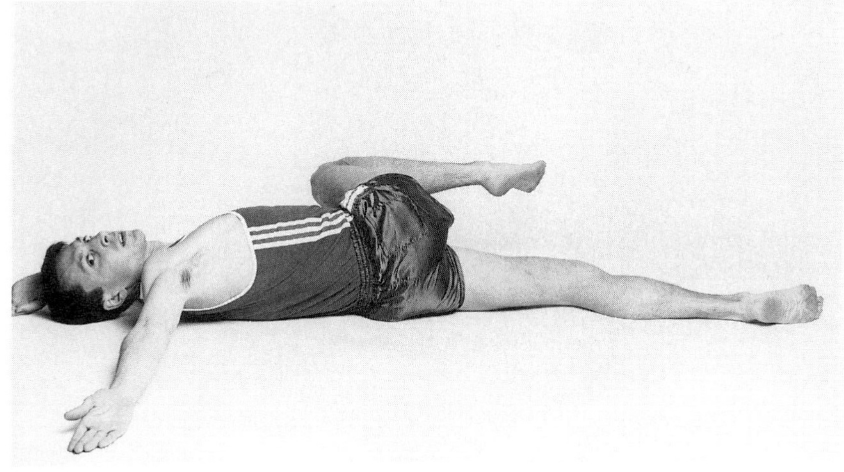

b

Fig. 5.11 Flexibility exercise – trunk rotation and pectoralis major stretch. (a) A subject with average flexibility. (b) An athlete with greater flexibility.

exercise is to allow the posterior aspect of the shoulder, and the elbow and forearm, to retain contact with the surface on which the patient lies. The exercise is then performed on the opposite side to a total of five repetitions each side. This exercise is particularly helpful in preparation for sports, such as swimming and golf, in which restricted thoracic rotation and tightness of external rotation of the shoulders have detrimental effects.

An alternative exercise for mobilization of the thoracolumbar spine combines flexion of the hips and knees in the supine position, and rolling of the knees to one side, then the other. This may be performed first with the feet on the floor, then with the feet raised (creating 90° flexion at the hips). Muscle toning is an added benefit, particularly if the exercise is performed slowly.

Cervicothoracic stretch

The round-shouldered posture, which is associated with hyperextension of the neck and loss of abduction at the shoulders, may be corrected by regular stretching – by retracting the shoulders and holding the arms aloft. Initially, the patient should attempt to 'stand tall', thereby reducing the proximal thoracic kyphosis and cervical lordosis. This facilitates the squaring of the shoulders, raising of the arms in abduction and, finally, extension of the shoulders with the arms fully upright. The same effect may be gained in the supine position by lifting the arms and attempting to place them on the floor above the head (Fig. 5.12).

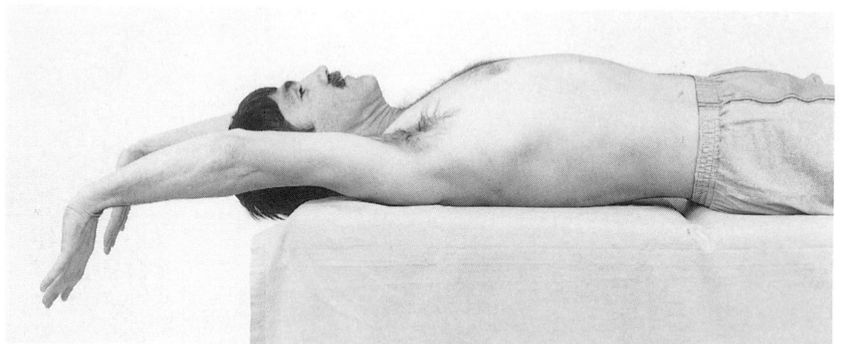

Fig. 5.12 Flexibility exercise – cervicothoracic stretch for the 'round back'.

Similarities between cervicothoracic stretch, pelvic tilting and double chinning (see below) will be noted: these exercises combine stretching of some muscle groups, toning of other groups, and flattening of excessive spinal curvatures.

Double chinning

This is a useful exercise to flatten the cervical lordosis, reduce the proximal thoracic kyphosis, tone the short muscles in the neck, and contribute to mobilization of the spinal joints. The patient should be instructed to retract the chin without nodding the head, creating self-mobilization at the proximal cervical joints (Fig. 5.13). If the patient squares the shoulders at the same time, there is a further mobilizing effect to the cervicothoracic junction and the proximal thoracic spine, and a toning of the shoulder fixators.

STRENGTHENING EXERCISES

Abdominal strengthening

Abdominal 'curls' are a most important part of the strength training programme. They may be performed isotonically or isometrically, but

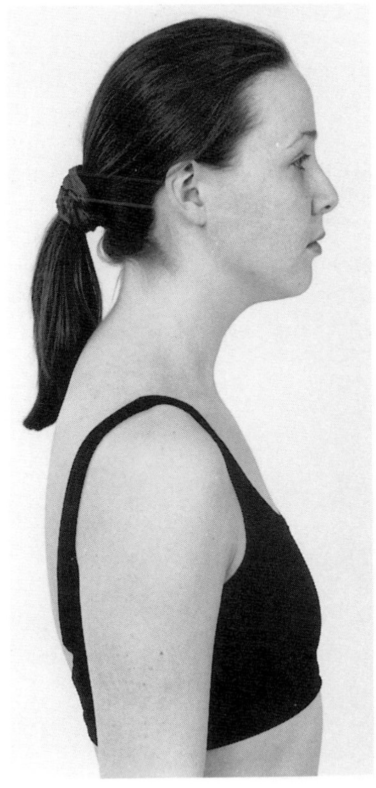

a

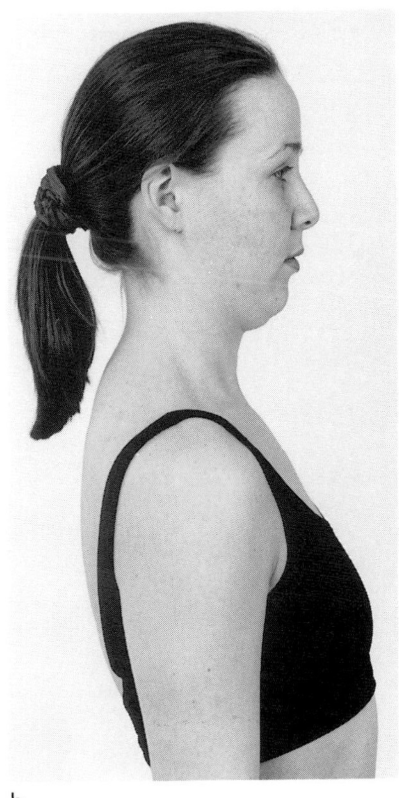

b

Fig. 5.13 Flexibility exercise – double chinning (self-mobilization at the proximal cervical joints). (a) Starting position. (b) Retraction of the chin.

should always be commenced with the hips in at least 30° flexion, preferably with the knees flexed in addition, in order to flatten the lumbar spine.

For a patient with weak abdominals, the programme should commence in the supine position with the hips and knees flexed and the feet flat on the floor (Fig. 5.14a) The head and shoulders should be raised approximately 6 in off the floor, and the hands slid along the floor towards the feet; the curled up position may be held for a slow count of three and then gradually released. Five repeats would be a suitable starter. Next, the same exercise may be repeated with the hands slid along the front of the thighs (Fig. 5.14b). The isometric element is useful as intradiscal pressure studies have demonstrated less increase in lumbar intradiscal pressure during isometric exercises compared with isotonic exercises (Nachemson and Elfstrom, 1970).

An alternative position is for both the hips and the knees to be flexed to 90°, and held in this position by hooking the legs over a chair, bed, couch or bench. From this position, the shoulders should be raised from the floor, when it is found that they cannot be raised excessively (Fig. 5.15); the patient should not link his hands behind his neck, as, occasionally, this may impose excessive strain on the cervical spine. Lifting both legs with the knees extended, and the head

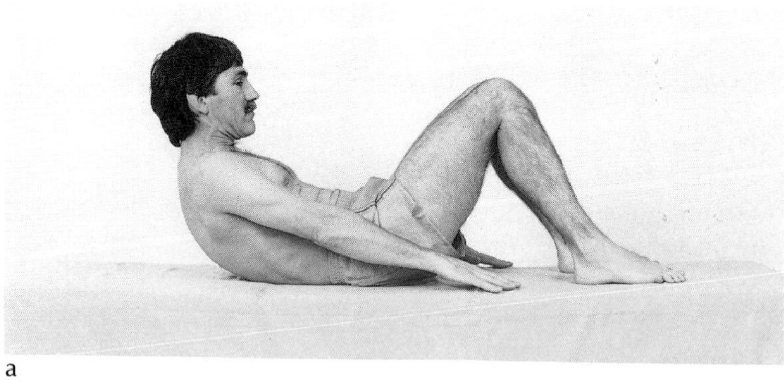
a

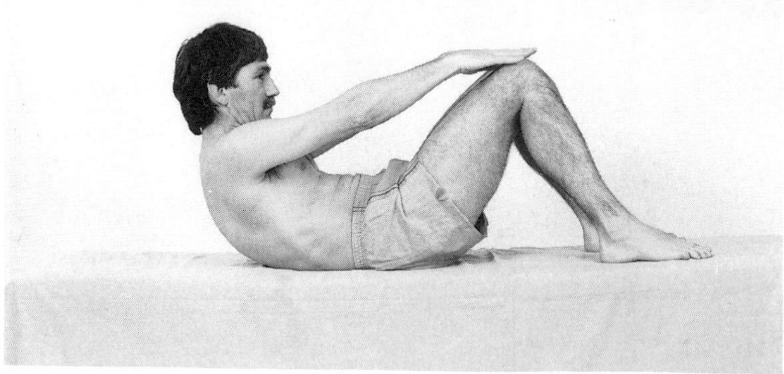
b

Fig. 5.14 Strengthening exercise – abdominal strengthening for a patient with weak abdominals. (a) Hands on the floor. (b) Hands on the front of the thighs.

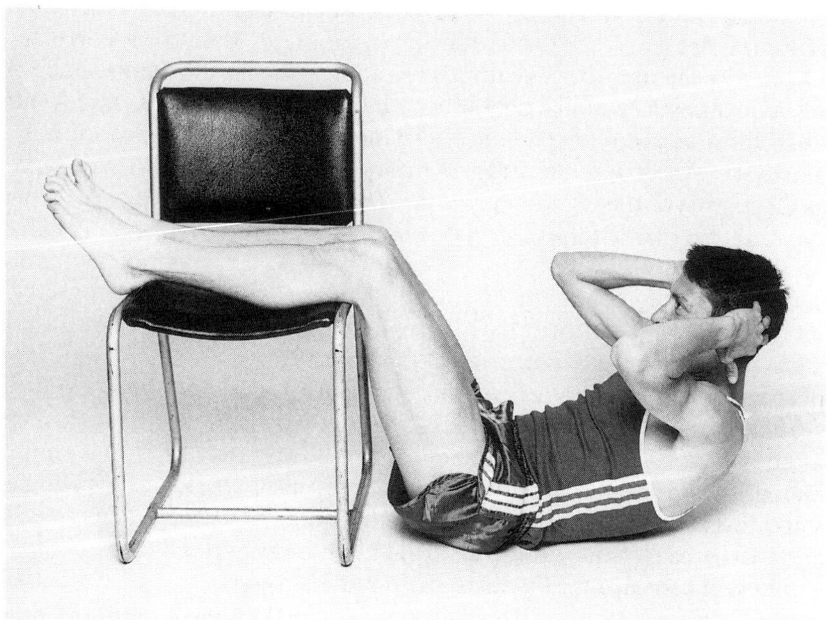

Fig. 5.15 Strengthening exercise – abdominal strengthening for an athlete.

and shoulders flat on the floor (in which position the lumbar spine is extended) should be reserved for the athlete who has no history of back problems, and who wishes to train the hip flexors additionally.

Glutei

Repetitive squeezing of the buttocks by the patient is an effective way of strengthening the glutei. Preferably, this should be part of a pelvic tilting programme which should be performed regularly in the upright position. Pelvic bridging (Fig. 5.16) also trains the glutei.

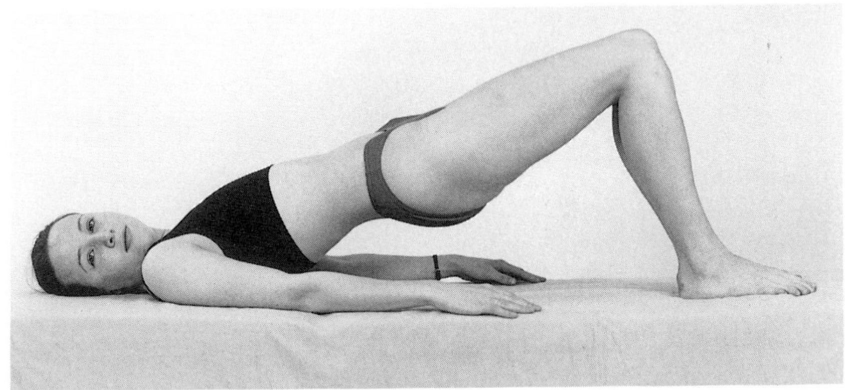

Fig. 5.16 Strengthening exercise – pelvic bridging (for the glutei).

Quadriceps

Weakness of the quadriceps, which is not uncommon in individuals who are not particularly active in middle age, should be corrected. Otherwise, it may be a contributory factor in the persistence of low back problems by compromising a sound 'bend and lift' technique. Due consideration should be given to the lumbar spine, to prevent excessive strain in extension, during isometric and isotonic quads exercises, as the back and pelvic muscles may be recruited unsuspectingly.

Lower trapezius/serratus anterior

The 'interscapular' muscles are prone to weakness; by contrast, pectoralis major, the upper portion of trapezius and the levator scapulae are prone to tightness. These muscle responses are an invariable finding when the shoulders become 'rounded', a common enough situation in the young, probably as a result of adolescent self-consciousness, as it is in the middle-aged and elderly, in whom the added stresses of family life and financial crises are contributory.

These interscapular muscles – rhomboids, serratus anterior and the lower portion of trapezius – retract and depress the scapula;

restoration of normal muscle tone and endurance is an important prerequisite for postural correction for the upper half of the body.

A particularly useful schedule of exercises is to be found in the section on 'underarms' in Callan Pinkney's *Callanetics for your Back* (1988), which incorporates postcontraction relaxation of the upper scapular fixators with toning exercises for the lower scapular fixators (the interscapular muscles). The crux of these exercises is isometric and isotonic contraction of the lower trapezius and associated fixators by depression and retraction of the shoulder girdle, combined with extension and internal rotation of the arms (Fig. 5.17).

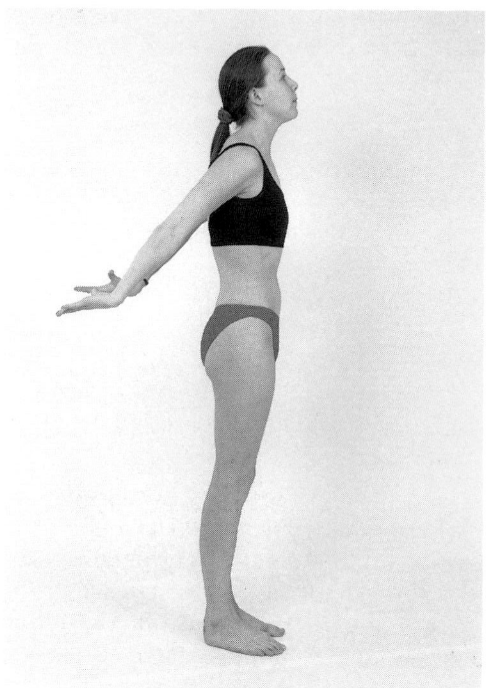

Fig. 5.17 Strengthening exercise – lower scapular fixators. Flattening of the lumbar lordosis may be carried out at the same time.

POSTURE AND KINETICS

It is clear that a spectrum of 'normality' exists throughout the population in respect to the convexity of the spinal curves. As a general rule, it is excessive stress upon the ligaments of the lumbar spine and sacroiliac joints which gives rise to backache when standing, as the promontory of the sacrum is rotated anteriorly and the lumbar spine becomes hyperlordotic – hence the emphasis upon pelvic tilting and abdominal strengthening exercises to flatten the lumbar lordosis. The lumbar lordosis may be reduced also by resting one foot upon a low stool or low bar rail (a feature of many public house bars which their users find accommodating). Reversal of lordosis by leaning forwards and resting the arms on a suitable support may be necessary, in the extreme case, for relief of pain in a patient with spinal stenosis.

The sitting position creates an entirely different set of circumstances, however. Not only is prolonged sitting painful in the majority of sufferers of backache (those with L3/4 disc protrusions and spinal stenotic syndromes being the exception), it contributes significantly to the development of neckache too. A more serious threat results from the biomechanical deformation of the lumbar intervertebral discs, and the loading of the supporting ligaments and muscles throughout the spine. During sitting, it is essential that *the lumbar lordosis is maintained*; as prolonged sitting, particularly at office desks and in automobiles, is unavoidable for many workers in Western civilised society, the

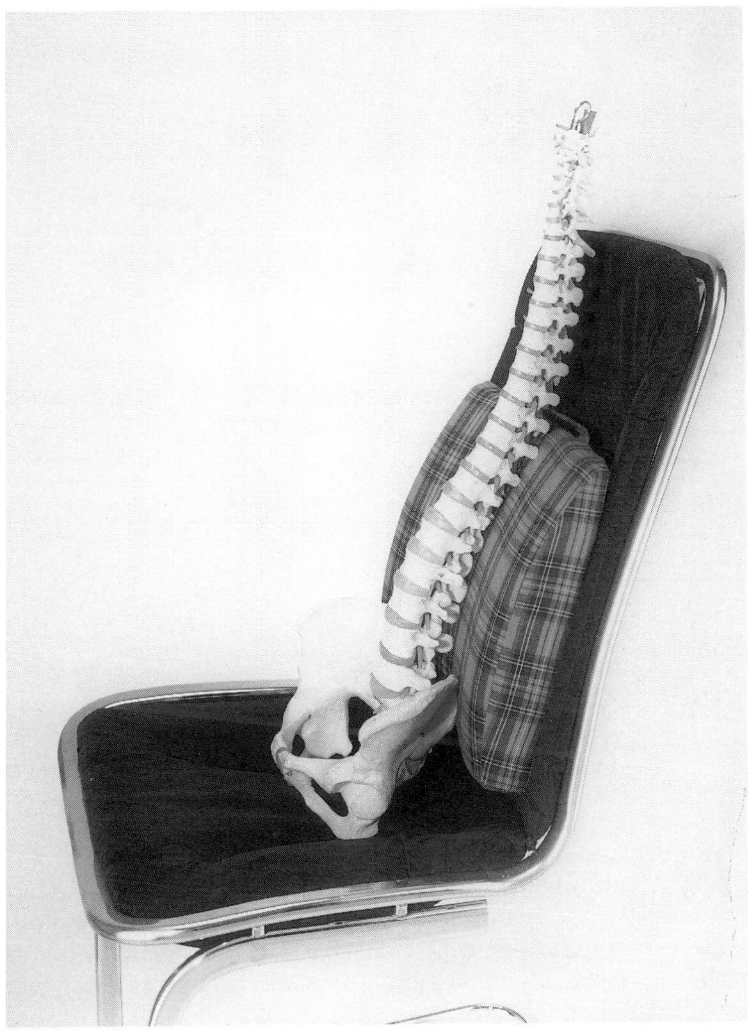

Fig. 5.18 The posture curve backrest, manufactured by F. Ashton Ltd.

lumbar spine should be given adequate support. Additionally, the position of the upper body in respect to the work-station should be addressed (see 'Ergonomics').

The standard of design of car and office seats continues to be very variable, despite considerable research over the past couple of decades. For seats which offer inadequate lumbar support, a backrest may be prescribed. A suitable backrest is the 'posture curve', manufactured by F. Ashton Ltd (Fig. 5.18). Alternatively, a lumbar (McKenzie) roll may be used. A good seat will offer an adjustable lumbar support.

In the office, some patients find additional benefit from a chair which offers forward angulation of the seat. This produces less hip flexion and less hamstring strain, and facilitates the maintenance of the lumbar lordosis as a result of less backwards rotation of the pelvis (Fig. 5.19). Such a sitting position approximates that found when riding horseback in which a good spinal posture is usually well maintained.

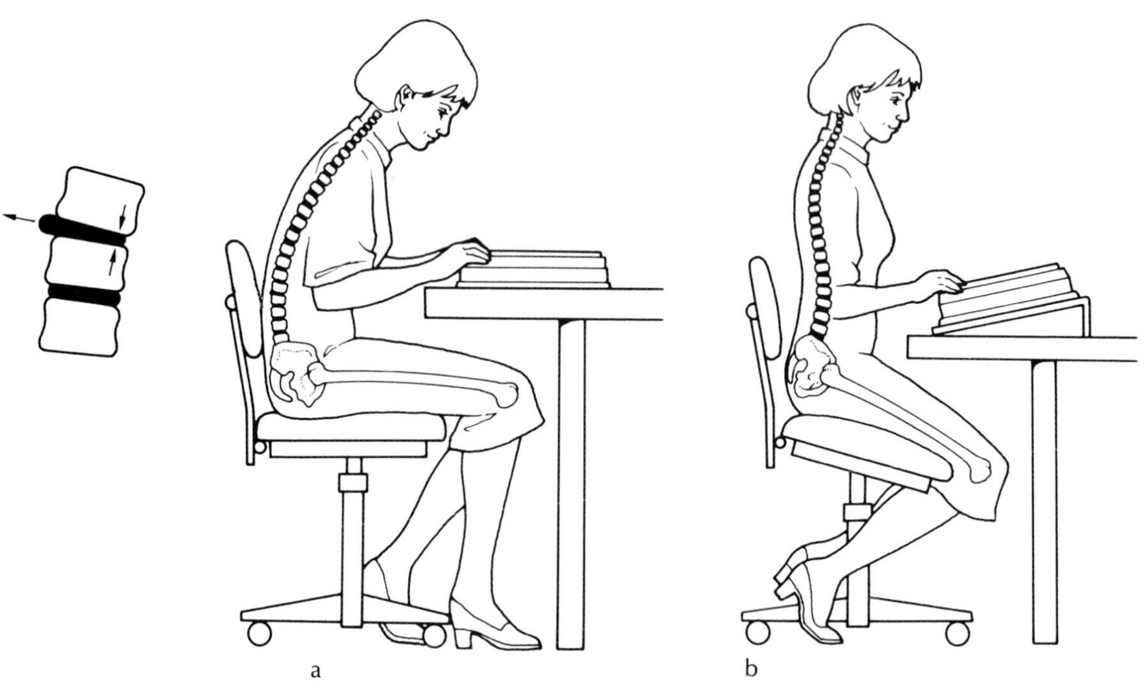

Fig. 5.19 (a) Poor sitting posture. (b) Improved posture using forward angulation of the seat.

Another method of producing less hip flexion is the use of a Balans chair, a Scandinavian design which relies upon the body weight being transferred forwards on to the knees (Fig. 5.20). It is comfortable for some, but does not appear to have become universally recognized. For obvious reasons, its use should be considered very carefully in patients with patellofemoral problems.

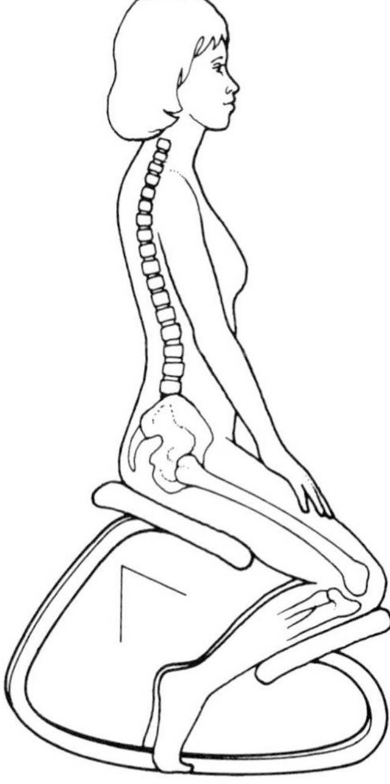

Fig. 5.20 The use of a Balans chair for maintenance of the lumbar lordosis.

ERGONOMICS

There has been an increasing awareness of the importance of ergonomics – in practical terms, the study of, and modifications to, the working environment – over recent years. Prior to 1992, the statutory obligations in the United Kingdom in respect to manual handling of loads and patient handling were incorporated in the Health and Safety at Work Act, 1974. The 1992 European Community regulations render all employers responsible for assessing risks in the workplace, and for ensuring the well-being of the workforce. Amongst other requirements, training in lifting techniques and the design of the work-station are paramount.

VDUs

Therapists and clinicians should be familiar with suggested optimum dimensions of the work-station (Fig. 5.21), and may be asked to inspect and advise. With respect to the incidence of neck and shoulder strains, and repetitive strain injury (RSI) in general, the height and angulation of the keyboard or work surface are critical. Conversion of a work surface for writing or graphic design, for instance to one of a draughtsman's board type, may be made by use of an adjustable unit such as the 'Posturite' magnetic sloping writing board (Fig. 5.22). This allows between 30° and 60° inclination, thereby improving the posture of the neck and shoulders considerably. For work with a

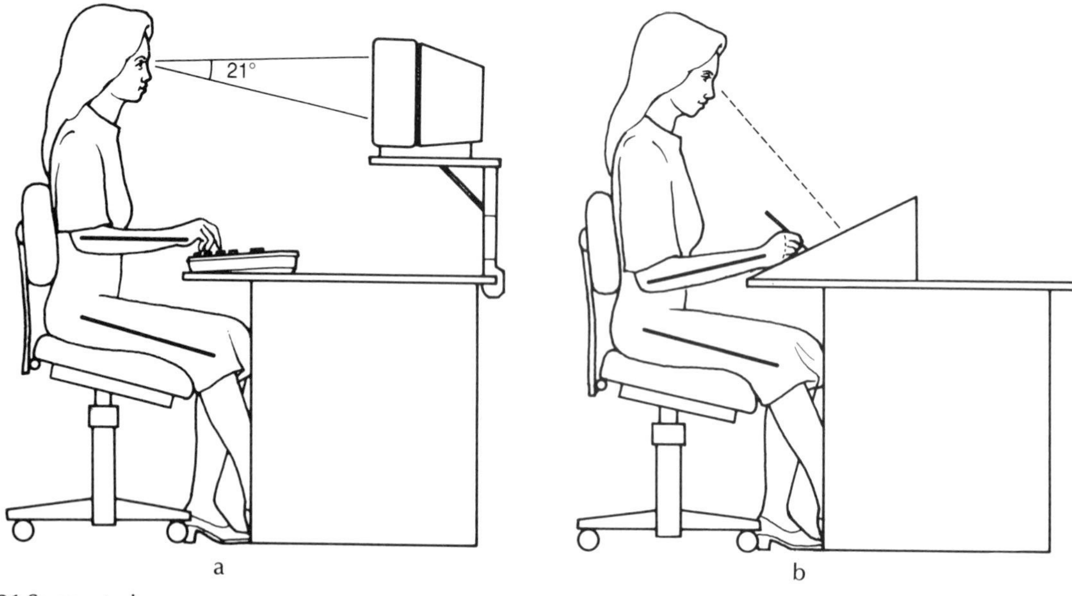

Fig. 5.21 Suggested optimum dimensions for the work-station.

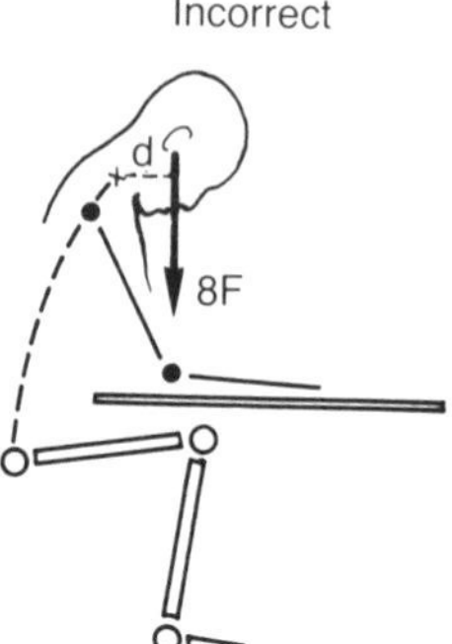

Note: The gravity force (F) increases the load moment as distance (d) increases.

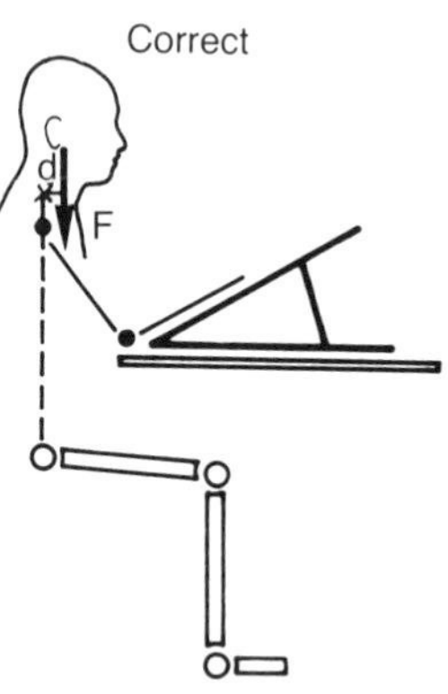

Fig. 5.22 Sitting posture improved by the use of a Posturite magnetic sloping writing board.

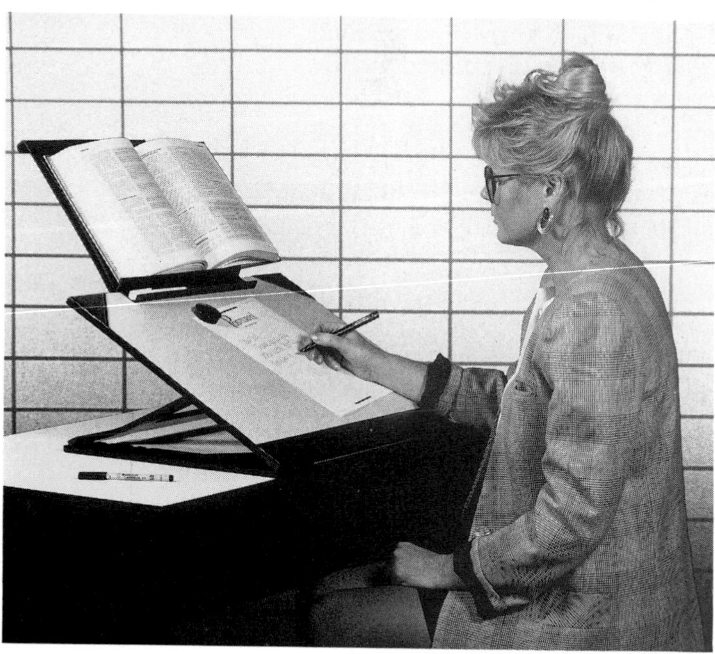

keyboard and screen, the screen height and angle should be adjustable so that the head remains upright, with the top of the screen at eye level.

Employees should be in receipt of appropriate advice such as:

- Feel comfortable while sitting.
- Take a 5–10 minute break from keyboard operation every 1–2 hours.
- Use a footstool or wedge, if appropriate.
- If necessary, try a different chair – for instance, one with a sloping seat.
- Do not rest wrists on the keyboard – try an armrest.

Other considerations for VDU operatives, outside the scope of this text, relate to the possible (though unproven) adverse effects on general health – visual, reproductive and stress related, for instance. Thus, factors such as space, noise, temperature, humidity and lighting may need to be considered, as well as ergonomics.

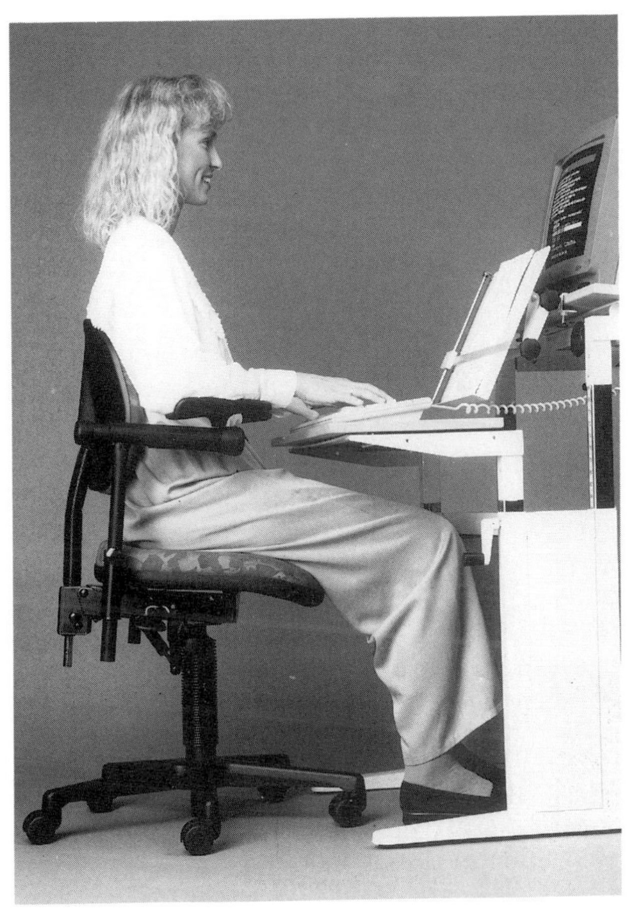

Fig. 5.23 A modern office chair may offer a built-in lumbar support, an adjustable forward-tilting seat, height-adjustable arm-rests and optional adjustable rocker action. (By permission of Advance Seating Designs.)

The choice of chair has considerable importance. To reduce the lumbar intradiscal pressures, the occupant should sit back in a chair type which offers an appropriate built-in lumbar support and an adjustable forward tilting seat (Fig. 5.23). Should the chair occupant not require a fixed typing position, an adjustable rocker action is very helpful. Height-adjustable armrests prevent excessive strain upon the neck and shoulder girdle muscles.

Manual handling

The new 'lifting at work' regulations demand that appropriate steps are taken to prevent back injuries. When manual handling is unavoidable, consideration should be given to:

- **Design of containers** – for instance, suitable handles to allow a good grip.
- **Cumulative weight** – muscle fatigue may result from repetitive lifting of relatively small weights.
- **Recommended maximum weights** for repeated lifting – for instance, research at the Ergonomic Research Unit, Robens Institute, University of Surrey, suggests that the following are appropriate for safe lifting:

1 Lifting at arms length – 10 kg (9 kg if aged 51–60).
2 Lifting with arms close to body – 16 kg (12 kg if aged 51–60).

- **Height** of work benches and shelving – for manipulation of loads, the most convenient height is 1.0–1.25 m from ground level.
- **Training** – may only be effective when combined with a safe and ergonomically suitable environment which will lessen the risk to health and safety (Stubbs *et al.*, 1983).

During kinetic load handling, the following points should be emphasized:

- Use a sound grip, not the finger tips.
- Maintain a straight back, with hips and knees flexed.
- Keep the head high, and tuck in the chin to help maintain a straight back.
- Keep the feet apart as wide as the hips, with one foot in advance of the other, pointing in the intended direction of travel.
- Keep the load close to the body.

Posters and pamphlets on lifting and patient handling are available from the National Back Pain Association, 31–33 Park Road, Teddington, Middlesex TW11 OAB (Fig. 5.24).

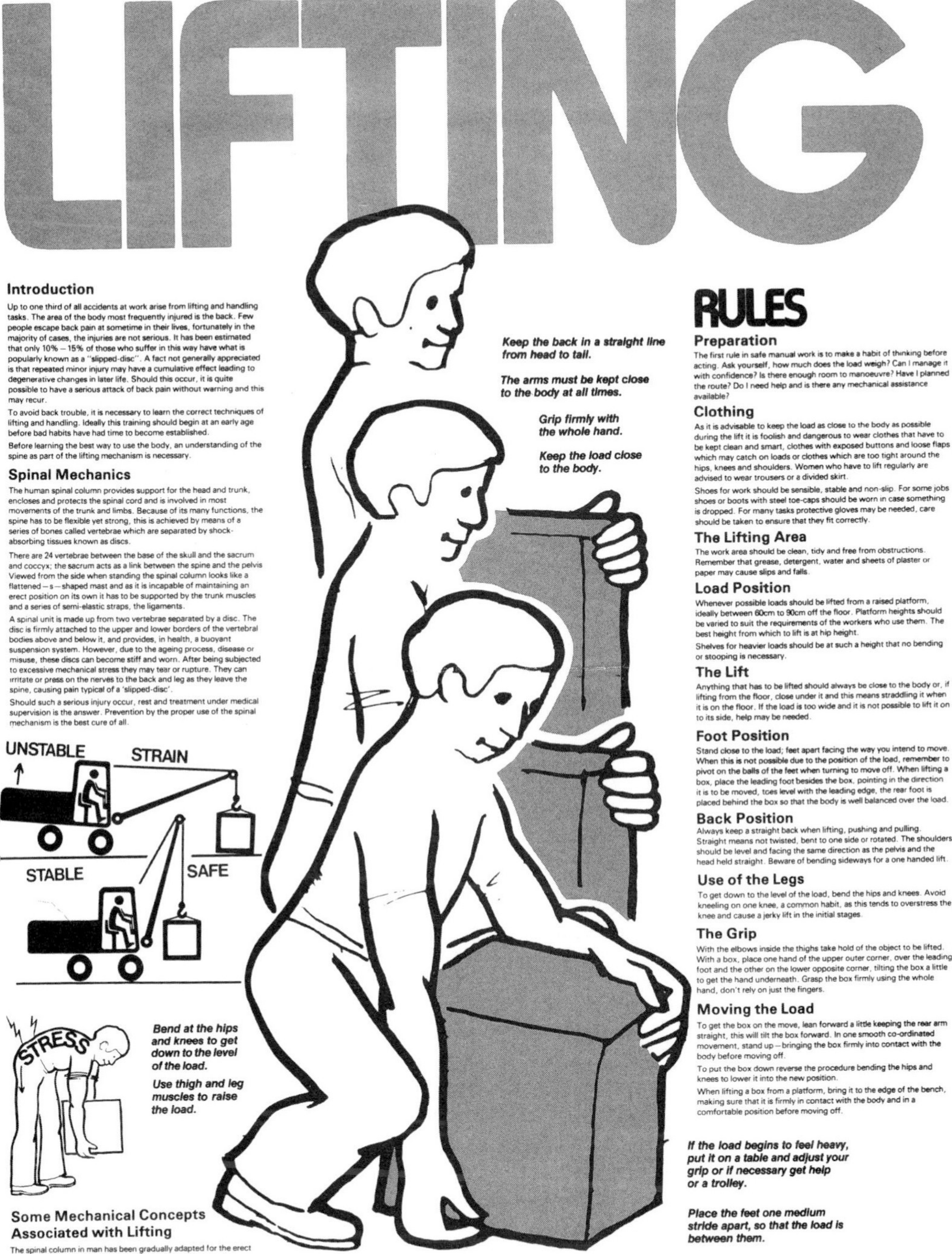

Fig. 5.24 A National Back Pain Association poster. (By permission of the National Back Pain Association, 1992.)

BEHAVIOUR MODIFICATION

Abnormal behavioural responses to chronic pain or disability may be observed frequently by physicians and therapists caring for sufferers from spinal pain. Such responses are not confined to those with inadequate personalities or those with strong neurotic traits, nor to those patients in whom the possibility of financial gain, for instance following RTAs, is a dominant factor. The presence of the gain factor, however, is an undoubted *inhibitor* to early progress despite appropriate management techniques.

The emphasis placed by the patient during the 'delivery' of the history upon the adverse effect of the illness on his lifestyle or well-being alerts the therapist. The expressionless facies, combined with the apparent lack of affect, are further guides during history taking. During examination, exaggerated responses are a consistent feature, though other observable behavioural characteristics include:

(a) reliance on props such as collars and walking sticks;
(b) abnormal and sometimes quite bizarre balance mechanisms;
(c) excessive difficulty performing ordinary tasks, such as undressing.

Reference has already been made in previous chapters to the extent to which the therapist's management strategies may be modified by a patient's behaviour. Should abnormal behaviour be found in response to chronic pain, a positive approach is required of the therapist. Courtesy demands a solicitous opening gambit, following which the emphasis should be firmly on the identification of areas of improvement followed by appropriate encouragement. To a great extent, evaluation of improvement is based on increased ability to perform day-to-day activities, as the somewhat histrionic response to examination is not surrendered easily and is not, therefore, the most appropriate parameter by which to judge early progress. Surreptitiously, increased praise and attention are directed towards the attainment of further goals; at the same time, abnormal behavioural characteristics are largely ignored by the therapist. Behavioural treatment of this type, focusing on reinforcement of healthy behaviour and attempting to eliminate sick behaviour, was developed by Mooney (1975) at Rancho Los Amigos Hospital.

Behavioural modification is also at the heart of the School for Bravery approach designed by Joyce Williams in Doncaster for patients with chronic pain and illness behaviour. She has found that the best results are gained when the medical profession has written off the patient, whose 'illness behaviour syndrome' is recorded on video. The medium of gymnasium activity is used to promote increased self-confidence and the transition from illness to wellness behaviour. The acquisition of increased fitness, and the identification by the patient of his ability to participate more fully in normal, acceptable social activities, is emphasized and rewarded by the therapist. An important principle is 'a deliberate move by the therapist away from the traditional professional caring expert-in-charge role to a relationship where the patient is seen as an equal adult who has a problem he is teaching himself to tackle and cope with' (Williams, 1989).

Of interest, from a psychoanalytical viewpoint, is that patients with such behavioural problems related to chronic pain almost invariably refute all suggestions that mental stress might play a role. They appear to be steadfast in this, litigation or no litigation. Despite this, the therapist-counsellor should promote a positive view on progress towards attainable goals, and seek assistance from a psychologist experienced in post-traumatic stress and depression should this be appropriate.

BACK SCHOOLS

Back schools were popularized in the 1970s in Sweden, since when favourable reports have been presented from, *inter alia*, Mattmiller (California 1980), Hall (Canada 1980), and Hayne (Derbyshire Royal Infirmary 1984). Although the emphasis in different centres has varied between ergonomic advice, attitudinal or behavioural changes, and increased fitness (Fisk *et al.*, 1983), the thrust has basically been to develop or increase self-confidence using a philosophy of self-help, so that patients take individual responsibility for managing and adjusting to their back conditions. Use is made of an admix of teaching and counselling principles, including formal lectures, audio-visual presentations, demonstrations, informal group interactions and practical sessions. A multidisciplinary team approach is advisable if resources allow.

Regrettably, there is a temptation to use back school as a 'last resort'; as such, a basic premise is that 'no more can be done' by doctors or therapists, at which stage it is often considered that, with the assistance of group therapy ('classes'), a more positive outlook and, as a result, less severe symptoms may be experienced by patients.

Two dangers, avoidable to greater or lesser degrees, are:

(a) that such a 'martyred' existence may be perpetuated if undue emphasis is placed on adjustment of lifestyle and accommodation to disability; and
(b) that individualized management strategies may be inappropriately or prematurely sacrificed, particularly if resources are very limited, or if, irritatingly (to the therapist), patients demonstrate behavioural traits such as lack of motivation and dependency.

Reference has already been made to management of back pain using a 'biopsychosocial' model rather than a disease model

(Waddell, 1987). Underlying this text is a basic assumption that the therapist should maintain a positive counselling role with an emphasis on encouragement and achievement of attainable targets. Aberg (1984) summarizes rehabilitation of the long-term low back pain patient as the successful combination of improved attitudes and behaviour with social, vocational and physical activity.

REFERENCES

Aberg, J. (1984) Evaluation of an advanced back pain rehabilitation programme. *Spine*, **9**, 317

Fisk, J.R., Dimonte, P. and Courington, S.McK. (1983) Back schools: past, present and future. *Clinical Orthopaedics and Related Research*, **179**, 18–23

Hall, H. (1980) The Canadian back education units. *Physiotherapy*, **66**, (4), 115–17

Hayne, C.R. (1984) Back schools and total back care programmes – a review. *Physiotherapy*, **70**(1), 14

Jull, G.A. and Janda, V. (1987) Muscles and motor control in low back pain: assessment and management. In *Physical Therapy of the Low Back*. (eds L.T. Twomey and J.R. Taylor), Churchill Livingstone, pp. 253–78

Mattmiller, A.W. (1980) The California back school. *Physiotherapy*, **66**(4), 118–22

Mooney, V. (1975) Alternative approaches for the patient beyond the help of surgery. *Orthopaedic Clinics of North America*, **6**, 331

Nachemson, A.L. and Elfstrom, G. (1970) Intradiscal dynamic pressure measurements in lumbar discs. *Scandinavian Journal of Rehabilitation Medicine*, Suppl. **1**, 1–40

Pinkney, Callan (1988) *Callanetics for your Back*, Ebury Press, London

Stubbs, D.A., Buckle, P.W., Hudson, M.P. *et al.* (1983) Patient handling and back pain in the nursing profession. Epidemiology and pilot methodology. *Ergonomics*, **26**(8), 755–65

Waddell, G. (1987). A new clinical model for the treatment of low back pain. *Spine*, **12**, 632–44

Williams, J.I. (1989) Illness behaviour to wellness behaviour: the School for Bravery approach. *Physiotherapy*, **75**(1), 2–7

Index